HOLISTIC HEALTHCARE

Possibilities and Challenges

HOLISTIC HEALTHCARE

Possibilities and Challenges

Edited by

Anne George, MD

Oluwatobi Samuel Oluwafemi, PhD

Blessy Joseph

APPLE ACADEMIC PRESS

Apple Academic Press Inc.
3333 Mistwell Crescent
Oakville, ON L6L 0A2
Canada

Apple Academic Press Inc.
9 Spinnaker Way
Waretown, NJ 08758
USA

First issued in paperback 2021

Exclusive worldwide distribution by CRC Press, a member of Taylor & Francis Group
No claim to original U.S. Government works

ISBN 13: 978-1-77463-621-3 (pbk)
ISBN 13: 978-1-77188-372-6 (hbk)

Library and Archives Canada Cataloguing in Publication

Holistic healthcare : possibilities and challenges / edited by Anne George, MD, Oluwafemi Samuel Oluwatobi, PhD, Blessy Joseph ; editorial board members, Sabu Thomas, PhD, Mathew Sebastian, MD, Raji V, PhD.

Includes bibliographical references and index.
Issued in print and electronic formats.

ISBN 978-1-77188-372-6 (hardcover).--ISBN 978-1-315-36624-1 (PDF)

1. Integrative medicine. 2. Holistic medicine. I. George, Anne, 1961-, author, editor II. Oluwafemi, Oluwatobi Samuel, editor III. Joseph, Blessy, editor

R733.H64 2017 615.5 C2016-907938-4 C2016-907939-2

Library of Congress Cataloging-in-Publication Data

Names: George, Anne, 1961- editor. | Oluwafemi, Oluwatobi Samuel, editor. | Joseph, Blessy, editor.
Title: Holistic healthcare : possibilities and challenges / editors, Anne George, Oluwatobi Samuel Oluwafemi, Blessy Joseph.
Description: Toronto ; New Jersey : Apple Academic Press, 2017. | Includes bibliographical references and index.
Identifiers: LCCN 2016055080 (print) | LCCN 2016055677 (ebook) | ISBN 9781771883726 (hardcover : alk. paper) | ISBN 9781315366241 (CRC Press/Taylor & Francis eBook) | ISBN 9781771883733 (AAP eBook) | ISBN 9781315366241 (ebook)
Subjects: | MESH: Integrative Medicine | Holistic Health
Classification: LCC R733 (print) | LCC R733 (ebook) | NLM WB 113 | DDC 610--dc23
LC record available at https://lccn.loc.gov/2016055080

Apple Academic Press also publishes its books in a variety of electronic formats. Some content that appears in print may not be available in electronic format. For information about Apple Academic Press products, visit our website at **www.appleacademicpress.com** and the CRC Press website at **www.crcpress.com**

ABOUT THE EDITORS

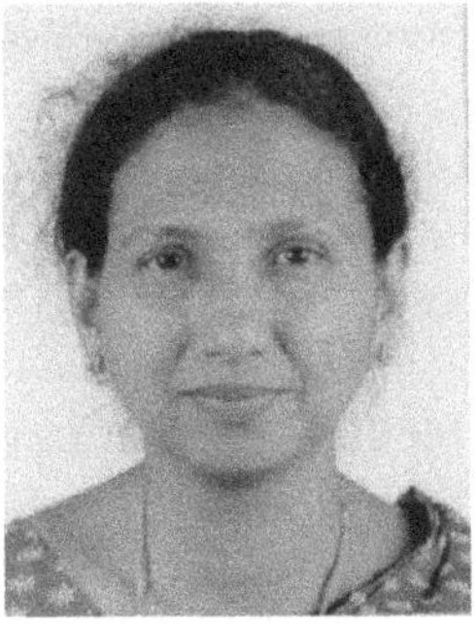

Anne George, MD, MBBS, DGO, Dip Acupuncture, is an Associate Professor in the Department of Anatomy at the Government Medical College, Kottayam, Kerala, India. She has organized several international conferences, is a fellow of the American Medical Society, and is a member of many international organizations. Dr. George has worked in several different international labs, which include the laboratories at Laval University, Quebec, Canada; Faculty of Medicine, University of Vienna, Vienna, Austria, and the Department of Immunology, Katholieke University of Leuven, Leuven, Belgium. Dr. George has edited many books and published research articles and reviews in international journals and has presented many papers at international conferences. Her major research interests human anatomy, polymeric scaffolds for tissue engineering, diabetes, nature cures, and diet and human health.

She received her MBBS Bachelor of Medicine and her Bachelor of Surgery from Trivandrum Medical College, University of Kerala, India. She acquired a DGO (Diploma in Obstetrics and Gynecology) from the University of Vienna, Austria; a Diploma of Acupuncture from the University of Vienna; and her MD from Kottayam Medical College, Mahatma Gandhi University, Kerala, India.

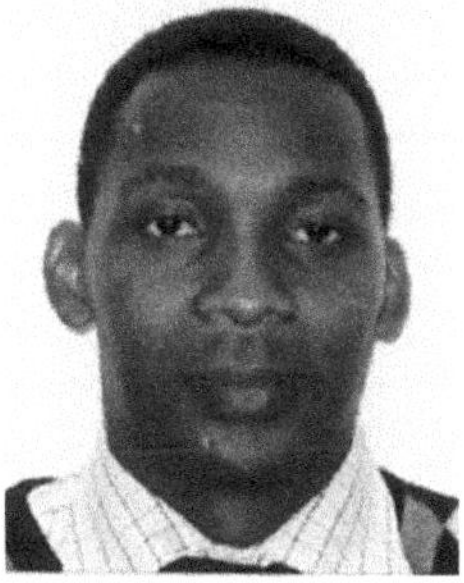

Oluwatobi Samuel Oluwafemi, PhD, is currently at Professor in the Department of Applied Chemistry at the University of Johannesburg, Doornfontein Campus, South Africa. Dr. Oluwatobi is an NRF-rated researcher and is actively involved in research in the area of nanotechnology. He has published many papers in internationally recognized journals and has presented at several professional meetings both locally and internationally. He is a fellow of many professional bodies, a reviewer for many international journals, and has received many awards for his excellent work in material research both local and international. His current research interests include green synthesis and application of nanoparticles in medicine, water treatment, polymer, LEDs, and sensors.

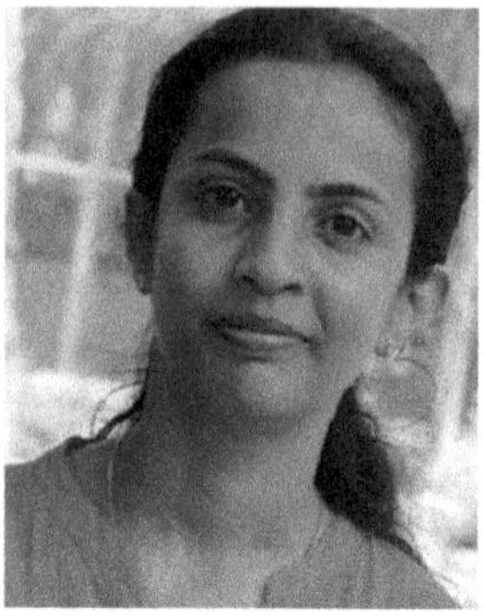

Blessy Joseph is a research fellow at the International and Inter University Centre for Nanoscience and Nanotechnology, Mahatma Gandhi University, Kottayam, Kerala, India. She received a bachelor's degree in Biotechnology and Biochemical Engineering and a Master's degree in Biotechnology and Biochemical Engineering (Molecular Medicine) from the University of Kerala, India. She has experience in green synthesis of gold nanoparticles for biomedical applications and is currently engaged in developing polymer based scaffolds for drug delivery applications at the International and Inter University Centre for Nanoscience and Nanotechnology. She is also interested in synthesizing various types of nanoparticles and evaluating their antibacterial and anticancer properties.

EDITORIAL BOARD MEMBERS

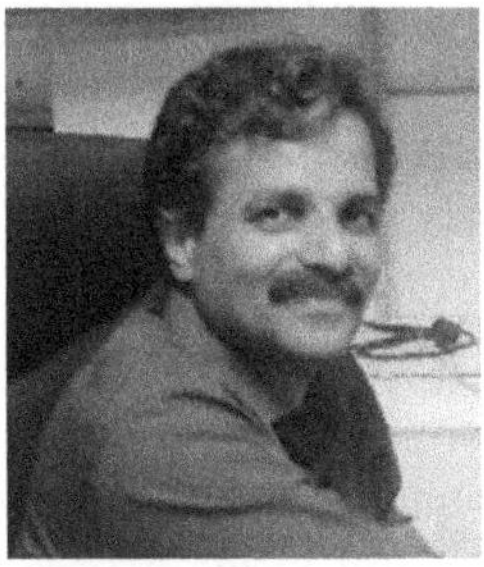

Sabu Thomas, PhD, is a Professor of Polymer Science and Engineering at the School of Chemical Sciences and Director of the International and Inter University Centre for Nanoscience and Nanotechnology at Mahatma Gandhi University, Kottayam, Kerala, India. He received his BSc degree (1980) in chemistry from the University of Kerala, a BTech (1983) in polymer science and rubber technology from the Cochin University of Science and Technology, and a PhD (1987) in polymer engineering from the Indian Institute of Technology, Kharagpur, India. The research activities of Professor Thomas include surfaces and interfaces in multiphase polymer blend and composite systems; phase separation in polymer blends; compatibilization of immiscible polymer blends; thermoplastic elastomers; phase transitions in polymers; nanostructured polymer blends; macro-, micro-, and nanocomposites; polymer rheology; recycling; reactive extrusion; processing–morphology–property relationships in multiphase polymer systems; double networking of elastomers; natural fibers and green composites; rubber vulcanization; interpenetrating polymer networks; diffusion; and transport and polymer scaffolds for tissue engineering. He has three patents to his credit and has received the coveted Sukumar Maithy Award as best polymer researcher in the country for the year 2008. Very recently Professor Thomas received the MRSI and CRSI medals for his excellent work. With over 720 publications to his credit and over 26811 citations, with an h-index of 78, Dr. Thomas has been ranked fifth in India as and published research articles and reviews in international one of the most productive scientists.

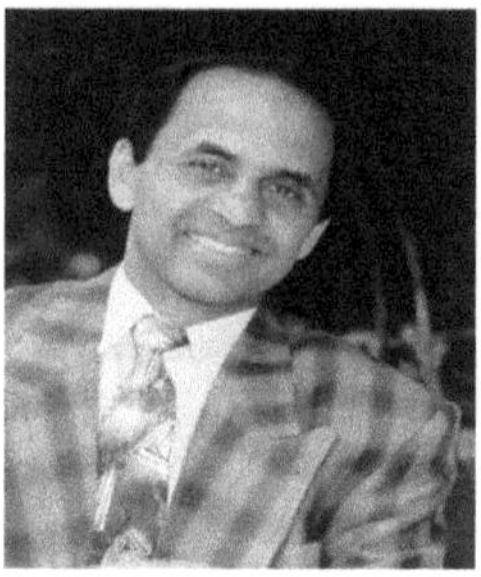

Sebastian Mathew, MD, is currently the Doctor in Charge at the Ayurveda and Vein Clinic in Klagenfurt, Austria, as well as a Consultant Surgeon at the Maria Hilf Clinic in Klagenfurt, Austria. He is a member of TAM Advisory Committee (Traditional Asian Medicine, Sector Ayurveda) of the Austrian Ministry of Health, and he has conducted an international Ayurveda congress in Klagenfurt, Austria, in 2010. He has several publications to his name. He was a missionary doctor in a Mugana Hospital, Bukoba in Tanzania, Africa (1976–1978). Dr. Mathew received his MBBS from Kottayam Medical College, University of Kerala, India. He acquired his MD in surgery in Austria. He underwent medical training in different hospitals in India, Germany, and Austria and holds several diplomas in acupuncture, neural therapy, manual therapy vascular diseases and Ayurveda.

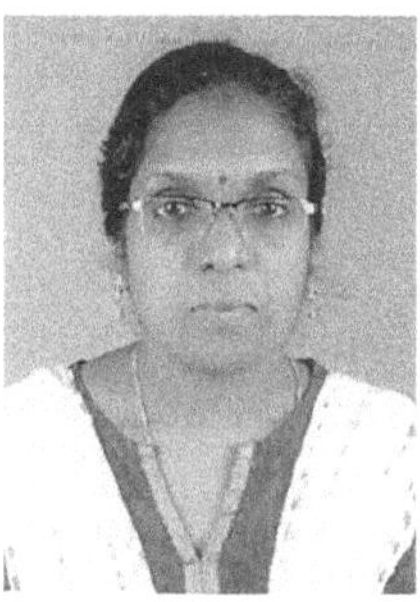

Raji V., PhD, is an Assistant Professor at the International and Inter University Centre for Nanoscience and Nanotechnology at Mahatma Gandhi University in Kerala, India. Her current research interests include synthesis and characterization of metal nanoparticles for drug delivery as well as imaging. She is also engaged in the synthesis of bioconjugated metal nanoparticles for photothermal therapy of cancer. She has several publications to her credit. Dr. Raji V obtained her PhD in biochemistry from the University of Kerala, India.

CONTENTS

LIST OF CONTRIBUTORS

Shama Aphale
Interactive Research School for Health Affairs (IRSHA), Bharati Vidyapeeth University, Katraj-Dhankawadi, Pune-Satara Road, Pune 411043, Maharashtra, India

Hemand Aravind
Department of Biotechnology, Navajyothi Sree Karunakara Guru Research Centre for Ayurveda and Siddha, Uzhavoor, Kottayam 686634, Kerala, India

Rashmi Deshpande
Interactive Research School for Health Affairs (IRSHA), Bharati Vidyapeeth University, Katraj-Dhankawadi, Pune-Satara Road, Pune 411043, Maharashtra, India

L. Dhivyalakshmi
Department of Biomedical Engineering, Sri Ramakrishna Engineering College, Anna University, Coimbatore, Tamil Nadu, India

Susana Dinis
Unus Research Center, Portugal

Gisala George
Department of Physical Education, Mercy College, Palakkad 678006, Kerala, India

Ruchika Kaul-Ghanekar
Interactive Research School for Health Affairs (IRSHA), Bharati Vidyapeeth University, Katraj-Dhankawadi, Pune-Satara Road, Pune 411043, Maharashtra, India

Anwar H. Gilani
College of Health Sciences, Mekelle University, PO Box 1871 Mekelle, Ethiopia

A. A. Mohamed Hatha
Department of Marine Biology, Microbiology and Biochemistry, School of Marine Sciences, Cochin University of Science and Technology, Cochin 682016, Kerala, India

G. Hema
Department of Biomedical Engineering, Sri Ramakrishna Engineering College, Anna University, Coimbatore, Tamil Nadu, India

Ann Holaday
Radiation Oncology, Cambridge University, Cambridge, UK

Tilak Kalra
Department of Chemical Engineering, Banaras Hindu University, Varanasi 221002, Uttar Pradesh, India

Ghislaine Madjou
International Institute of Management, Cotonou, Republic of Benin

J. N. Mishra
Faculty of Ayurveda, Lucknow University, Lucknow 226007, Uttar Pradesh, India

T. K. Mukundan
S.N.M. College, Maliankara, Kerala

Indu M. Nair
School of Environmental Sciences, Mahatma Gandhi University, P.D. Hills, Kottayam 686562, Kerala, India

Sowmya Narayanan
Department of Biomedical Engineering, Sri Ramakrishna Engineering College, Anna University, Coimbatore, Tamil Nadu, India

Jeane Yonkeu Ngogang
Departement de Biochimie, Faculte des Sciences Biomedicales, Université des Montagnes, Bangangte, Ouest, Republic of Cameroon

K. A. Treasa Nimy
PG Department of Zoology and Aquaculture, St. Albert's College, Banerji Road, Ernakulam 682018, Kerala, India

V. Vijaya Padma
Translational Research Laboratory, Department of Biotechnology, Bharathiar University, Coimbatore 641046, Tamil Nadu, India

Savita Pandita
Interactive Research School for Health Affairs (IRSHA), Bharati Vidyapeeth University, Katraj-Dhankawadi, Pune-Satara Road, Pune 411043, Maharashtra, India

Vincent Terrence Rebello
PG Department of Zoology and Aquaculture, St. Albert's College, Banerji Road, Ernakulam 682018, Kerala, India

S. Saranya
Translational Research Laboratory, Department of Biotechnology, Bharathiar University, Coimbatore 641046, Tamil Nadu, India

Ernest Tambo
Sydney Brenner Institute for Molecular Bioscience, Wits 21st Century Centre of Excellence, University of the Witwatersrand, Johannesburg, South Africa

Emmanuel Mouafo Tekwu
Laboratory for Tuberculosis Research (LTR), Biotechnology Centre-Nkolbisson, Faculty of Sciences, University of Yaoundé I, Yaoundé, Republic of Cameroon

Emmanuel Chidiebere Ugwu
Department of Human Biochemistry, Faculty of Basic Medical Sciences, Nnamdi Azikiwe University, Awka, Nnewi Campus, Nigeria
National Institute of Parasitic Diseases, Chinese Center for Diseases Control and Prevention & WHO Collaborating Center on Malaria, Schisostomiasis and Filariasis, Shanghai 200025, PR China

Søren Ventegodt
Quality of Life Research Center, Copenhagen, Denmark Research Clinic for Holistic Medicine, Copenhagen, Denmark Nordic School of Holistic Medicine, Copenhagen, Denmark

Mariya Yeldhos
Department of Biomedical Engineering, Sri Ramakrishna Engineering College, Anna University, Coimbatore, Tamil Nadu, India

LIST OF ABBREVIATIONS

A	ampicillin
ADHD	attention-deficit hyperactivity disorder
AFRO	African Regional Office
AH	*Aeromonas hydrophila*
Ak	amikacin
AKT	serine/threonine-protein kinases
AT/CAM	African traditional complementary and alternative medicine
AVE	audiovisual entrainment
B	bladder
B	bulb
BS	*Bacillus subtilis*
C	chloramphenicol
CAM	complementary and alternative medicine
CBT	cognitive behavioral therapy
CDK	cyclin-dependent kinases
Cf	ciprofloxacin
CHM	clinical holistic medicine
CIN	cervical intraepithelial neoplasia
CM	conventional medicine
COX-2	cycloxygenases-2
CP	cyclophosphamide
CTC	crush, tear, curl
CVD	cardiovascular diseases
DALY	disability-adjusted life year
E	erythromycin
EC	*Escherichia coli*
EGCG	epigallocatechin gallate
EGFR	epidermal growth factor receptor
ERK	extracellular signal-regulated kinase
EU	European Union
EUSART	enhanced universal asynchronous receiver transmitter
Fl	flower
Fr	fruit

G	gentamycin
G+ve	gram positive
GAP	good assurance practices
GB	gall bladder
GMP	good manufacturing practice
GSP	good standard practices
GV	governing vessel
HALY	health-adjusted life year
HER	human epidermal growth factor receptor
HIF-1α	hypoxia-inducible factor-1α
HIV/AIDS	human immuno-deficient virus/acquired immuno-deficiency syndrome
HPA	hypothalamic-pituitary-adrenal-axis
HPV	human papilloma virus
HRT	hormone replacement therapy
HSIL	high grade squamous intraepithelial lesions
HTCM	herbal and traditional Chinese medicine
I	intermediate
IARC	International Agency for Research on Cancer
IPR	intellectual property rights
IRSHA	Interactive Research School for Health Affairs
JAMA	Journal of the American Medical Association
K	kanamycin
L	lincomycin
LED	light emitting diode
LSIL	low grade squamous intraepithelial lesions
LTPP	long-term psychodynamic psychotherapy
LTR	Laboratory for Tuberculosis Research
MAPK	mitogen-activated protein kinase
MDGs	millennium development goals
MHA	Mueller–Hinton agar
MI	myocardial infarction
MMPs	matrix metalloproteinase
MOH	Ministry of Health
mTOR	mammalian target of rapamycin
Na	nalidixic acid
Nf	nitrofurantoin
NF-κB	nuclear factor κB

NHP	National Health Policy
NNHs	number needed to harm
Nv	novobiocin
P	penicillin
pRb	phospho Rb
PRP	platelet-rich plasma
PSMs	plant secondary metabolites
QALY	quality-adjusted life year
QOL	quality of life
R	resistant
R&D	research and development
Raf	rapidly accelerated fibrosarcoma
Ras	rat sarcoma
Rb	retinoblastoma
RCT	randomized clinical trial
Rh	rhizome
RTK	receptor tyrosine kinase
S	streptomycin
SA	*Staphylococcus aureus*
SATM	standardized African traditional medicines
SB	*Salmonella bovis*
SBa	*Salmonella bareilly*
SCN	suprachiasmatic nucleus
SE	*Salmonella enteritidis*
SIL	squamous intraepithelial lesions
SM	*Salmonella mgulani*
SP	*Salmonella paratyphi*
SS	*Salmonella senftenberg*
ST	*Salmonella typhimurium*
STD	sexually transmitted diseases
STPP	short-term psychodynamic psychotherapy
SW	*Salmonella worthington*
SWe	*Salmonella weltevreden*
T	tetracycline
TB	tuberculosis
TCM	traditional Chinese medicine
TIM	traditional Indian medicine
TRAIPR	trade-related aspects of intellectual property rights

UN	United Nations
USDA	United States Department of Agriculture
Va	vancomycin
VBAC	vaginal birth after caesarean
VC	*Vibrio cholera*
VED	vascular endothelial dysfunction
VEGF	vascular endothelial growth factor
VV	*Vibrio vulnificus*
WHO	World Health Organization

PREFACE

"The cure of the part should not be attempted without treatment of the whole."

—Plato

The United Nations World Health Organization (WHO) defines health as "a state of complete physical, mental, and social well being and not merely the absence of disease or infirmity." Holistic medicine is a form of healing that considers the whole person-body, mind, spirit, and emotions. Holistic healing is the art of maintaining a proper balance between the physical, social, and emotional dimensions of well-being. Thus, holistic medicine can be considered as the key to optimal health and wellness. The holistic practitioners strongly believe that our body has a remarkable healing capacity, when given the proper foundation. Hence, they educate the patients on ways to improve their health and thus make them active participants of healing process. In holistic healing, the treatment or health program is tailored to meet the specific needs of the patient. For effective healing, three factors should be taken into account—"stay healthy, prevent disease and manage illness." It is apparent that for attaining personal well-being, a healthy diet along with a proper balance between mental and social aspects is equally important. Times have changed. Today, to deal tactfully, with the vicissitudes of life, one has to be emotionally strong and positive in attitude. Accompanied by proper guidance, holistic healing provides relaxing and energizing effect to patients.

The main scope of this book is to provide an overview about holistic medicine and to spread awareness about the healing power of natural therapies. In Chapter 1, the author along with relevant experimental data, states that holistic medicine is the safest and effective medicine for all clinical conditions. Chapter 2 gives an insight about the traditional medical practices in African countries. The obstacles of integrating African traditional/CAM into health care delivery systems are also carefully discussed. Chapter 3 details the importance of the management of body postures.

The advantages of Integrative pharmacology are described in Chapter 4. Chapter 5 focuses on the positive aspects of Yoga. Chapters 6 and 7 focus on the antibacterial properties of medicinally relevant plants against selected bacteria. The anti-platelet aggregation property of a tribal medicinal plant from Western Ghats is demonstrated in Chapter 8. Chapter 9 introduces the role of medicinal plants in targeting important signaling pathways in case of cervical cancer. A portable and user-friendly device for drug-free treatment of insomnia is suggested in Chapter 10. Chapter 11 provides a detailed review about the cardioprotective efficacy of various phytochemicals from medicinal plants. Chapter 12 describes a successful keloid management technique based on the knowledge from Sushrut. The importance of Ayurveda is detailed in Chapter 13.

This book will hopefully be helpful to researchers, scientists, students, and other experts in the field of holistic medicine. Publishing of this book would not have been possible without the help of authors. We are greatly thankful to all the authors for their valuable contributions. We would like to extend our sincere thanks to the publisher Apple Academy Press for publishing this book and for their guidance throughout. Special thanks to Prof. Soren Ventegodt for his constant support.

Holistic healing has significantly improved the quality of life around the globe. Nature plays a vital role in human health and well-being. Natural healing remedies, to study the underlying cause of disease are being explored nowadays. Medicinal plants are powerful natural healers and are very affordable and effective. This book *"Holistic Healthcare: Possibilities and Challenges"* provides valuable insights into the healing power of nature. Hopefully, having read this book, the reader will be suitably equipped to better understand the therapeutic relevance of natural remedies.

In wrapping up, holistic medicine is the language of healing that helps to improve the quality of life. The harmony of body and soul contributes to holistic healing. Hence, holistic health is a life style to be followed for attaining good health.

—Blessy Joseph

CHAPTER 1

A TOUR AROUND THE WORLD'S MEDICAL SYSTEMS USING EVIDENCE-BASED MEDICINE TO POINT OUT WHAT IS THE BEST MEDICINE: HOLISTIC MIND–BODY MEDICINE IS SAFEST AND MOST EFFECTIVE FOR MOST CLINICAL CONDITIONS

SØREN VENTEGODT*

Quality of Life Research Center, Copenhagen, Denmark Research Clinic for Holistic Medicine, Copenhagen, Denmark Nordic School of Holistic Medicine, Copenhagen, Denmark

E-mail: ventegodt@livskvalitet.org

CONTENTS

ABSTRACT

Aim: To examine the conditions for good medical science and to compare cost-benefit and cost-effectiveness of all types of evidences-based medicine, both pharmaceuticals and non-drug complementary and alternative medicine (CAM) for all clinical conditions.

Method: Calculating therapeutic value (TV = Total number needed to harm (NNH_{total})/Number needed to treat (NNT)) and cost per cured patient (year 1–50) for 10 different types of evidence-based medicine. Cost is presented as EURO (€) per cured patient, EURO per quality-adjusted life year (QALY), EURO per health-adjusted life year (HALY), and number of harmed patients per cured patient. The cost of one year of treatment was set to €2000 and the difference between healthy to 20% (quality of life (QOL), self-rated health).

Results: We found the most effective CAM-types (mind–body medicine, holistic medicine, Shamanism) to be 100 times as cost-effective and 10,000 times less harmful compared to pharmaceuticals. The 50 years' estimated cost for one patient cured was for drugs €1,000,000; physical therapy €100,000; psychotherapy €100,000; mind–body medicine €50,000; holistic mind–body medicine €20,000; and one-session shamanistic healing with hallucinogenic drugs €2000. CAM is more efficient than drugs and has no side effects and adverse events, whereas treatment with drugs always has adverse effects and events.

Interpretation: To be useful, medicine must have significant therapeutic value (good benefit-to-harm ratio: TV ≥ 1) and documented long-term effect and safety. Holistic mind–body medicine seems to be the safest and most effective of all types of medicine for almost all clinical conditions. The shift from drugs to non-drug CAM would improve health and quality of life radically in society and reduce harm to patients and the cost of healthcare to a small fraction. Strict laws should be introduced immediately in all countries to stop the pharmaceutical industry from promoting drugs without therapeutic value, and from repressing CAM.

1.1 WHAT IS EVIDENCE-BASED MEDICINE?

Evidence-based medicine is medicine based on scientific evidence of high quality. Medicine is everything that is intended for healing or prevention of physical and mental disease, discomfort, suffering, pour sexual, social, work etc. functioning, general unhappiness or any other aspect of our "global quality of life." What quality of life (QOL) truly is remains a deep mystery for science; countless efforts of reducing this concept to something more practical and measurable have failed miserably. Therefore, medicine at its core remains a mystery also: It is simply philosophically unclear what you intend to improve. In the end of the analyses you want to improve the human being him- or herself, which is basically impossible, unless we let go of our own personality and conditioning, all our properties, and all our bonds to the world, as recommended by the spiritual mystics and religious leaders like Krishna, Buddha, and Jesus.

Medicine of the mind and the body remains an interest of small souls; greater souls would address the health of the spirit; unfortunately, spiritual health and self-insight often comes from suffering, poverty, and physical and mental illnesses which therefore should not be alleviated.

Medicine comes as magical rites, behavioral advices, magical amulets or potions, chemical drugs, physical interventions, like surgery or radiation therapy, physical therapy like massage and acupressure, and many different kinds of talk therapy. Even religious interventions like prayers, healings, meditation, and religious and philosophical teachings must be classified as medicine in the broadest meaning of this word.

The root of all these problems is of course that we do not, in scientific terms, understand consciousness itself, which gives rise to all our experiences, good and bad.

Table 1.1 gives a classification of medicines (including complementary and alternative medicine (CAM) and biomedicine) into 10 principal classes.

The next important question is "what scientific evidence is?" It is almost as difficult to answer as to the question about what medicine is. All sciences use axioms which cannot be proven. Therefore, all sciences are basically religion. That is even the case with pure mathematics, and much more the case with chemistry and physics, and even more with life sciences like biology and medicine, where life, consciousness, and happiness becomes core issues in spite of our almost total lack of scientific understanding of these subjects.

In science, the concept of true and false is essential, but how can any statement based on mind be absolutely true? It can only be relatively true, so the art of science is to make it simple and so, related to reality that we can be somewhat happy that our statement is at least true in a relative sense.

TABLE 1.1 Classification of Medicine (Including CAM and Biomedicine) into 10 Principal Classes: Classes 1 and 2 are Chemical Medicines; 3–10 are Informational Medicines.

1. Chemical medicine (biomedicine with bioactive molecules).
2. Chemical CAM (flower medicine, herbal medicine, diets, minerals, vitamins etc.).
3. Body-medicine (low-energy types: massage, reflexology, physical therapy, physiotherapy, spa, sauna etc.; high-energy types: chiropractics etc.).
4. Mind-medicine (psychotherapy—psychodynamic, cognitive, gestalt etc.—psychoanalysis, meditation, no-touch sexology, couching, healing music etc.).
5. Spirit-medicine (philosophical interventions, energy medicine, prayers, spiritual healing (i.e., Reichi), Shamanism, spiritual CAM (i.e., crystal healing) etc.).
6. Mind–body medicine (acupuncture, acupressure, homeopathy, manual sexology, body-psychotherapy, Reichian bodywork, Rosen therapy, ergo therapy etc.).
7. Body–spirit medicine (prayer involving physical activity like in Tibetan Buddhist-style meditation, pilgrimage etc.).
8. Holistic body-mind-spirit medicine—including existential therapy (holistic medicine, clinical medicine, clinical holistic medicine, holistic body-psychotherapy, holistic bodywork, the sexological examination, holistic mind–body medicine, biodynamic body-psychotherapy, tantric bodywork and massage, holistic sexology, Native American rituals).
9. Chemical body-mind-spirit medicine (Shamanism with peyote, Ayahuasca, magic mushrooms, Grof's LSD psychotherapy etc.)
10. Social and environmental medicine (coaching, work-related personal development programs, stress management, leadership training, gardening, aesthetic architecture, Feng Shui etc.)

If consider a medicine and ask if a cure is helpful to a clinical condition, we need to test the cure on patients, and see if their condition improves. This is lovely simple. If you have a simple measure like pain, we can make the patient rate his pain before and after treatment and we can immediately see if we help the patients. If we test the cure on 20 patients with comparable pains, we can even calculate a mean for the improvement and say that our cure is so and so helpful for his kind of pain.

So, simple before-and-after studies using simple measures for simple and well-defined states of illness and suffering gives us relatively true measures for effectivity and safety of medicine.

But, the methods used for testing medicines today are not like that. They are highly complex procedures where many things can be adjusted until the wished-for results are created. The famous randomized clinical trial (RCT) is an example of such a method, which is not even relatively true. According the many critiques, it is nowadays only used by pharmacological companies to market poisonous chemicals as effective and safe medicine.[1]

In general, the more complex a thing is made, the less transparent it is, and the less it has to do with reality, the less true it is.

1.2 TWO MAJOR COMPONENTS OF GOOD SCIENTIFIC MEDICINE: GOOD THEORY AND GOOD CLINICAL DOCUMENTATION

Human beings are bio-psycho-social beings[2]; while science is quite clear and simple when it comes to chemistry, physics, and biology, it gets quite unclear and flimsy when it comes to psychology, and really messy when it comes to the social dimensions of man.

Good medicine theory is of course interdisciplinary; it describes man as a bio-psycho-social being and disease as a disturbance in the wholeness, not in one of its parts. When you get sick, the symptoms are often in your body, but the cause is in your psyche; and if you explore your mental dimension you will find that it is highly dependent on you social reality.

If you look at the immune system, its immunological defense power comes from the inner balance of the organism[3]; but this balance is hard to describe in scientific terms. We know that staying healthy is closely related to quality of life and happiness; you can say that happiness is the best medicine.

The biological and cellular order is highly sensitive to the state of mind of the person; but happiness goes even deeper: happiness goes to the roots of you being and stretches out to you most remote of your relationships. Your happiness vibrates though you whole existence. Happiness is a mystery in itself; there is no really good science about happiness, so to include happiness in the scientific theory of medicine has been and remains a real challenge. This work is simply not done yet. We have a lot of research to do here in the future! What we can say for sure is that a simple chemical model for life is totally inadequate to explain health, disease, bad thriving, and healing.

When it comes to scientific documentation of the clinical effect of medicine, we have even bigger problems, for what is a good test of clinical effect? We know by now that the RCT, which everybody 30 years ago believed to be the final solution to the problem of how to test pharmacological medicine, is so faulty and flawed that it cannot be taken as scientific documentation.[4]

One problem is that the active placebo effect of poisonous drugs in the RCT as it is designed today turns all poisonous drugs tested by the method into effective medicine with exactly the specific action the test aims to explore.[1,4] This is a hopeless situation; the blinding is always broken by the toxic effects of the drugs, and the pharmaceutical companies are producing "medicines" which only have toxic effects.[1,4–6] A number of Cochrane studies have recently documented that many of the drug-groups we are using are without significant beneficial effects and poisonous.[1,5,6] Yet, 100 million people or so are taking these drugs every day in the belief that they are helpful.[1] And because of the active placebo, they are helpful for a short while. But this is like peeing your pants to get heat: It only helps for a very short time; then it gets really annoying.

The consequence of the lack of a valid test method for pharmacological drugs has been devastating. According to leading experts in the Cochrane Collaboration, millions of patients are getting poisoned with severe consequences for their health every year; and thousands of these patients are even dying from the poisoning.[1] Especially, the psychiatric patients are burdened by the toxic effects of drugs.[1,6]

In evidence-based medicine, you need to look at the quality of the scientific evidence. The best scientific evidence, like the meta-analyses made by independent researchers, that is, the Cochrane reviews from the 3000 fairly independent physicians and researchers in the international Cochrane Collaboration, has systematically shown that drugs are of little help for patients and almost always very harmful. Even the best of pharmacological medicines has surprisingly little effect; if you look at how many patients you need to treat for one being helped (the number needed to treat (NNT)) it is normally 20 patients or more[7] (and often 100 or more for serious diseases like cancer and schizophrenia).

An NNT of 20 means that if a doctor gives such a drug to a patient, the likelihood for the patient to be helped is 0.05, or only 5%! If NNT = 100, only 1% of the patients are helped. And the people who are helped are most often NOT cured. They only have a few symptoms of the disease. Hence, this is the situation of the pharmacological medicines we have today. At the same time, adverse effects are so normal that in average, every patient will have a harmful effect from taking a drug.[8] Honestly, it is not worth being a doctor with such poor results. Therefore, many doctors burn out and loose the joy of work while they year after year see that their patients systematically are not improving.

So, how is it with evidence-based CAM—alternative medicine, non-drug medicine—call it what you like? Today, hundreds of meta-analyses and Cochrane reviews have shown that there are *no significant side effects of non-drug medicine*[9,10]—with high-energy manipulations (chiropractic) as a rare exception. So you can safely go to any psychotherapist or body worker. Talk and touch therapy are just safe.[10] That is good to know.

But is CAM effective? Well, in general, alternative medicine is not effective. Sorry. If you look at all that we do to help and cure, this broad spectrum of activities we call CAM are mostly NOT helpful. A number of scientific studies of prayers and positive thinking, diets, exercises, breathing exercises, yoga, meditation, art therapy, herbal medicine etc. have proven these types of CAM to be without significant positive effect for the patient.[9] Therefore, in general, CAM cures are not working.

With this said, there are some types of talk and touch therapy that has been proven extremely effective. These are methods that at the same time focus on (a) feelings and emotions including sexuality, (b) understanding and self-exploration including almost all types of self-inquiry, and (c) letting go of negative beliefs, attitudes, thoughts, philosophies, concepts etc.—that is, mind-work that empties your mind from all its mental contents and structures, and all our identifications.[11–16]

Psychodynamic psychotherapy—that is, talk therapy with focus on emotions and sexuality—have been proven extremely effective; 95% have been helped and the help is often a cure.[17–19] Holistic medicine has recently been found extremely effective in the USA for cancer and coronary heart disease, with around 80% of the patients helped within 3–6 month.[20–22] These are amazing results.

Similar results have been found for a number of existentially oriented talk-and-touch therapies.[23,24] Methods that combine talk-and-touch therapy to help the patient FEEL, UNDERSTAND, and LET GO of negative beliefs have in general been found very effective, with amazing NNT numbers (1 or 2) and totally harmless. And the wonderful thing is that these methods seem to help a wide range of clinical conditions—almost all types of patients can be helped.[25] And these results are also found in meta-analyses made by independent researchers.

See, this is good, evidence-based medicine. So we have after all come a long way in medicine.

1.3 ADVICES TO THE PERSON WHO WANTS TO SEEK HOLISTIC MEDICINE/THERAPY

The true problem of therapy is that some people just seem to have what it takes to become a therapist; they are good from the beginning of their practice even without education and training and they become only a little better as years go by.[26] And then, there are the other group of therapists; the hardworking people with good intentions and little talent who will do much but accomplish little.[27]

As we have not been able to teach these therapists how to become good therapist, we obviously do not understand what it is that makes a good therapist.

In my experience, it is about love. Some people simply love other people. These people can help almost everybody—because of their love as Buber points out.[28] They don't judge; they don't create a distance to their clients or patients. They just accept, acknowledge, care, and support whoever comes to them.[29]

You cannot learn to love. If you do not love other people, you cannot be trained to do so. So at the end of the day, it all comes down to this simple thing: if you want to be a therapist ask if you love other people. If you do not and you still want to become therapist, you might want to look at your motives. Being a bad therapist will not serve the world. But if you love other people, just start today and open your practice. You will without doubt succeed.

Maybe you will wonder how these things fit together: that some methods seem to work, but that people cannot learn therapy. It seems that people with a talent for therapy are simply attracted to effective methods that focus on important issues like the meaning of life.[30]

It takes a lot of love to work with people's feelings and sexuality; to help the sick and insane to explore their innermost secrets and to work patiently endless numbers of hours to help neurotic people to let go of untrue believes.[27]

If you are troubled and in search for a good therapist yourself, do not waste your time reading science. Go and look for somebody who can love and serve you. Find a therapist with whom you have a good chemistry, a person you can feel you can trust and love yourself. If you can find such a person, this is your best change for getting the help you need to change your life.

Everybody can heal, everybody can become happy. But to heal from a serious disease, we need to change from a very deep place within ourselves. Facilitating this inner change that in the end will transform our whole being and experience of life is what all effective medicine is about.[31]

1.4 HOLISTIC MEDICINE AROUND THE WORLD

What has been the most amazing thing for me on my journey through the universe of medicine has been the way different cultures have implemented medicine traditions.

It has been astonishing for me to travel around different continents, just to learn that the Native American shamans, the African Sangomas, and the Indian sages have understood very much the same thing about the human nature: that we—the false self, the ego, or call it our personality or conditioning—is the fundamental cause of almost all human suffering. Our ignorance, called our unconsciousness in Western science, is causing our problems.

And the cure is almost the same in all cultures: feel the feelings you have oppressed, understand what happened to you since you are not your true and wonderful self these days, and let go of all the negative learning and untrue beliefs you have picked up through your life.

Good healers are always loving and companionate human beings with deep self-insight and enormous spaciousness.

In eastern philosophy, that is, in the tradition of Sri Ramana Maharshi,[32] consciousness about the self is the door to happiness ("eternal bliss"). In premodern religion, the shaman is one with the universe, and all his or her doing expresses the will of the Great Spirit. In existential philosophy, as formulated by Kierkegaard and Sartre, happiness rises from the personal choice, and only by choosing the true can a person be truly happy.

Ramana[32] asked one fundamental question: "Who am I?" To answer this question, a simple method of intuitive introspection is used. One simply observes all phenomena that one can observe from the perspective of the heart, both internally and externally; and systematically asks, "Am I this?"

The outer world of objects is soon seen as non-self. The thoughts, feelings, the body, all mental images, memory, anticipations, intentions, desires, attachments etc. are also watched, and little by little, also seen as non-self. In the end all phenomena is acknowledged as non-self, including all concepts and words, all knowledge and all mental structures, ideas and perceptions.

The second, quite logic, question is then: "If I am none of these, then who am I?" Answer: "After negating all of the above mentioned as 'not this,' 'not this,' that awareness which alone remains—that I am."[32] The third questions is, "What is the nature of awareness?" Answer: "The nature of awareness is existence-consciousness-bliss." This is often called Sat-Shit-Ananda. The fourth question is, "When will the realization of the self be gained?" Answer: "When the world which is what-is-seen has been removed, there will be realization of the self which is the seer."

This is basically it. The rest is for your own experience. The state of being present in truth, or inner self, cannot be described; being, happiness and knowledge is what seem to appear in consciousness of the one who finds it and dwells in it. And even the idea of finding it is illusory: It is already and always there. You just need to realize it; you just need to wake up at this level. Then you know that you have been this all the time. The problem is that it is a quality-less state, often describes as emptiness, the great void, or Sunya(ta). It is a non-phenomenon, and the recognition is non-phenomenal. This does not make sense to the mind at all. You cannot understand it mentally. That is the problem. Experience can go deeper that though; consciousness is earlier than thought; it came first. Therefore, it cannot be understood by thought.

The traditional value of being conscious is, from the eastern point of view, that one can break the conditionings that make human slave of past. This is called personal freedom, or "enlightenment."

If you happen to pass South Africa, it is worth the trouble to go to Johannesburg to meet the Traditional Healers Organization, where the leaders are experts in even the more dark and bizarre aspects of traditional African healing. This story is also about consciousness but seen from the brutal side of life: These people are going blindly with the life force.

In Africa, many people believe that there are healing properties associated with the organs of the body. Animal organs have some healing power, but human organs are the most powerful for healing humans.

Of the organs, the genitals are considered the most powerful for healing. The younger the person is, the more powerful is the healing power of the organ. The organ is most powerful for healing if it is removed alive, and the more painful the removal is, the more powerful medicine can be made from the organs.

Therefore, when a number of children, mostly girls, where found killed, obviously after torture and mutilation, with their genitals cut away, seemingly while the children were still alive, this left little doubt in the local population that this was the Sangomas harvesting the necessary ingredients for their magical brews.

The superstitions related to Muthi killings have a number of horrible expressions in South Africa, Botswana, and the related countries, that is, rape of young virgin girls which is generally believed in many parts of the black population to be able to cure AIDS. This leads to thousands of rapes of children in Africa every year.

The local population has been reacting to the Sangomas since the systematic and frequent Muthi killings—14 killings in one region in only one year—have been given a lot of media attention in South Africa. In many regions, healers have been robbed, lost their houses and property which has been taken over by angry neighbors, they have been beaten, raped, and in a number of cases, stoned or burned to dead in classical witch-fires.

It seems that the Indian sages and the African Sangomas live in different universes, and yet both are human beings, and both must obey the laws of the universe when they do what they can to heal and help their fellow man. Consciousness and the life force seem to be the two fundamental forces in every single human being, and only when we come to terms with them can we be healthy and happy.

1.5 COMPARATIVE ANALYSIS OF COST-BENEFIT AND COST-EFFECTIVENESS OF ALL TYPES OF EVIDENCE-BASED MEDICINE FOR ALL CLINICAL CONDITIONS

We have suggested that the five major categories of CAM used by National Center for Complementary and Alternative Medicine (NCCAM) are revised into a 10-class system for evidence-based medicine in general,[33] as we agree to the viewpoint often presented in *Journal of the American*

Medical Association (JAMA) that CAM and biomedicine must be one integrated medical system of evidence-based medicine[34] (Table 1.1).

We are now able using simple and reliable science to examine the cost-benefit and cost-efficiency of the 10 different types of evidence-based medicine. We want to look at the benefit-to-harm ratio (often called therapeutic value), the cost of the production of quality of life and self-rated health and the cost of health in patient-damage.

1.6 METHODS

Today, there are three major population health measures permitting morbidity and mortality to be simultaneously evaluated: quality-adjusted life years (QALYs), health-adjusted life years (HALYs), and disability-adjusted life years (DALYs). In this paper, we will only estimate QALYs and HALYs.

The method is estimating the general numbers from meta-analyses, preferably Cochrane reviews, and, when possible, meta-meta-analyses covering one or more of the different types of evidence-based medicine. We will include estimates from the leading medical journals of typical numbers of NNTs and number needed to harm (NNHs). To make such a highest level analysis where we look at all types of medicine for all clinical conditions, we will need to simplify matters.

The prize of pharmaceutical drugs will be calculated from the Danish cost of drugs to more than two million chronic patients in Denmark using biomedicine; this number might be high compared to the number in developing countries were medicine often is sold cheaper. The prize of CAM treatments are also coming from Danish circumstances, where a year of therapy often is about 20 sessions costing around €2000; in developing countries the prize is often a tenth of that. The calculation of QALY and HALY is using the knowledge on normal loss of quality of life and self-rated health when people get ill in Denmark; and have a lot of social security to some extend compensating for loss of quality of life and health, the prize per QALY and HALY might be lower in less developed countries.

As our results are calculated based on estimate numbers, we must admit having an uncertainty of ±100%; we believe our results to be correct within a factor three. As the differences between the different types of medicine are often a factor 10 or 100, this large uncertainty is still acceptable.

As the biggest problem in medical research today is bias from economic interests, we have avoided sources that might be strongly biased, like RCTs from pharmaceutical industry, overoptimistic estimates in reviews from CAM-journals not represented in MedLine/ www.PubMed.gov etc.

Actually the process of limiting bias has been our biggest problem, forcing us to leaving out most of the sources often used in this type of analyses, like statistics made by public organs headed by people close to the pharmaceutical industry. Such statistics seems mostly to be extremely biased in favor of biomedicine.

There are many fundamental problems in biomedicine we could have addressed to make this study more thorough; there are problems from the practical use of drugs with low compliance, wrong diagnosis, errors in prescriptions and over medication; there are problems with the RCTs at its very roots making the NNT and NNH numbers from industrial testing difficult to trust, and this paper is after all based on numbers coming from the pharmaceutical industries' use of the RCT in testing its products. So, we know that we are only scratching the surface of the problems in this paper.

We have wanted things to be so simple that complexity of things could not allow us to bias the paper our self; what happens in any complex procedure is that you unconsciously take things in the direction you wish or expect, and only by making things so simple that there are no steps to twist or manipulate, you can truly avoid bias. We believe that the simplicity of our calculations and estimates has leaded us to trustworthy, fairly unbiased results.

Our main source of information is the Cochrane library. In former papers, where we have analyzed aspects of one of the 10 types of medicines, we have had several hundred references. In this paper, we are using the whole Cochrane library as reference. To make the reference list of acceptable length we are only listing complementary material used in the study in the reference list.

1.7 RESULTS

Based on the Cochrane library we have evaluated the benefit and harm from pharmaceutical drugs and the different CAM systems. We have looked at the likelihood to benefit using NNT, the likelihood to be harmed by the different adverse effects/side effects by using NNH, and the total likelihood to get one side effect/adverse reaction or adverse event (NNH_{total}) and from this we have calculated the ratio "benefit to harm" called the therapeutic value of the treatment ($TV = NNH_{total}/NNT$),[25,8,35] for the 10 different types of medicine, see Table 1.2.

TABLE 1.2 Typical Numbers for Effect and Harm, and the *Benefit-to-Harm* Ratio for 10 Classes of Evidence-Based Medicine (NNTs, NNHs, NNH_{total} and TVs) (Estimated from Cochrane Reviews of RCTs and from Clinical Studies with Chronic Patients).[25,8,35,10,9,37,3]

CAM class	Short-term effect (0–6 months)	Long-term effect (6–24 months)	Side effects/ adverse events	Total risk of harm	Therapeutic value TV = NNH_{total}/ NNT
	NNT	NNT	NNH	NNH_{total}	TV (6–24 months)
Class 1—Biomedicine (pharmaceuticals)	20 (5–50)	50 (5–100)	1–5	1–3	1–0.01
Class 2—CAM (Chemical CAM)	≥20	≥50	25 (allergy)	25	0.5
Class 3a—CAM (Physical therapy, low-energy i.e., massage, therapeutic touch)	2–4	6	>1,000,000	>1,000,000	167,000
Class 3b—CAM (Physical therapy, high-energy i.e., chiropractic treatment)	2–4	6	1000 (fractures)	1000	167
Class 4—CAM (psychotherapy)*	3	6	>1,000,000	>1,000,000	167,000
Class 5—CAM (spiritual therapy)	>10	>20	>1,000,000	>1,000,000	50,000
Class 6—CAM (mind–body medicine)	2	4	>1,000,000	>1,000,000	250,000
Class 7—CAM (body–spirit medicine)	Not known	Not known	>1,000,000	>1,000,000	Not known

TABLE 1.2 *(Continued)*

CAM class	Short-term effect (0–6 months)	Long-term effect (6–24 months)	Side effects/ adverse events	Total risk of harm	Therapeutic value TV = NNH_{total}/ NNT
	NNT	NNT	NNH	NNH_{total}	TV (6–24 months)
Class 8—CAM (holistic mind–body medicine)	2	1–2**	>1,000,000	>1,000,000	500,000–1,000,000
Class 9—CAM (Shamanism with drugs etc.)***	1	1	>1000	>1000	>1000
Class 10—CAM (Social medicine)	1	10	>1,000,000	>1,000,000	100,000

*Some types of psychotherapy have short-term NNTs of 2–3 (short-term psychodynamic *psychotherapy* (STPP)) and long term NNTs of 1–2 (long-term psychodynamic *psychotherapy* (LTPP)) for mental, somatic and sexual health problems.[3,10] **The effect of clinical holistic medicine and similar medical systems seem to continue to increase though time.[11] NNT: number needed to treat, NNH: number needed to harm, NNH_{total}: total likelihood of getting one side effect/adverse effect or adverse event. TV: therapeutic value, which here means benefit-to-harm ratio. For a treatment to be of true value to patients, it must be efficient, with a low NNT, and a high TV. ***Adverse effects: Mostly brief reactive psychoses are only seen with mentally ill patients.[10]

While for a long time, thanks to the many Cochrane reviews, it has been easy to find NNT and NNH for most pharmaceutical drugs, it has been more difficult to establish these for the many different types of holistic and alternative medicine (CAM), and the relative harm of non-drug medicine had to be estimated from the number of reported cases in the literature.[10] Recently, more than hundred Cochrane reviews have been made on a large number of CAM-types for a large number of clinical conditions, and NCCAM, the US research center for CAM, has published a number of reports on five major categories of CAM, allowing us for a far better estimate of NNHs and NNTs[36,9] (Table 1.2). For example, NCCAM has evaluated the number of patients treated every year in the USA with massage therapy (therapeutic touch) and the number of patients experiencing significant side effects from such treatments; NCCAM found that 20,000,000 adults and 700,000 children are treated every year with very few patients harmed,[9] allowing us to estimate NNH > 1,000,000 for massage and similar types of therapeutic touch. Of the 145 Cochrane reviews of CAM analyzed by "Committee on the Use of Complementary and Alternative Medicine by the American Public,"[9] 38.4% of the reviews showed a positive or possibly positive (12.4%) effect. These Cochrane reviews documented typical NNTs of 2–30, depending on CAM type, and typical NNHs of 1000–1,000,000. Typical NNTs and NNHs for the 10 types of evidence-based medicine are presented in Table 1.2.[25,35]

Two things are especially interesting for patient: (a) How efficient is the medicine? This is best known from NNT telling how likely it is that the patient will benefit from the treatment. (b) How harmful is the medicine? The absolute harm is important but even more important is the benefit-to-harm ratio. Many patients will feel that a treatment is of therapeutic value if its advantages (statistically) dominate its disadvantages. The benefit-to-harm ratio is simplest expressed by the ratio $TV = NNH_{total}/NNT$, where NNH_{total} is the total likelihood of getting a side/adverse effect or adverse event. Typical values of NNH_{total} and TV can also be found in Table 1.2.

In general, chemical medicine, whether biomedical drugs or CAM (herbs, aromatic oils, diet changes etc.) have high NNH_{total} and low TVs. The effect of chemical CAM seems to be less than pharmaceutical drugs, but it is a lot safer.

If you manipulate the biological informational system of the patient (for the scientific concept of biological information, see Ref.[12]) instead of body chemistry, you seem to avoid side/adverse effects and adverse events. Some types of CAM have a low efficacy, but still the TV is high because of the relative safeness. Some types of CAM are both efficient and safe. Holistic mind–body medicine seems to be as safe as other kinds of CAM but more efficient and they have the highest TV. Interestingly, there are adverse effects of the drugs traditionally used in Shamanism,[10] giving shamanistic medicine the lowest TV of all CAM treatments; but if you look at the cost during a 50-year life span, Shamanism ends up looking the best of all known treatments (Table 1.6). As we do not want to return to Shamanism, we would like to give our tribute to the premodern medicine. Indigenous people often know much about medicine.

The cost of different drugs and different CAM treatment varies a great deal. Within every class of evidence-based medicine, there are expensive and cheap alternatives. We have found it fair to set both a pharmaceutical and a CAM treatment to €2000 per year, knowing that praying is cheaper and cancer-chemotherapy is more expensive. If you know the NNT-number and the cost of one patient treated, you can find the cost for one patient cured (or at least treated successfully) by multiplying these numbers (Cost of one patient cured = NNT × yearly treatment cost) (Table 1.3). The next year, the cured patients will not cost anything but the patient not cured will still cost the yearly treatment cost. In this way, we can estimate the 10 and 50 years' cost of one patient cured (Table 1.3). If the NNT is very high, very few patients get cured and most become chronic patient. This is the case for pharmaceutical drugs, so here the calculation is simple: The cost as times goes by is calculated as *yearly cost* × *time*. If all or most patients are cured in one or a few years, the calculation is similarly simple: The total treatment cost is the one-year treatment cost. When patients get better little by little, as in psychotherapy, a more complicated estimate must be made, accounting for the current recovery of patients. Our estimates of all ten classes are found in Table 1.3. Due to lack of data, we could not make estimates for Classes 5 and 7.

If there are many adverse effects and events, they cost sick days, hospitalization etc. We know that drugs are always poisonous to some extent, and that it is estimated that there are now 100,000 deaths a year in US hospitals directly caused by pharmaceutical drugs.[38,39,40] This is a huge cost but we have only included the direct cost to the drugs in our estimate. The true cost is likely to be several times larger.

A popular effect measure is QALY, or quality-adjusted life years. The idea is simple: Survival has in itself no value; if you survive but suffer to an extreme extent, it might be better if the doctor had not saved you in the first place. The secure that the patient gets value for money, the cost per QALY must be calculated. As quality of life in general is 20% lower for ill people than for healthy,[41] we can make a simple estimate of cost/QALY, presented in Table 1.4. The principles of the estimate are simple: If a patient is cured right away and stays healthy, and would have become a chronic patient without treatment, the cost for one cured patient is multiplied with the time the patient's health is improved. As very few patients are cured with biomedicine, the cost of one QALY becomes astronomic as the treatment continues for life without results—which is normally the case in Denmark where we have socialized biomedicine, free or very cheap for all chronic patients. On the other hand, QALY-unit with an efficient CAM cure, which normally has an extra plus that patients not only stays healthy but also improves health through time (as they have learned the basic principles for human development), will as times go by be relatively cheaper. For every past year, the quality of life and health is already paid, as shown in Table 1.4. Interestingly one-session shamanistic healing is far the cheapest kind of medicine, presumably explaining its great popularity in almost all premodern cultures. In one-session healing, you are normally taken unto a daylong journey of guided self-exploration where you come to understand how you make yourself ill by the way you live and look at things. It is thus a life-style and philosophy of life intervention. From a theoretical point of view, it might actually work.

TABLE 1.3 Accumulated Cost (Number of Patient with Side Effects/Adverse Effects and Adverse Events) for One Patient Cured through Time (Year 1, 10 and 50) for 10 Classes of Evidence-Based Medicine.

Continuous treatment (only stopped if the patients gets cured)	Cost per patient-year	Accumulated cost (€)		
	per treated patient	per cured patient	per cured patient	per cured patient
	First year	First year	Year 10	Year 50
Medicine with drugs (chemical medicine)				
Class 1—chemical medicine*	2000	≥100,000	≥200,000	≥ 1,000,000
Class 2—CAM (chemical CAM)	2000	>100,000	>200,000	>1,000,000
Non-drug CAM (informational medicine)				
Class 3—CAM (physical therapy)	2000	12,000	60,000	100,000
Class 4—CAM (psychotherapy)	2000	12,000	60,000	100,000
Class 5—CAM (spiritual therapy)	Not known	Not known	Not known	Not known
Class 6—CAM (mind–body medicine)	2000	8000	30,000	50,000
Class 7—body–spirit medicine				
Class 8—CAM (holistic mind–body medicine)	2000	5000	10,000	20,000
Class 9—CAM (Shamanism with drugs)	500	600	800	2000
Class 10—CAM (social/environmental medicine)	5,000	50,000	350,000	500,000

*Cost of biomedical examination, hospitalization, and treatment of adverse effects and events not included (estimated round numbers, see text).

TABLE 1.4 Accumulated Cost of One Quality-Adjusted Life Year (QALY) through Time (Year 1, 10 and 50) for 10 Classes of Evidence-Based Medicine.

Continuous treatment (only stopped if the patients gets cured)	QOL improvement from treatment (%) if successful	Prize of one QALY calculated from NNT and accumulated cost (Table 1.3)		
	Global QOL	per cured patient First year	per cured patient Year 10	per cured patient Year 50
Medicine with drugs (chemical medicine)				
Class 1—chemical medicine*	20%	500,000	≥1,000,000	≥5,000,000
Class 2—CAM (chemical CAM)	20%	>500,000	>1,000,000	>5,000,000
Non-drug CAM (informational medicine)				
Class 3—CAM (physical therapy)	20%	60,000	300,000	60,000
Class 4—CAM (psychotherapy)	20%	60,000	300,000	60,000
Class 5—CAM (spiritual therapy)	20%	Not known	Not known	Not known
Class 6—CAM (mind–body medicine)	20%	40,000	180,000	40,000
Class 7—CAM body–spirit medicine	20%	Not known	Not known	Not known
Class 8—CAM (holistic mind–body medicine)	20%	25,000	50,000	10,000
Class 9—CAM (Shamanism with drugs)	20%	3000	4000	800
Class 10—CAM (social/ environmental medicine)	20%	250,000	1,750,000	2,500,000

*Cost of biomedical examination, hospitalization, and treatment of adverse effects and events not included (estimated round numbers, see text).

Instead of QALYs, WHO often recommends the use of HALYs (and DALYs), which is exactly the same, only with health (most often self-rated health) instead of quality of life. We know that the strongest measure of health is self-rated health,[42–45] and we also know that sick people experience there health very much the same way as they experience their quality of life[41] allowing us again to use a difference of 20% between healthy and ill people. This gives us Table 1.5, showing that mind–body medicine gives lots of health for the money, while chemical medicine and social medicine does not.

TABLE 1.5 Accumulated Cost of One Health-Adjusted Life Year (HALY) through Time (Year 1, 10 and 50) for 10 Classes of Evidence-Based Medicine.

Continuous treatment (only stopped if the patients gets cured)	Health improvement from treatment (%) if successful	Prize of one HALY calculated from NNT and accumulated cost (Table 1.3)		
	Self-rated health	per cured patient First year	per cured patient Year 10	per cured patient Year 50
Medicine with drugs				
Class 1—chemical medicine*	20%	500,000	≥1,000,000	≥ 5,000,000
Class 2—CAM (chemical CAM)	20%	>500,000	>1,000,000	>5,000,000
Non-drug CAM				
Class 3—CAM (physical therapy)	20%	60,000	300,000	60,000
Class 4—CAM (psychotherapy)	20%	60,000	300,000	60,000
Class 5—CAM (spiritual therapy)	20%	Not known	Not known	Not known
Class 6—CAM (mind–body medicine)	20%	40,000	180,000	40,000
Class 7—CAM body–spirit medicine	20%	Not known	Not known	Not known
Class 8—CAM (holistic mind–body medicine)	20%	25,000	50,000	10,000
Class 9—CAM (Shamanism with drugs)	20%	3000	4000	800
Class 10—CAM (social/ environmental medicine)	20%	250,000	1,750,000	2,500,000

*Cost of biomedical examination, hospitalization, and treatment of adverse effects and events not included (estimated round numbers, see text).

The harm caused by the 10 different types of evidence-based medicine as times goes by has been estimated in Table 1.6. Patients using biomedicine for years without being cured, as is normally the case, are accumulating the harmful adverse effects and events caused by the pharmaceutical drugs. Non-drug CAM does not cause significant harm. The hallucinogenic drugs have some rare but significant adverse effects but, as shamanistic medicine is often very efficient with result that lasts for life due to increase self-awareness and self-insight, the harm inflicted over a life-span becomes similar to the level of harm inflicted by the other CAM systems, indicating that we might be more open to the potential benefits of premodern medicine and drug-induced one session healing, like Grof's LSD therapy.[46]

TABLE 1.6 Accumulated Harm through Time (Year 1, 10 and 50) for 10 Classes of Evidence-Based Medicine—Prize for One Patient Cured.

Continuous treatment (only stopped if the patient gets cured)	Number of patients harmed for one patient cured	Accumulated harm (number of patients harmed per patient cured)		
	Self-rated health	per cured patient	per cured patient	per cured patient
	NNH_{total}	First year	Year 10	Year 50
Medicine with drugs				
Class 1—chemical medicine	3	17	25	50
Class 2—CAM (chemical CAM)	25	2	4	5
Non-drug CAM				
Class 3a—CAM (physical therapy, Low E)	1,000,000	0.00001	0.0001	0.001
Class 3b—CAM (physical therapy, high efficacy)	1000	0.002	0.01	0.1
Class 4—CAM (psychotherapy)	1,000,000	0.00001	0.0001	0.001
Class 5—CAM (spiritual therapy)	1,000,000	Not known	Not known	Not known
Class 6—CAM (mind–body medicine)	1,000,000	0.00001	0.0001	0.001

TABLE 1.6 *(Continued)*

Continuous treatment (only stopped if the patient gets cured)	Number of patients harmed for one patient cured	Accumulated harm (number of patients harmed per patient cured)		
	Self-rated health	per cured patient	per cured patient	per cured patient
	NNH_{total}	First year	Year 10	Year 50
Class 7—CAM body–spirit medicine	1,000,000	Not known	Not known	Not known
Class 8—CAM (holistic mind–body medicine)	1,000,000	0.00001	0.0001	0.001
Class 9—CAM (Shamanism with drugs)	1000	0.001	0.001	0.001
Class 10—CAM (social/environmental medicine)	1,000,000	0.00001	0.0001	0.001

1.8 DISCUSSION

For a society, the most important thing is to choose a medicine that is affordable, which in general benefits the patients, without harming them. Table 1.6 shows the sad consequences of the large NNH and NNH_{total} numbers of the chemical medicine in the long run. As one of three patients are harmed every year with pharmaceutical drugs, and treatment often continues for life when the patient is not cured, the consequence is that almost every patient is harmed in the end, and 50 patients are harmed for every single, chronic patient helped or cured. In Denmark, over 2 million chronic patients out of a population of 5 millions uses drugs for about €6 billion per year (or €2–3000 per chronically ill patient, confirming the prize of drugs used in Table 1.3). It is clear for us that the same money spent on the most efficient types of non-drug CAM (group 3, 4, 6, and 8) would do immensely more for the populations' health.

As this is not new, one wonders why chemical medicine is so much used, and why mind–body medicine is not part of the official health system. One likely explanation is the close connection between pharmaceutical industry, the physicians, and the public health system—often called the "medico-industrial complex." This system is often seen to actively work against CAM, repressing CAM researchers and effectively by all means keeping CAM out of the political scene.[47]

Drugs obviously turn patients into chronic patients instead of curing them. Half the population of the Western world today is chronically ill, seemingly because of strong political and financial interests in biomedicine, leading to massive oppression of CAM in favor of drugs.

The shift from drugs to CAM would improve health radically in the society and reduce the cost of healthcare to a small fraction. Strict laws should be introduced immediately in all countries to stop the pharmaceutical industry and its collaborates from promoting drugs without evidence of therapeutic value (the ratio, benefits: harm larger being no less than 1) and long-term effect and patient safety, and from repressing CAM.

1.9 CONCLUSION

Strong economic and political interest seem to control medicine in Denmark and many other countries, making the pharmaceutical drugs often used, in spite of better and safer alternative for almost all clinical conditions (see Ref.[3,10] for comprehensive lists of clinical conditions that can be helped or cured with mind–body medicine).

People who still doubt the reality of the low cost, high efficacy and safety of CAM presented in this review are encouraged to study Dean Ornish's cure for coronary heart disease. It was this well-documented CAM cure for a serious disease that made us believe in its potentials.[20,21]

We have seen that the 10 different types of evidence-based medicine have very different profiles when it comes to efficacy, cost per cured patient, cost per QALY, cost per HALY, and cost per harmed patients. In general, chemical medicine as well as biomedicine is expensive and harmful in the long run, while CAM that is, massage therapy and psychotherapy is safe.

The best types of CAM, like mind–body medicine, holistic mind–body medicine (i.e., the classical Hippocratic medicine, often called clinical holistic medicine/CHM) are 50.000 times less harmful and 100 times more efficient in producing health and happiness (quality of life). The cost of one cured chronic patient is about €1,000,000 with pharmaceutical drugs and €100,000 or less with the efficient types of CAM.

Surprisingly, we found premodern medicine—Shamanism—to win the race in the end. While the drugs used often have some rare adverse effects, the efficacy of traditional one-session healing might make shamanistic medicine the cheapest, safest, and most effective in the end. While we do not advocate the back-propagation to premodern times, we find it very interesting that such a medicine exists, inspiring us all to continue our quest for a still better medicine.

ACKNOWLEDGMENTS

The Danish Quality of Life Survey, Quality of Life Research Center and the Research Clinic for Holistic Medicine, Copenhagen, was from 1987 till today, supported by grants from the 1991 Pharmacy Foundation, the Goodwill-fonden, the JL-Foundation, E. Danielsen and Wife's Foundation, Emmerick Meyer's Trust, the Frimodt-Heineken Foundation, the Hede Nielsen Family Foundation, Petrus Andersens Fond, Wholesaler CP Frederiksens Study Trust, Else and Mogens Wedell-Wedellsborg's Foundation, and IMK Almene Fond. The research in quality of life and scientific complementary and holistic medicine was approved by the Copenhagen Scientific Ethical Committee under the numbers (KF)V. 100.1762-90, (KF)V. 100.2123/91, (KF)V. 01-502/93, (KF)V. 01-026/97, (KF)V. 01-162/97, (KF)V. 01-198/97, and further correspondence. We declare no conflicts of interest.

This chapter in the last sections quotes texts taken from chapters from the six volumes "Textbook on Evidence-Based Holistic Mind-Body Medicine"[11–16] and recent scientific papers by the author.

KEYWORDS

- **holistic medicine**
- **CAM**
- **cost-efficacy**
- **quality of life**
- **mind–body medicine**
- **biomedicine**
- **non-drug medicine**
- **side effects**

- **adverse effects**
- **therapeutic value**
- **evidence-based medicine**
- **medical politics**
- **law**
- **QALY**
- **HALY**
- **all clinical conditions**
- **CEA**
- **CBA**

REFERENCES

1. Gøtzsche, P. *Deadly Medicines and Organised Crime: How Big Pharma Has Corrupted Healthcare*; Radcliffe: New York, **2013.**
2. Ventegodt, S.; Flensborg-Madsen, T.; Andersen, N. J.; Nielsen, M.; Mohammed, M.; Merrick, J. Global Quality of Life (QOL), Health and Ability are Primarily Determined by Our Consciousness. Research Findings from Denmark 1991–2004. *Soc. Indic. Res.* **2005,** *71,* 87–122.
3. Ventegodt, S.; Omar, H.; Merrick, J. Quality of Life as Medicine: Interventions That Induce Salutogenesis. A Review of the Literature. *Soc. Indic. Res.* **2009,** DOI: 10.1007/s11205-010-9621-8.
4. Ventegodt, S.; Andersen, N. J.; Brom, B.; Merrick, J.; Greydanus, D. E. Evidence-Based Medicine: Four Fundamental Problems with the Randomised Clinical Trial (RCT) Used to Document Chemical Medicine. *Int. J. Adolesc. Med. Health.* **2009,** *21*(4), 485–496.
5. Boutron, I.; Estellat, C.; Guittet, L.; Dechartres, A.; Sackett, D. L.; Hróbjartsson, A.; Ravaud, P. Methods of Blinding in Reports of Randomized Controlled Trials Assessing Pharmacologic Treatments: A Systematic Review. *PLoS Med.* **2006,** *3*(10), e425.
6. Gøtzsche, P. C. Psychiatry Has Gone Astray. We would be Much Better off if we took Away All Psychotropic Drugs from the Market. The Physicians are Not Able to Handle Them. [Psykiatripåafveje. Vi ville være langt bedre stillet, hvis alle psykofarmaka blev fjernet fra markedet. Lægerne er ikke i stand til at håndtere dem. Kroniken.] Politiken, January 6, 2014.
7. Smith, R. The Drugs Don't Work. *BMJ.* **2003,** *327*(7428), 0–h.
8. Ventegodt, S.; Merrick, J. Therapeutic Value (TV) of Treatments with Pharmaceutical Drugs. Rough Estimates for All Clinical Conditions Based on Cochrane Reviews and

the Ratio: Number Needed to Harm/Number Needed to Treat (TV = NNH_{total}/NNT). *BMJ.* Nov 15, 2010. http://www.bmj.com/content/341/bmj.c5715.full/reply#bmj_el_244738 (accessed November 16, 2010).

9. *Committee on the Use of Complementary and Alternative Medicine by the American Public. Complementary and Alternative Medicine (CAM) in the United States;* National Academies Press: Washington, DC, 2005.
10. Ventegodt, S.; Merrick, J. A Review of Side Effects and Adverse Events of Non-Drug Medicine (Nonpharmaceutical Complementary and Alternative Medicine): Psychotherapy, Mind-Body Medicine and Clinical Holistic Medicine. *J. Complement. Integr. Med.* **2009,** *6*(1), 16.
11. Ventegodt, S.; Merrick, J. *Textbook on Evidence-Based Holistic Mind-Body Medicine: Basic Philosophy and Ethics of Traditional Hippocratic Medicine;* Nova Science: New York, 2012.
12. Ventegodt, S.; Merrick, J. *Textbook on Evidence-Based Holistic Mind-Body Medicine: Basic Principles of Healing in Traditional Hippocratic Medicine;* Nova Science: New York, 2012.
13. Ventegodt, S.; Merrick, J. *Textbook on Evidence-Based Holistic Mind-Body Medicine: Healing the mind in Traditional Hippocratic Medicine;* Nova Science: New York, 2012.
14. Ventegodt, S.; Merrick, J. *Textbook on Evidence-Based Holistic Mind-Body Medicine: Holistic Practice of Traditional Hippocratic Medicine;* Nova Science: New York, 2013.
15. Ventegodt, S.; Merrick, J. *Textbook on Evidence-Based Holistic Mind-Body Medicine: Research, Philosophy, Economy and Politics of Traditional Hippocratic Medicine;* Nova Science: New York, 2013.
16. Ventegodt, S.; Merrick, J. *Textbook on Evidence-Based Holistic Mind-Body Medicine: Sexology and Traditional Hippocratic Medicine;* Nova Science: New York, 2013.
17. Leichsenring, F.; Rabung, S.; Leibing, E. The Efficacy of Short-Term Psychodynamic Psychotherapy in Specific Psychiatric Disorders: A Meta-Analysis. *Arch Gen Psychiatry.* **2004,** *61*(12), 1208–1216.
18. Leichsenring, F. Are Psychodynamic and Psychoanalytic Therapies Effective?: A Review of Empirical Data. *Int. J. Psychoanal.* **2005,** *86*(Pt 3), 841–868.
19. Leichsenring, F.; Leibing, E. Psychodynamic Psychotherapy: A Systematic Review of Techniques, Indications and Empirical Evidence. *Psychol. Psychother.* **2007,** *80*(Pt 2), 217–228.
20. Ornish, D.; Brown, S. E.; Scherwitz, L. W.; Billings, J. H.; Armstrong, W. T. et al. Can Lifestyle Changes Reverse Coronary Heart Disease? The Lifestyle Heart Trial. *Lancet.* **1990,** *336*(8708), 129–133.
21. Ornish, D.; Scherwitz, L. W.; Billings, J. H.; Brown, S. E.; Gould, K. L. et al. Intensive Lifestyle Changes For Reversal of Coronary Heart Disease. *JAMA.* **1998,** *280*(23), 2001–2007.
22. Frattaroli, J.; Weidner, G.; Dnistrian, A. M.; Kemp, C.; Daubenmier, J. J.; Marlin, R. O.; Crutchfield, L.; Yglecias, L.; Carroll, P. R.; Ornish, D. Clinical Events in Prostate Cancer Lifestyle Trial: Results from Two Years of Follow-Up. *Urology.* **2008** (Dec), *72*(6), 1319–1323. Epub 2008 Jul 7.

23. Allmer, C.; Ventegodt, S.; Kandel, I.; Merrick, J. Positive Effects, Side Effects, and Adverse Events of Clinical Holistic Medicine. A Review of Gerda Boyesen's Nonpharmaceutical Mind-Body Medicine (Biodynamic Body-Psychotherapy) at Two Centers in the United Kingdom and Germany. *Int. J. Adolesc. Med. Health.* **2009** (Jul–Sep), *21*(3), 281–297.
24. Ventegodt, S.; Merrick, J. Meta-Analysis of Positive Effects, Side Effects and Adverse Events of Holistic Mind-Body Medicine (Clinical Holistic Medicine): Experience from Denmark, Sweden, United Kingdom and Germany. *Int. J. Adolesc. Med. Health.* **2009** (Oct–Dec), *21*(4), 441–456.
25. Ventegodt, S.; Andersen, N. J.; Kandel, I.; Merrick, J. Comparative Analysis of Cost-Effectiveness of Non-Drug Medicine (Non-Pharmaceutical Holistic, Complementary and Alternative Medicine/CAM) and Biomedicine (Pharmaceutical Drugs) for All Clinical Conditions. *Int. J. Disabil. Hum. Dev.* **2009,** *8*(3), 245–256.
26. Goleman, D. *Healing Emotions: Conversations with the Dalai Lama on the Mindfulness, Emotions, and Health;* Mind and Life Institute: Boston, MA, 1997.
27. Kierkegaard, S. A. *The Sickness unto Death;* Princeton University Press: Princeton, NJ, 1983.
28. Buber, M. *I and Thou;* Charles Scribner: New York, 1970.
29. Maslow, A. H. *Toward A Psychology of Being.* Van Nostrand: New York, 1962.
30. Frankl, V. *Man's Search for Meaning;* Pocket Books: New York, 1985.
31. Antonovsky, A. *Unravelling the Mystery of Health. How People Manage Stress and Stay Well.* Jossey-Bass: San Francisco, 1987.
32. *Who Am I? The Teachings of Bhagavan Sri Ramanamaharshi.* Sri Ramanasramam: Tiruvannamalai, India, 2010.
33. Ventegodt, S.; Merrick, S. Developing NCCAMS Five Category System for CAM into a New 10 Class Categorical System for All Types of Medicine, Based on Four Levels of Human Existence: Molecules, Body, Mind And Spirit. In preparation.
34. Fontanarosa, P.; Lundberg, G. Alternative Medicine Meets Science. *JAMA.* **1998,** *280,*1618–1619.
35. Ventegodt, S.; Merrick, J. Therapeutic Value (TV) of Alternative Medicine (Non-Drug CAM). Rough Estimates for All Clinical Conditions Based on Cochrane Reviews and the Ratio: Number Needed to Harm/Number Needed to Treat (TV = NNH_{total}/NNT). *BMJ.* Nov 15, 2010. URL: http://www.bmj.com/content/341/bmj.c5715. full/reply#bmj_el_244740
36. URL: http://nccam.nih.gov/
37. National Center for Complementary and Alternative Medicine. *Massage Therapy: An Introduction;* NCCAM: Bethesda, MD; Publication No. D327, 2006.
38. Ventegodt, S.; Thegler, S.; Andreasen, T.; Struve, F.; Enevoldsen, L.; Bassaine, L. et al. Clinical Holistic Medicine: Psychodynamic Short-Time Therapy Complemented with Bodywork. A Clinical Follow-Up Study of 109 Patients. *Scientific World J.* **2006,** *6,* 2220–2238.
39. Ventegodt, S.; Hermansen, T. D.; Flensborg-Madsen, T.; Nielsen, M. L.; Clausen, B.; Merrick, J. Human Development V: Biochemistry Unable to Explain the Emergence of Biological Form (Morphogenesis) and Therefore a New Principle as Source of Biological Information is Needed. *Scientific World J.* **2006,** *6,* 1359–1367.

40. Lazarou, J.; Pomeranz, B. H.; Corey, P. N. Incidence of Adverse Drug Reactions in Hospitalized Patients: A Meta-Analysis of Prospective Studies. *JAMA*. **1998,** *279*(15), 1200–1205.
41. Ventegodt, S. Quality of Life in Denmark. Results from a Population Survey. Forskningscentrets Forlag: Copenhagen, 1995.
42. Long, M. J.; McQueen, D. A.; Bangalore, VG; Schurman, J. R. 2nd. Using Self-Assessed Health to Predict Patient Outcomes after Total Knee Replacement. *Clin. Orthop. Relat. Res.* **2005,** *434,* 189–192.
43. Idler, E. L.; Russell, L. B.; Davis, D. Survival, Functional Limitations, and Self-Rated Health in the NHANES I Epidemiologic Follow-Up Study, 1992. First National Health and Nutrition Examination Survey. *Am. J. Epidemiol.* **2000,** *152*(9), 874–883.
44. Idler, E. L.; Kasl, S. Health Perceptions and Survival: Do Global Evaluations of Health Status Really Predict Mortality? *J. Gerontol.* **1991,** *46*(2), S55–S65.
45. Burström, B.; Fredlund, P. Self Rated Health: Is it As Good a Predictor of Subsequent Mortality among Adults in Lower As well As in Higher Social Classes. *J. Epidemiol. Commun. Health.* **2001,** *55*(11), 836–840.
46. Grof, S. *LSD Psychotherapy: Exploring the Frontiers of the Hidden Mind;* Hunter House: Alameda, CA, 1980.
47. Ventegodt, S.; Andersen, N. J.; Kandel, I. Bio- and Alternative Medicine in Conflict. Human Rights Protection of the Alternative Therapist. *J. Altern. Med. Res.* **2009,** *1*(2), 189–202.

CHAPTER 2

AFRICAN TRADITIONAL AND ALTERNATIVE MEDICINE IMPLEMENTATION INTO PRIMARY HEALTHCARE SYSTEMS IN AFRICA: BOTTLENECKS AND PROSPECTS

ERNEST TAMBO[1,4,7*], EMMANUEL CHIDIEBERE UGWU[2], GHISLAINE MADJOU[3,4], EMMANUEL MOUAFO TEKWU[5], ANWAR H. GILANI[6], and JEANNE YONKEU NGOGANG[7]

[1]*Sydney Brenner Institute for Molecular Bioscience, Wits 21st Century Centre of Excellence, University of the Witwatersrand, Johannesburg, South Africa*

[2]*Department of Human Biochemistry, Faculty of Basic Medical Sciences, Nnamdi Azikiwe University, Awka, Nnewi Campus, Nigeria*

[3]*Department of management, International Institute of Management, Cotonou, Republic of Benin*

[4]*Africa Disease Intelligence and Surveillance, Communications and Response, (Africa DISCOR), Institute, Yaoundé, Cameroon*

[5]*Laboratory for Tuberculosis Research (LTR), Biotechnology Centre-Nkolbisson & Faculty of Sciences, University of Yaoundé I, Yaoundé, Republic of Cameroon*

[6]*College of Health Sciences, Mekelle University, PO Box 1871 Mekelle, Ethiopia*

[7]*Department of Biochemistry and Pharmaceutical, Higher Institute of Health Sciences, Université des Montagnes, Bangangte, Republic of Cameroon*

[*]*Corresponding author. E-mail: tambo0711@gmail.com*

CONTENTS

ABSTRACT

Despite the growing consumers, African Traditional, Complementary, and Alternative Medicine (AT/CAM) is at the crossroads of competences and responsibilities of being integrated and implemented into primary healthcare delivery system in most African countries. A systematic review was undertaken using web knowledge and national health policy programs to gather relevant information till December 2014. The objective was to overview the regional policy and regulations of AT/CAM for attaining sustainable optimal potential of safe and effective practices in primary healthcare.

A total of 78.26% (36/46) countries in the continent had formulated national policies, 45.65% (21/46) countries have developed legal frameworks for traditional medicine practice while 39.13% (18/46) have national codes of ethics to enhance the safety, efficacy, and quality of services provided to patients. Only 32.60% (15/46) had developed national strategic plans for implementation of their policies and national traditional medicine offices have been established in 84.78% (39/46) countries. Twenty-four (56.17%) countries have traditional medicine programs in their ministries of health, and have established national expert committees to support the development and implementation of policies, strategies, and plans but challenged by the high levels of fragmentation within the system, and inappropriate financial incentives for providers are to blame for the relatively low health care value.

The paper highlights integrated health system mechanisms and delivery approaches in optimizing the benefits of African traditional medicine in alleviating public health burden, and improving primary healthcare system and health system research through intense communication between researchers, policy makers, and policy implementers in Africa.

2.1 INTRODUCTION

The potential of traditional medicines to overcome the increased drug resistance to antimicrobial agents and vectors, by providing cost-effective, easily accessible and available drugs and thereby improving the public health in African communities has been recognized.[1,2] Recent studies have showed the importance of integrating African Traditional, Complementary, and Alternative Medicines (AT/CAM) and practices into healthcare delivery systems based on the biological and pharmacological basis of various types of AT/CAM therapies and challenges in sustainability of natural biodiversity resources.[2–4] There is a general recognition that AT/CAM, the medicines once described as primitive, could be beneficial to mankind as they have their roots in ancient traditional medicine practices from various cultural, historic and ethnic origins.[6,7] It was estimated that about 70–80% of the population in developing countries depends on traditional medicine for their primary health care needs and management of both communicable and non-communicable diseases such as malaria, diabetes, cardiovascular, depression, asthma, cancer, HIV/AIDS, hypertension, and tuberculosis,[6–13] either due to consistency with indigenous cultures and tradition and/or accessibility, affordability, availability, cost-effective, or misconceptions of therapeutic effectiveness/toxicity and outcomes of same.[13–15]

Nowadays, African traditional medical practices have gained significant recognition and public acceptance, and also they have been integrated into health services in some African countries. Yet its implementation in a wider range for the benefits of the majority of people in the endemic, tropical, and industrialized countries for primary healthcare needs has not been realized. However, growing consumer demands and promotion of AT/CAM services and integration of proven medicinal plants into national drug policies has outpaced the development of policies by governments and health systems. Excessive mortality, morbidity, and disability due to diseases such as HIV/AIDS, malaria, tuberculosis, sickle-cell anemia and chronic diseases/disorders have been decreased greatly due to conventional therapies coupled with AT/CAM, thus prospects of reducing the health disparities and increasing the health coverage and economic well-being of communities and perhaps development of health systems.[6,8,10,12,15,16] Therefore, it is important to build a sustainable integrated model that can serve as a unified framework for guidance and health care decision-policy on the uses of AT/CAM therapies within a given context. Factors essential in the integration of AT/CAM into the primary healthcare system and practices, and should be embedded in theories, beliefs and experiences which belong to different peoples, communities perceived as a fundamental feature of their own identity and is often closely intertwined with lifestyles, cultural frameworks and social regulations, as well as domestic legislation and implications directly linked with promotion of cultural diversity, African beliefs and myths.[9,17–20]

We aimed to overview and analyze the regional integrated AT/CAM implementation, regulation of policy and practices in primary healthcare delivery system, and to understand sustainable implementation mechanisms within the framework of the global strategy, and plan of action on public health and innovation and in scaling up appropriate health strategies optimal – related Millennium Development Goals(MDGs) using the AT/CAM approach for strengthening health systems through renewed commitment and support of all member countries and globally.

2.2 REVIEW OF TRADITIONAL MEDICINE IN AFRICAN COUNTRIES

AT/CAM can be studied for several perspectives, including anthropology, botany, anthropology and sociology of religion and more recently, medical sciences.[14] In 1976 and then adopted in 1985 by AFRO members, traditional medicine was defined by experts at the World Health Organization's (WHO) meeting in Brazzaville in Africa as follows:

"The sum total of all the knowledge and practices, whether explicable or not, used in diagnosis, prevention and elimination of physical, mental and social imbalance and relying exclusively on practical experience and observation handed down from generation to generation, whether verbally or in writing. Traditional medicine might also be considered to be the sum total of practices, measures, ingredients and procedures of all kinds, whether material or not, which from time immemorial had enabled the African to guard against disease, alleviate his sufferings and to cure himself. Traditional medicine might also be considered as a solid amalgamation of dynamic medical knowhow and ancestral medicine."

The methods of this review were based on recommendations from systematic review for evidence-based clinical practice with adaptations for the review's broader health systems and policy related questions, and the overall principle of replicability.[1,4]

Early involvement of decision makers was instrumental to ensure the relevance of the literature review. Identification of primary topics of interest; these included the definitions, models and outcomes of planning and implementation, and the characteristics of successfully integrated systems.[3,6] Two focus groups provided direction for the research questions which were then validated for decision makers. These groups comprised senior management, planners, medical leaders, directors, and managers of programs from within African healthcare centers and institutions, senior policy advisors with the provincial department of health, and others.[4,6,7] They represented portfolios across the continuum of care including acute care, community, primary care, rural jurisdictions, urban centers, and public health in order to identify recent innovations in the implementation of integrated systems outside healthcare that may be applicable to the healthcare context.

Articles were obtained for abstracts with summary scores ≥5 out of 9 (health sciences and business). These articles were reviewed to determine appropriateness and included if they would, or were likely to, inform the research questions, resulting in 120AT/CAM health science and practices articles. Each of these 120 articles was rated by two independent researchers for quality, using criteria for empirical or non-empirical studies. A review of the bibliographies of these articles provided an additional 36 articles which provided historical context. A second search of the integrated AT/CAM health sciences databases yielded additional 22 relevant articles to December 2014 which was included in the review.

2.3 OUTCOMES MEASUREMENTS

A search of the literature was undertaken to capture non peer-reviewed literature relevant to the review. Sources included conference proceedings, government, health associations' and agencies' websites. A Google™ search was also conducted using the same search terms as were used for the peer-reviewed health systems literature search. A process similar to that used for the peer-reviewed literature determined inclusion of articles. Approximately 178 documents were identified, 26.40% (47/178) were judged to be relevant to implementation mechanisms review and was integrated into the draft report. The majority of these documents were obtained from government and health association websites. We reviewed studies based on the relevance of outcome (measurement of at least one of a list of political, financial, behavioral or biologic, pharmacological or clinical outcomes on ailments/infections) and detailed the design methodology in AT/CAM implementation.

In terms of regulation, African traditional or complementary and alternative medicines quality and safety criteria must obey the limits for heavy metals and microbial contamination, absence of steroids and other adulterants, prohibition of herbs with adverse effect and should be in compliance with Good Manufacturing Practice(GMP).The list of qualified AT/CAM included (a) traditional health forum/group; (b) traditional health professional; (c) herbalist; (d) any other health professional; (e) traditional healer; (f) religious or spiritual advisor (e.g., minister, priest, Alfa, or rabbi); (g) any other healer (e.g., chiropractor or spiritualist). For the purpose of this study AT/CAM health implementation of service utilization was assessed. The literature was reviewed for evidence of effectiveness and outcomes of integrated health systems. Few studies (17.1%) reported on the impact of integration and ended to focus on perceived benefits rather than empirically derived outcomes at the system level, studies reported conflicting results and financial performance whereas others found no improvement in new skills and knowledge performance, organizational structures, or lack of professional cultures. Shared culture and increased co-operation, teamwork and communication with other health personnel and health agencies are believed to benefit healthcare professionals versus social care philosophies.

The overall prevalence data on the uses and integration of AT/CAM were evaluated. Further analyzes categorized AT/CAM users, where users are those individuals/patients reporting the use of one or more AT/CAM substances in the reported study, depending on the specific analysis being conducted AT/CAM use was calculated and bivariate associations between the variables and any use of AT/CAM from previous papers were investigated. Multivariate logistic regression was used to estimate the influence of each independent variable on the odds of using herbs and AT/CAM; included in the analyses were all variables significant at $p < 0.05$ in bivariate analysis. The 95% confidence intervals for odds ratios and p values obtained by logistic regression were obtained using SPSS software, version 14.0 (Chicago, IL, USA).

2.4 BOTTLENECKS IN AT/CAM IMPLEMENTATION ACROSS AFRICA

Although, there have been progress in the integration and implementation of ATM in most African countries, the progress has been rather slow.[2,3,5,8] Africans remain challenged by inherent complexity of health care policy implementation and the multiple variables such as the heavy burden of communicable diseases such as HIV, malaria and other parasitic diseases, pneumonia, diarrhea, tuberculosis and outbreaks (Ebola, Influenza)associated poverty vicious cycle.[4,5,7,9] Contemporary, this situation has been complicated with the rising threat and burden of chronic diseases such as diabetes, hypertension, cardiovascular and mental diseases that persistently torment lives, co-morbidity and mortality in most African countries.[1,3] Lowering costs and improving health outcomes faces many roadblocks and shared governance, untested programs, African health care culture, program monitoring and evaluation as high maternal and child mortality.[1] Also, rapid demographic changes and urbanization, underutilization of public healthcare, ineffective health support systems for poor population, increasing privatization of health facilities, migration of medical professionals, environmental changes and related epidemics are some other major public health concerns with social and economic consequences.[1,3,5,9] Sustainable implementation steps need to be articulated through continuous communication, sharing information, collaboration, co-ordination and organization of forums, enforcement of regulations and responsibilities in addressing these barriers.

2.5 DIFFERENTIAL STAGES OF AT/CAM INTEGRATION IN HEALTH SYSTEMS AND SERVICES IN AFRICA

The data analyzed on the implementation of integrated AT/CAM into the health care delivery system showed increasing trends in population demands and needs across Africa, but varied from one country to another depending on the population size, degree of tie to cultural belief and practices and disease severity. The results showed based on consumer population, that AT/CAM is an important contributor in the health care delivery in Africa, covering a wide range of conditions from ailments, cardiovascular diseases, complex of supernatural or psychosocial problems, acute/chronic diseases, pain management, cancer, respiratory diseases, HIV and other sexually transmitted infections, and other diseases therapy. Countries in African sub-region are at different stages of integration of AT/CAM in health systems and services (Legend 2.1).

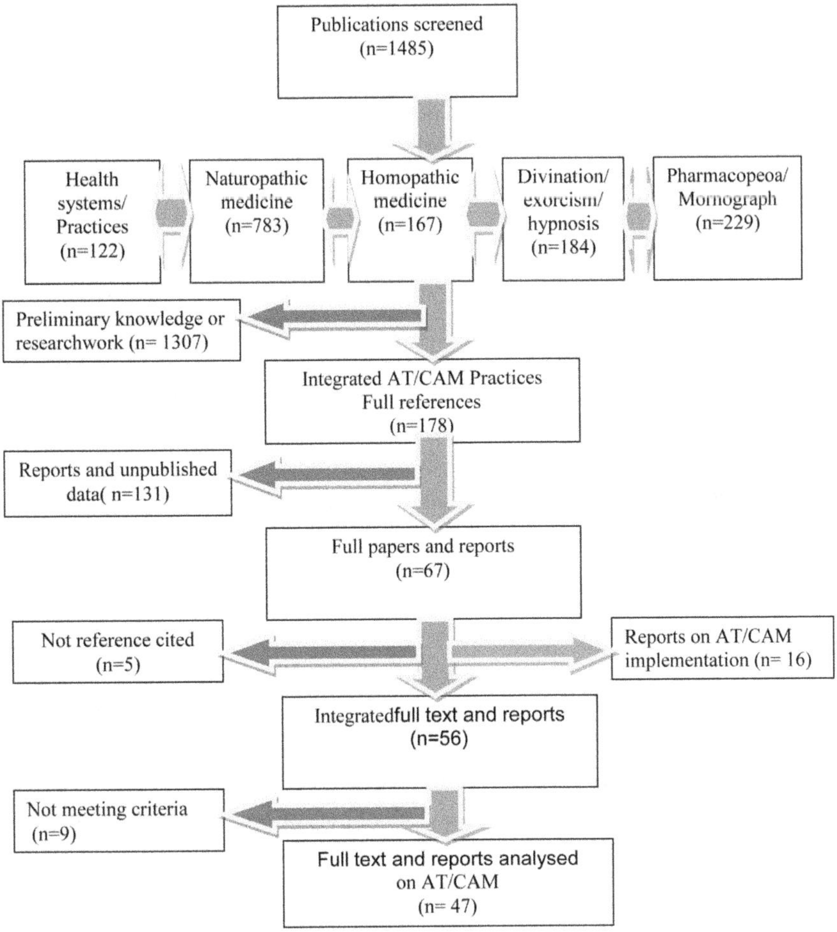

LEGEND 2.1 Flow chart of screened publications on implementation of integrated AT/CAM in Africa.

2.6 INCREASING POLITICAL COMMITMENT AND INVESTMENT IN AT/CAM INTEGRATION IN AFRICA

Our results showed that during the decade, the political commitment and support by 78.26% (36/46) out of 46 WHO member states in the African region have formulated national traditional medicine policies and regulatory frameworks to ensure the efficacy, safety and quality of traditional medicines and the regulation of the practice of traditional health practitioners. A total of 56.52% (26/46) have developed a legal framework for AT/CAM with more than half having national codes. Overall 32.61% (15/46) countries have established the national strategic plans, structures, programs and offices in their ministries of health to institutionalize traditional medicine in health care systems. Also, 84.78% (39/46) countries have put in place AT/CAM offices in ministries of health to support the development of traditional medicine while 52.17% (24/46) have AT/CAM programs and experts committees (Fig. 2.1).Substantial progress on AT/CAM political commitment and funding support has been achieved by the adopted various declarations at the African Summit of Heads of States and Governments in 2000 by increasing progressively in reaching 15% health budget allocation (Table 2.1). Emphasis has been placed at the consistent and long term scaling up for impact political and financial support, critical in achieving communal actions toward health promotion and disease prevention and control, the most efficient and sustainable and affordable health interventions of ensuring better, equitable health outcomes, ensuring accountability and benefits to populations regardless of their ethnicity, geographical location, level of education and economic status. Key strategic priorities and leadership, natural and alternative medicine task force on AT/CAM should be strengthened in increasing funding and results oriented goals in maximizing on the best expertise and practices from national programs and partners' experiences, facilitating national and regional co-ordination and regular exchange of views, and critically review strategic framework of interventions. Also, advocate for additional interest and expertise from international partners in mobilizing funds to rapidly scaling up research and development (R&D) and delivery interventions where appropriate, and addressing key technical and operational challenges to further achieving ambitious impact goals, as 2001–2010 was tagged "Decade of African Traditional Medicine."

Implementation of African traditional and complementary medicine in primary health care in hospitals and remotes rural health centers requires the establishment of policy implementation, legal and regulatory bodies and frameworks in providing a platform for evidence based practice within the framework of national health policies and health legislation oversee by the ministries of health across African countries (Fig. 2.1).

TABLE 2.1 List of WHO-MemberAfricanCountries with ATCAM Platform, National Policies, and Strategic Implementation Programs.

Region	Country	ATCAM policy	Legal framework	National office	Strategic implementation	Expert committee	ATCAM development	GMP/QA
Southern Africa	South Africa	✓	✓	✓	✓	✓	✓	✓
	Angola	✓	✓	✓	✓	✓	✓	
	Namibia	✓	✓	✓	✓	✓	✓	
	Mozambique	✓	✓	✓	✓	✓	✓	*
	Swaziland	✓	✓	✓	✓	✓	✓	*
Central Africa	Cameroon	✓	✓	✓	✓	✓	✓	*
	Gabon	✓	✓	✓	✓	✓	✓	*
	Equatorial Guinea	✓	✓	✓	✓	✓	✓	*
	Congo DR	✓	✓	✓	✓	✓	✓	*
	RCA	✓	✓	✓	✓	✓	✓	*
Western Africa	Ghana	✓	✓	✓	✓	✓	✓	*
	Nigeria	✓	✓	✓	✓	✓	✓	*
	Mali	✓	✓	✓	✓	✓	✓	*
	Gambia	✓	✓	✓	✓	✓	✓	*
	Senegal	✓	✓	✓	✓	✓	✓	*
Eastern Africa	Ethiopia	✓	✓	✓	✓	✓	✓	*
	Kenya	✓	✓	✓	✓	✓	✓	*
	Tanzania	✓	✓	✓	✓	✓	✓	*
	Zambia	✓	✓	✓	✓	✓	✓	*
	Uganda	✓	✓	✓	✓	✓	✓	*

TABLE 2.1 *(Continued)*

Region	Country	ATCAM policy	Legal framework	National office	Strategic implementation	Expert committee	ATCAM development	GMP/QA
Northern Africa	Morocco	✓	✓	✓	✓	✓	✓	*
	Mauritania	✓	✓	✓	✓	✓	✓	*
	Sudan	✓	✓	✓	x	x	x	*
	South Sudan	x	x	x	x	x	x	*

Note: V=Yes,* = in process, x = not.

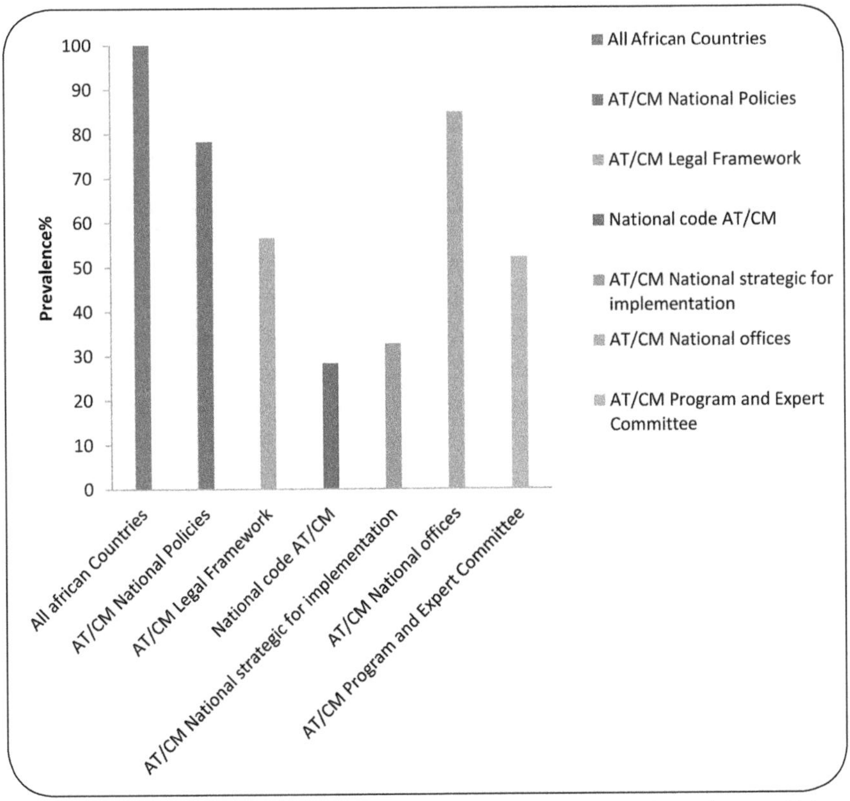

FIGURE 2.1 The African traditional, complementary and alternative medicines regulation framework in member state African countries.

Only 66 countries out of 213 WHO member states have traditional medicine policies, while around 43 states have some kind of legislation and 20 member states are in the process of establishing some regulatory policies.[21] In Africa, integrating ATM/CAM into modern health care with national institute of traditional medicine grew from 37% (17/46) countries in 1990, up to 62 and 77% in 2007 and 2012, respectively (Table 2.1). Countries such as India and China have purposively sought to develop the traditional medicine sector in order to strengthen their traditional medical heritage and at the same time provide comprehensive, integrated, appropriate, and effective essential health services, design their models of delivery to their people. It is also a response to capitalize on the economic opportunity arising from an increasing global demand for herbal products in achieving the MDGs and related targets.[5,21]

2.7 NURTURING AT/CAM INNOVATIVE EDUCATIONAL CAPACITY BUILDING AND RESEARCH FOR DEVELOPMENT

Education and training are among the key ingredients required for the institutionalization of traditional medicine in national health systems. AT/CAM is based on holistic approach to the management of the patient involving the body, soul and spirit using plants, animals and minerals resources and acquired fruitful dialogue between traditional practitioners and clinicians on knowledge and skills through observation, spiritual revelation personal experience, training and direct information from their predecessors. The overall assessment showed that 52.86% addressing naturopathic aspect of traditional medicine and health care delivery system, and more than 41% teaching and training centers have been set up in Africa with only 8.22% in health systems. The most commonly prescribed naturopathic therapeutics included botanical medicines (51%), vitamins (41%), minerals (39%), homeopathy (29%), and allergy treatments (13%) (Fig. 2.2), which are consistent with previous studies.[7,8,10,16] The need for the establishment AT/CAM curriculum in educational system at secondary and tertiary levels, training of health personnel its various fields and scaling up impact pilot/multicenter research and evaluation needs has seen substantial health gains and advances in public health, health centers and health technology and economic wealth are of immense importance in Africa countries, but yet to totally be translated into increased health status by improving the health system benchmarks for Africans and effective qualitative research outcomes rather than process and the financial benefits. Such organization relies on main bodies, national R&D institute or centers in medicinal compounds, natural products good manufacturing compliance and sales of AT/CAM Act and regulatory authority, and AT/CAM Act and council/departments with multi-tiered collaboration including the ministries of health, sciences, technology, research and innovation, and communications on appropriate information dissemination to the public, fidelity in good clinical practices, education schemes, and training.[7,12]

Promoting and conducting innovative research designs can provide information for health care providers and patients on the best clinical, functional, and quality of life and outcomes for everyday users in routine practice settings. Evidence-based validation on the quality, safety and efficacy of traditional medicine used is crucial for the prevention and management of priority diseases such as HIV/AIDS, malaria, sickle cell anemia, diabetes, and hypertension. WHO has developed guidelines on research methodologies and is supporting countries in this process. It also requires prompt management of case, monitoring and evaluation assessment, monitoring and scoring of interventions performance or effectiveness for evidence based targeted and contextual adaptations in time and space. It was observed that institutionalization of African traditional medicines in health systems could be a key pillar in the promotion and development, health systems strengthening and capacity-building, appropriate education and training of populations and care practitioners on adherence to acceptable of safety and quality standards of products and practice. Advocacy and mobilization on the right to AT/CAM medicines for prevention and treatment that are safe and efficacious, as well as regulation of the traditional healing profession and African traditional medicine processes and strategies can help in strengthening the community health systems against marginalized traditional healers and traditional medicines, and their value against cultural and medical imperialism and the power of multinational pharmaceutical industry. Therefore, there is an urgent need to scale investment and support of traditional healers and African traditional medicines not only by governments, but also by civil society and the private sector including pharmaceutical firms cannot be over emphasized.

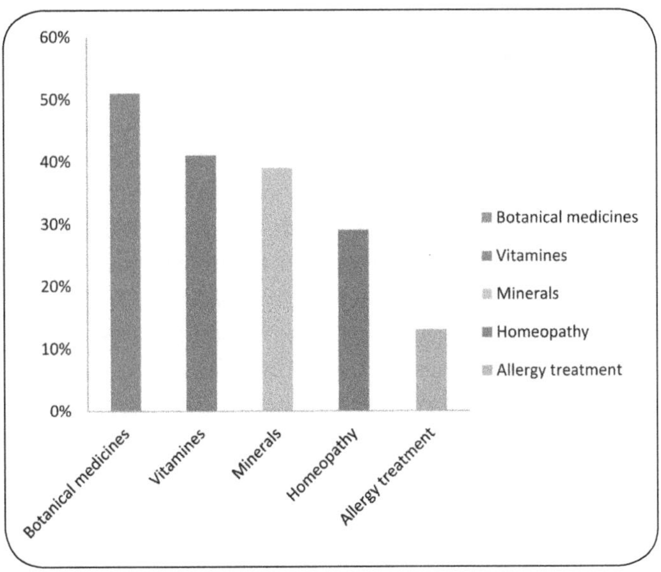

FIGURE 2.2 Commonly prescribed AT/CAM therapeutics in African countries.

2.8 FOSTERING AT/CAM MODERNIZATION TOWARD INDIVIDUALIZED DISEASE PREVENTION AND MANAGEMENT

On the basis of the evidence-based interventional methods used for healing, maintaining health, therapies used in traditional medicine can be differentiated into the following categories. *Medication therapies* using herbal medicines and/or medicines based on animal parts and/or minerals was reported in 58.3%. *Non-medication therapies* using physical (massages), mental (meditation, hypnosis) and spiritual (exorcism, magic-religious) therapies or a combination was 22.7% and *Mixed therapies* combining medication and non-medication therapies was 19%. The need has since been expressed for industrial drug production from medicinal and aromatic plants in Africa in order to increase the economic and health potentials as well as the social benefits from our natural resources. To date, over 30% of the pharmaceutical products manufactured in Egypt are plant-derived, for example, *Ammi visnaga, Glycyrrhiza glabra, Aloe vera,* and so forth. Rwanda and Zimbabwe also produce pharmaceuticals from plants' essential oils. In Burundi, makes available both orthodox and traditional drugs for the hospital dispensaries. In the centre for scientific research into plant medicine established in Ghana since 1973, pilot drug production is carried out to provide well-formulated, stable, standardized, and safe preparations from plants for clinical evaluation, utilization, and monitoring in a clinical setting. Similarly, in the Centre for Research on Pharmacopoeia and Traditional Medicine in Rwanda, *Datura stramonium*; *Eucalyptus globulus, Capsicum frutescens,* and *Plantago lanceolata* are prepared in the Dispensary of traditional medicine where they are administered for antispasmodic, pulmonary disinfectant, counter-irritant, and antitussive activities, respectively. And also in South Africa and West Africa, several herbal products have been formulated for the management of HIV/AIDS, as tea bags for use as follows: Dysenteral (*Euphorbia hirta* for dysentery), Laxa cassia (*Cassia italica* for constipation), and Hepatisane (*Combretum micranthum* for constipation).[9,22] Whereas, in many developed countries, certain Complementary and Alternative Medical therapies (CAM) are popular; about 48% in Australia, 50% in Canada, 42% in the USA, 40% in Belgium, 65% in India, and 75% in France in contrast to 80% in African countries.[14] Although many populations in developing countries are reported as depending heavily on ATM help to meet their health care needs, accelerating the development of local production of traditional and complementary medicines in alleviate the burden of diseases and to improve access to health care for the African region present crucial challenges and ethical issues.[3,23,24]

Moving African health agenda forward with integrated traditional and complementary medicine and individualized care, enhancing international technical co-operation and exchanges relevant to AT/CAM and progressive monitoring and evaluation as advances and modernization of AT/CAM healthcare services and practices continuous implementation in national strategy for integrated health systems in primary health care in most African countries with obvious benefits require multi-sectorial and trans-disciplinary collaborations and partnerships in the integrated approaches.[25] Countries such as South Africa, Burkina Faso, Madagascar, Cameroon, Mali, and Tanzania have made partnership arrangements with traditional health practitioners and the private sector as equal partners because trust among collaborators is crucial, and this holds the key to the success of integrating AT/CAM.[6] WHO has developed memorandum of understanding between biomedical researchers and traditional health practitioners, which countries can adapt to their local situations in fostering synergies between the various stakeholders involved in health development.[2,5] Each country needs to find and develop systems of harmony and fairness between traditional and orthodox practices of health care in the universal context to ensure sustainability and social acceptance of both systems of primary health care delivery coverage to the majority of the population. Also networking amongst public health researchers would further strengthen such AT/CAM complete integration and implementation in national health programs and community practices.[24,26] Clinical evaluation of AT/CAM interventions at all levels and kinds of evidence in supporting patient-flow and personalized care, advanced accessibility, general prevention, and community systems; prenatal and patient safety co-operation in workforce development and skills empowerment, health education, community and clinical pharmacy services are needed.

2.9 REGULATION, PROTECTION, AND BIOPIRACY LAWS

The crucial challenge to address remains that of recognizing and improving medicines regulation for public interest comprises of three integral aspects: quality, safety, and efficacy in medical practices – regardless of the experience and context. Formulation of national policy and legal and regulatory frameworks have to build on a AT/CAM Act on product manufacturing and procurement with a drug control authority, practices and training, and research units coordinated by the AT/CAM council and departments: a regulatory framework for the protection of Intellectual Property Rights (IPR) and indigenous knowledge of traditional medicines in the WHO African region. Some African countries have formulated national policies, legal frameworks, and regulations including mechanisms for registration of traditional medicinal products, established national expert committees, national programs and national offices and developed training programs for various cadres of health workers. WHO is supporting this process in member states through the provision of guidance in these policy issues.[12]

Beyond the differences in traditional and western systems, most countries have set up national AT/CAM national policy, laws and regulation with diverse approaches to licensing, dispensing, manufacturing and trading, also working on testing safety and production standards. Some African countries are attainting to tackle challenges in enacting laws to protect indigenous knowledge through the establishment of phytomedicine data sharing and database platforms to protect local resources including Ghana, South Africa, Nigeria, and Tanzania. AT/CAM knowledge, culture, and biological resources, conservation of plants, marine and animals sources of AT/CAM development with participation of all relevant agencies are necessary. In addition, guide to intellectual property management are priority items on the agenda of member states to protect indigenous knowledge about traditional medicine and ensuring professionalism of practitioners through education, enhancing public safety and healthcare practices, empower patients so that they can take responsibility and assist in regulating the practitioners.[9] Furthermore, efficient utilization of government resources by establishing an enabling economic, regulatory and political environments for local production of traditional medicines as well as develop industries that can produce standardized remedies to increase access with the technological advancement, dissemination of appropriate information to the general public to empower them with knowledge and skills for the proper use of traditional medicines with case reporting system registration (on-line), standards/codes of practice, practitioner (APC), regulation in phases, self-regulation, and statutory regulations.

2.10 STRENGTHENING INTEGRATED HEALTH SYSTEMS IN AFRICA

The primary health care integrated into best practice health model within each African country implies seamless responsible co-ordination of care within their communities, within healthcare organizations, and within their internal and external systems, based on care models for appropriate evidence-based options or interventions. Develop comprehensive policies and plans for health workforce development within the context of national health policies and plans so as to translate the noble intention into viable quantifiable services and products within specified time frames. The purpose of the plan of action could be to provide general framework to guide member states in formulating their national strategies. Infrastructures improvement are required to effectively co-ordinate and implement various activities on AT/CAM especially in areas related to the practitioners, culturally innovative education, resources capacity both human and material development are vital in order to carry out and accomplish institutionalization strategies, perform adequate scientific proof, precise diagnosis and dosage, standardized medicines and practices and policy by the National Pharmaceutical Control Bureau, and research practitioners in a formalized system of education (e.g., Bachelor ATCAM, Naturopathy, etc) and annual regional AT/CAM conferences/seminars to give access to appropriate knowledge, monographs and compendium. Evidence guided plans for standardization of raw materials, effective conservation of medicinal plants, encourage industrial participation, control production, distribution, import and export of TM products, compliance to sustainable and effective GAP, GSP, GMP, and IPR. Also promotion of standard practices of AT/CAM in accordance to standard regulations and ethics particularly in the primary health care delivery system and a number of countries have developed national herbal pharmacopoeias to document medicinal plants that have been found to be effective and to further ensure their safety, efficacy and quality.[14]

Also, elaboration of national policies and plans on health technologies are essential when they are evidence-based, cost-effective, and meet essential public health needs within the context of overall national health policies and plans and also strengthen national pharmacovigilance systems for health technologies on herbal medicines with availability and access to reliable and affordable laboratory and diagnostic services. In addition progressively build sustainable capacity in pharmaceuticals management as a fundamental component of functional and reliable health systems priority areas and strategic activities, include sensitization, legislation, institutional arrangements, information, education and communication, resource mobilization, setting directions for research and training, cultivation and conservation of medicinal plants, protection of traditional medical knowledge, local production of commercial quantities of Standardized African Traditional Medicines (SATM), partnerships as well as evaluation, monitoring and reporting, standardization of training and practice, registration of practitioners, licensing manufacturers, increase supervision of manufacturers with regards to hygiene and safety.[18] Advocate reporting of adverse events to a regulatory body, formal review of existing herbs, better labeling of herbal medicines, R&D funding research-based instructional or settings. WHO produced guidelines for research help improving standards of evidence, encouraging scientific research quality control methods, safety, and efficacy as well as increasing capacity in research of AT/CAM, herbal medicine formulary.[3] Empowering communities and ensuring their involvement in the governance of health services through appropriate capacity-building, establishing and strengthening community and health service interaction to enhance needs-based and demand-driven provision of AT/CAM health services, including reorienting the health service delivery system.

2.11 CONCLUSION

Implementation of integrated AT/CAM into healthcare delivery in African countries requires understanding of determinants socio-political and legislative, economical determinants and frameworks, but also traditional and modern practitioners must acknowledge their areas of strengths and weaknesses from which they operate and be recognized as equal and complementary partners. Sustained implementation efforts of the great potentials of integrated AT/CAM in healthcare delivery system are promising in addressing public health burden, complementing health needs, and disparities in primary healthcare system and communities in Africa and in achieving global health initiatives.

COMPETING INTERESTS

The authors declare that they have no competing interest.

AUTHORS' CONTRIBUTIONS

TE designed and conducted the research. TE executed, analyzed, and drafted the manuscript. UCE, TEM, GM AG and JYN provided additional literature information and improved the manuscript. All authors read and approved the final version of the manuscript.

ACKNOWLEDGMENTS

We wish to thank Madjou Ghislaine for the research ideas and for providing additional search information on African medicine. TE is a recipient of China-Africa Sciences and Technology Partnership Program, Postdoctoral Science Foundation, Ministry of Science and Technology, and Ministry of Human Resources and Social Security of China, and National Institute of Parasitic Disease, Chinese Center for Disease Control and Prevention, Shanghai 200025, PR China and Vice-Chancellor Postdoctoral fellowship at University of Pretoria.

KEYWORDS

- **health**
- **delivery system**
- **challenges**
- **implications**
- **Africa**
- **traditional**
- **complementary**
- **medicine**
- **integrated**

REFERENCES

1. Van den Geest, S. Is There a Role for Traditional Medicine in Basic Health Services in Africa? A Plea fora Community Perspective. *Trop. Med. Intl. Health.* **1997,** *2*(9), 903–911.
2. Peltzer, K.; Simbayi, L.; Banyini, M.; Kekana, Q. Utilization and Practice of Traditional/Complementary/Alternative Medicine (TM/CAM) in South Africa. *Afr. J. Tradit. Complement. Altern. Med.* **2009,** *6*(2), 175–185.
3. Van Der Geest, S. Integration or Fatal Embrace? The Uneasy Relationship between Indigenous and Western Medicine. *Curare.* **1985,** *8*(*1*), 9–14.
4. WHO. *Plan of Action on the Africa Union Decade of Traditional Medicine (2001–2010),* 2nd Ordinary Session of the Conference of African Ministers of Health(CAMH2) Gaborone, Botswana, Oct 10–14, 2005.
5. WHO. *General Guidelines for Methodologies on Research and Evaluation of Traditional Medicine,* 2000. WHO/EDM/TRM/2000.1.
6. Ernst, E. Prevalence of Use of Complementary/Alternative Medicine: A Systematic Review. *Bull. World Health Organ.* **2000,** *78*(2), 252–257.
7. Fokunang, C. N.; Ndikum, V.; Tabi, O. Y.; Jiofack, R. B.; Ngameni, B.; Guedje, N. M.; Tembe-Fokunang, E. A.; Tomkins, P.; Barkwan, S.; Kechia, F.; Asongalem, E.; Ngoupayou, J.; Torimiro, N. J.; Gonsu, K. H.; Sielinou, V.; Ngadjui, B. T.; Angwafor, III, F.; Nkongmeneck, A.; Abena, O. M.; Ngogang, J.; Asonganyi, T.; Colizzi, V.; Lohoue, J.; Kamsu-Kom. Traditional Medicine: Past, Present and Future Research and Development Prospects and Integration in the National Health System of Cameroon. *Afr. J. Tradit. Complement. Altern. Med.* **2011**, *8*(3), 284–295.
8. Sofowora, A. Recent Trends in Research into African Medicinal Plants. *J. Ethnopharmacol.* **1993a,** *38,* 209–214.
9. WAHO. TM Workshop Report. *Situational Analysis of the Level of Development of Traditional Medicine in the ECOWAS Member States;* 2008.
10. Elujoba A. A.; Odeleye, O. M.; Ogunyemi, C. M. Traditional Medicine Development for Medical and Dental Primary Care Delivery System in Africa. *Afr. J. Tradit. Complement Altern. Med.* **2005,** *2*(1), 46–61.
11. Bishaw, M. Promoting Traditional Medicine in Ethiopia: A Brief Historical Review of Government Policy. *J. Soc. Sci. Med.* **1991,** *33*(2), 193–200.
12. *The World Medicines Situation 2011,* Traditional Medicines: Global Situation, Issues and Challenges. World Health Organization: Geneva, 2011; pp 2.
13. Cocks, M.; Møller, V. Use of Indigenous and Indigenised Medicines to Enhance Personal Well-Being: A South African Case Study. *Soc. Sci. Med.* **2002,** *54*(3), 387–397.
14. WHO. *Promoting the Role of Traditional Medicine in Health Systems: A Strategy for the African Region;* WHO Regional Office for Africa: Temporary Location, Harare, Zimbabwe, 2001(Document AFR/RC50/9 and Resolution 2001, AFR/RC50/R3).
15. Kamagaté, M.; Die-Kacou, H.; Balayssac, E.; Yavo, J. C.; Daubret, P. T.; Kakou-Augustine, K.; Gboignon, V. M. Clinical Trials Using Medicinal Plants: Bibliographical Review and Methodological Analysis. *Therapie.* **2005,** *60*(4), 413–418.
16. Houessou, L. G.; Lougbegnon, T. O.; Gbesso, F. G.; Anagonou, L. E.; Sinsin, B. Ethno-Botanical Study of the African Star Apple (Chrysophyllumalbidum G. Don)

in the Southern Benin (West Africa). *J. Ethnobiol. Ethnomed.* **2012,** *8*(40). Doi: 10.1186/1746-4269-8-40.

17. Langwick, S. From Non-Aligned Medicines to Market-Based Herbals: China's Relationship to the Shifting Politics of Traditional Medicine in Tanzania. *Med. Anthropol.* **2010,** *29*(1), 15–43.
18. Kofi-Tsekpo, M. Institutionalization of African Traditional Medicine in Health Care Systems in Africa. *Afr. J. Health. Sci.* **2004,** *11*(1–2), i–ii.
19. Stangeland, T.; Dhillion, S. S.; Reksten, H. Recognition and Development of Traditional Medicine in Tanzania. *J. Ethnopharmacol.* **2008,** *117*(2), 290–299.
20. Gavriilidis, G.; Östergren, P. O. Evaluating a Traditional Medicine Policy in South Africa: Phase 1 Development of a Policy Assessment Tool. *Glob. Health Action.* **2012,** *5,* 17271.
21. Bodeker, G. Lessons on Integration from the Developing World's Experience. *British. Med. J.* **2001,** *322,* 164–167.
22. Bodeker, G.; Burford, G. *Traditional, Complementary and Alternative Medicine Policy and Public Health Perspectives,* Imperial College Press: London, 2007; pp 9–38.
23. Nwokocha, E. E. Traditional Healthcare Delivery Systems in the 21st Century Nigeria: Moving Beyond Misconceptions. *World Health Popul.* **2008,** *10*(1), 23–33.
24. Bichmann, W. Primary Health Care and Traditional Medicine—Considering the Background of Changing Health Care Concepts in Africa. *J. Soc. Sci. Med. Med. Anth.* **1979,** *13,* 175–182.
25. Nelms, L. W.; Gorski, J. The Role of the African Traditional Healer in Women's Health. *J. Transcult. Nurs.* **2006,** *17*(2), 184–189.
26. Bodeker, G.; Ong, C. K.; Grundy, C.; Burford, G.; Shein, K. *WHO Global Atlas of Traditional, Complementary and Alternative Medicine;* World Health Organization: Kobe, 2005.

CHAPTER 3

POSTURES

TILAK KALRA*

Acupuncturist-6 Moona Avenue, Baulkham Hills, NSW Australia -2153

**E-mail: kalratilak@hotmail.com*

CONTENTS

ABSTRACT

Lack of maintenance of correct postures can lead to deteriorating health effects like obesity, heart diseases, and diabetes. Good postures are inevitable for attaining a healthy life. Correct postures helps us to be fit and gives relaxation to the mind and body. Sitting and standing with proper posture helps to work more efficiently. Poor postures can lead to abnormalities in spine and also affect the functionalities of other body parts as time proceeds. Best sleeping, sitting, and standing positions are discussed in this chapter.

3.1 INTRODUCTION

About 20 years ago, a lady came to see me for pain in the abdomen area, saying that she passed out due to pain. She told me that endoscopy, ultrasound of organs, CT scan of the lumber, and blood test did not reveal any abnormality. She told me "10 years ago when she gave birth to her son, she tore muscles around coccyx." This started me thinking and I concluded that it had to do with her sitting posture. I noticed that she sat in a position where there was no pressure on her tailbone. I recommended her to buy a hemorrhoid ring and sit straight. I also treated her for muscular pain and after three treatments, she has been fine till today. This experience has led me to check the postures of all patients since that time.

Posture is defined as the characteristic of how a person holds his or her body while standing, sitting, sleeping, or working.[1] We spend at least one third of our life sleeping or lying in bed. Studies have shown that deprivation of sleep or having poor, sleep can lead to deteriorating health outcomes including coronary heart disease, obesity, and diabetes. It can also lead to lack of concentration, tension headaches, and migraines. Sleeping with a bad posture[2] can lead to headaches and also reduced cervical, lumber, and hip functionality. The Better Sleep Council has said that there are basically three main sleeping positions with different variations of each. The best sleeping postures and their benefits are discussed in this chapter. Those who are working on computers or sitting in front of a screen and are not sitting correctly, could result in long-term pain and disability. The correct sitting position in front of a computer screen is discussed. Incorrect standing posture can lead to some long-term serious issues later in life.[4]

Incorrect standing posture will affect the neck and shoulders; and later on can create breathing problems. The correct postures are discussed.

3.2 SLEEPING POSITIONS

During the early years of my practice, I treated many patients for headaches and migraines. My success rate in this area had been very high and it would take 3–5 sittings to alleviate the condition. There was one patient who was coming regularly for treatment and was not responding as well to the treatment. After further investigation, I found out that he used to sleep on his stomach. Once that was changed, his headaches were alleviated. From there on, I investigated various sleeping positions and how these positions affect the human body.

Before I discuss sleeping positions, it is important to note that the quality of sleep is also very important. One needs a good sleep for 6–8 hours in order to charge ones bodies, to be ready for work the next day. I will discuss here one part of the equation, which will help patients who toss and turn between 1 and 3 hours or more before they fall sleep. When one cannot fall asleep within 30 min, then their brain is active and they start thinking about the day's work and worrying about the next day. The aim is stop one's mind wandering by a simple technique. If a person starts counting into the multiplication of 3, that is, 3, 6, 9, 12, 15…, or 1000, 999, 998, 997, 996…they will not be thinking about his work or any other thing. Their mind will be concentrating on this exercise and they will fall into sleep in a very short span of time. My experience is that this exercise helps at least 80% of patients.

During the last 20 years, I have noticed that persons who sleep on their stomachs tend to have headaches and cervical dystrophy. Based on my experience, I have discussed various sleeping positions.

3.2.1 SLEEPING ON THE BACK

Sleeping on the back with arms on the side is considered a good position as long as high pillows are not used. It is considered a good position to sleep for those who have back problems. Variations are where you keep your arms, that is, whether they are on the tummy, sides, or above the head. One can also keep a pillow under the knees to relieve pressure on the lower back. Figures 3.1 and 3.2 show one without the pillow while the other with the pillow. Pillow supports the neck, which is very important. Back sleepers tend to snore more and invariably suffer from sleep apnea.

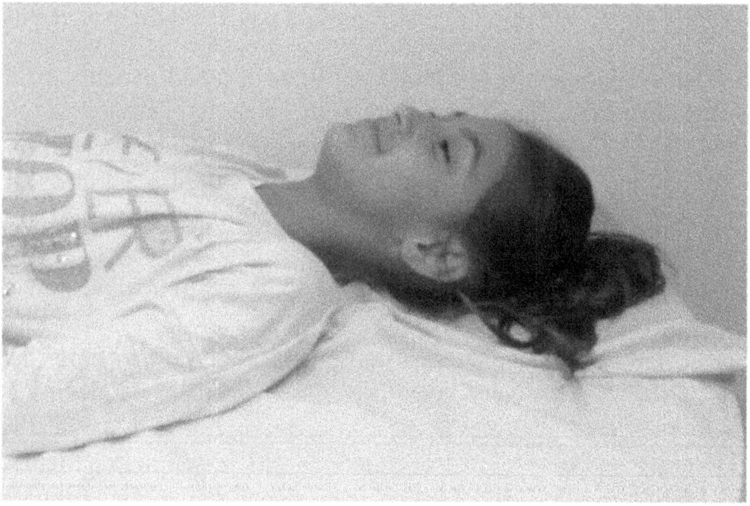

FIGURE 3.1 Sleeping on the back.

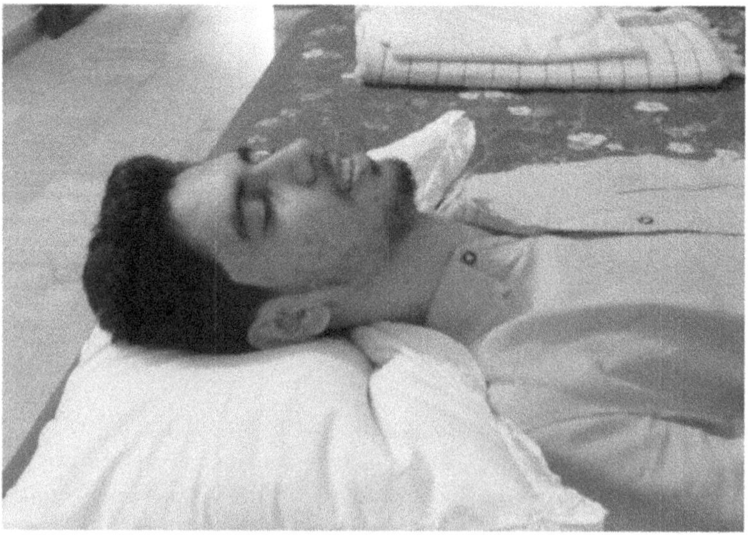

FIGURE 3.2 Sleeping on the back with neck support.

3.2.2 SLEEPING ON THE STOMACH

Sleeping on the stomach is not a good position to sleep because your neck is twisted toward left or right. This can lead to neck problems over time. It can also lead to back pain because the curvature of the back is not supported. This can also affect breathing. People who sleep on their stomach report increased restlessness caused by frequent tossing and turning in an effort to get comfortable. They generally suffer with headaches. This can also lead to Asthma in some cases. This is shown in Figure 3.3.

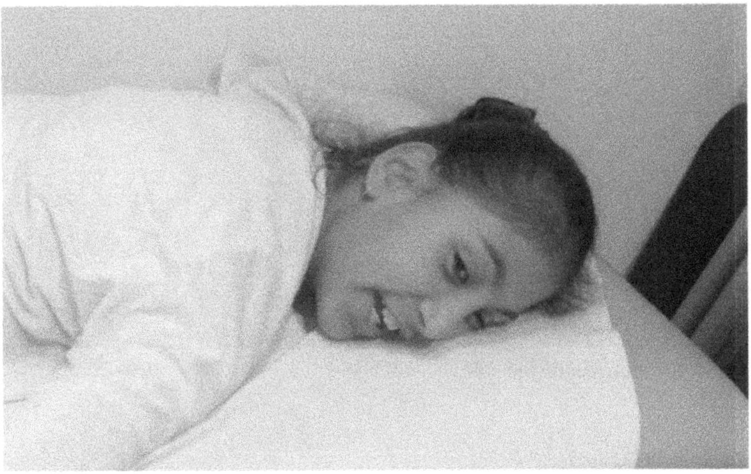

FIGURE 3.3 Sleeping on the stomach.

3.2.3 SLEEPING ON THE LEFT OR RIGHT SIDE

Sleeping on the side is a good sleeping position provided one keeps the back reasonably straight and knees together. Variations can be placing hands under the neck or pillow and/or at right angle to the body as shown in Figure 3.4. Another variation is placing ones upper leg similar to COMA position as shown in Figure 3.5. In the later case, the person is twisting his lower back, which can lead to lower back and hip problems. It can cause some discomfort in the shoulder. The other variation of sleeping on the side is in fetal position as shown in Figure 3.6; this can lead to curvature of the spine including scoliosis. This may create significant problems later in life. Based on my experience, I have discussed the various positions of sleeping. Sleep specialists recommend sleeping on your side in order to rest more comfortably and decrease the likelihood of interrupted sleep. The most comfortable position involves bending the knees slightly upwards toward the chest as shown in Figure 3.4.

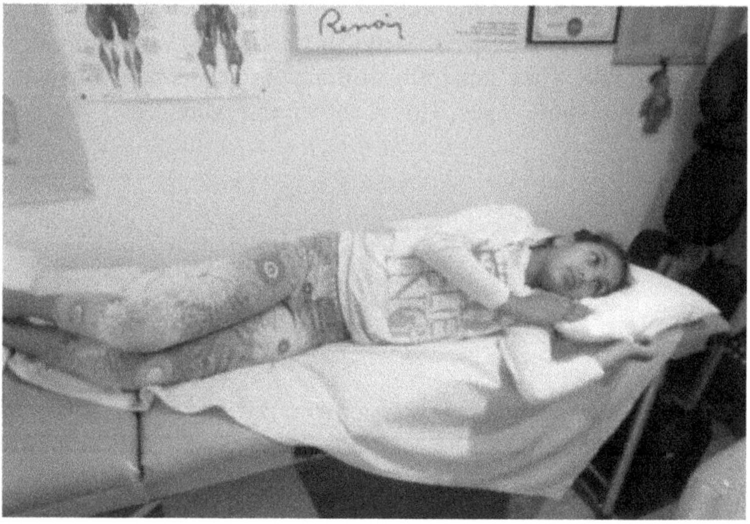

FIGURE 3.4 Sleeping on the side.

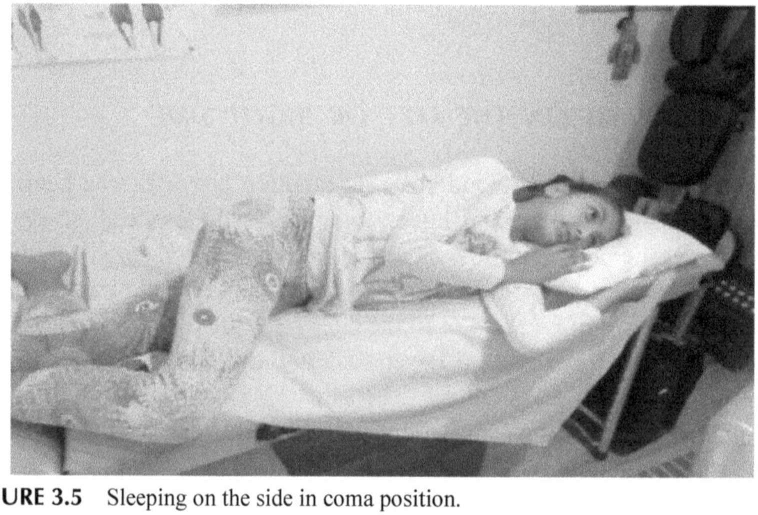

FIGURE 3.5 Sleeping on the side in coma position.

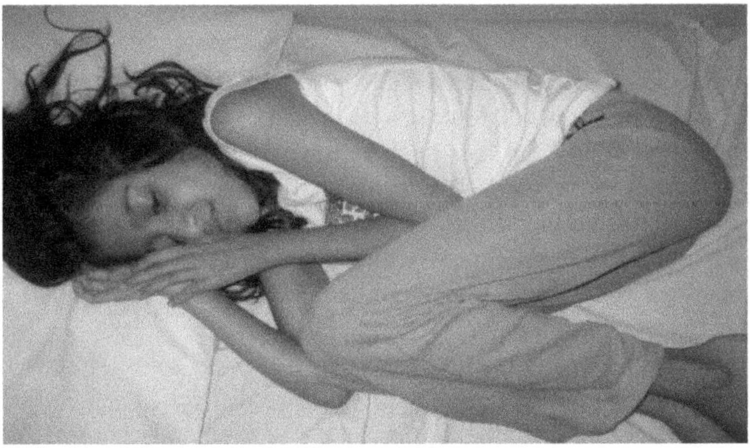

FIGURE 3.6 Sleeping on the side in fetal position

Although Sleeping on the side is decidedly the best position, we all do move during our sleep in particular as we age. One can also use a pillow in between the knees and it will help placing the knees together Figure 3.7. Use of a pillow is also very important. Using a big pillow can be harmful for your neck. Supporting your neck with a pillow is very important as shown in Figure 3.7.

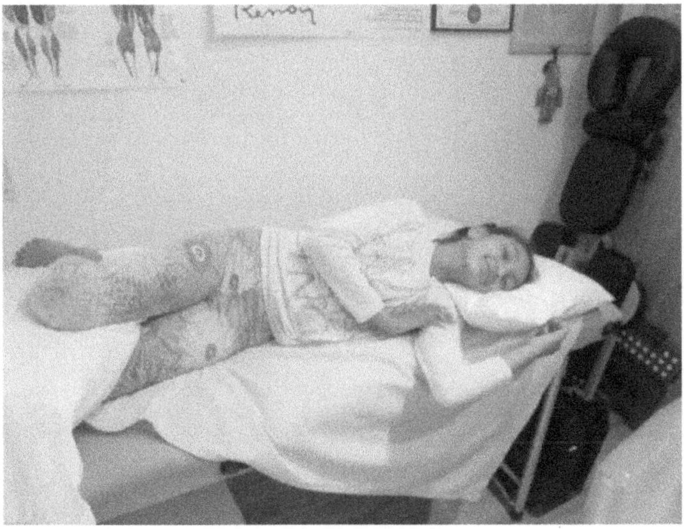

FIGURE 3.7 Sleeping on the side with neck support.

3.3 SITTING POSTURE

If your job requires sitting and without any support for your back then you should sit up straight with your torso balanced over your hips.[3] The height of seat should allow your legs to slope toward the floor at angle of about 10–15 degrees. Your knees should never be higher than your hips. This will allow fluid and blood flow freely. Your feet should rest in a comfortable position and you should move them regularly. Your sitting posture has an impact on your health. You should adjust your chairs to support good postures.[4]

Reading and writing requires sitting forward over a desk. In this situation, you should adjust your seat to tilt in forward direction and you should keep your hands on the table. In this case, you should place a small towel under your elbows so that you are not lifting you hand upwards. This is further explained in the next section.

Most of us spend our day in a sitting position. These days, we spend lot of time in front of a screen either a TV or a computer. The most common positions are shown in Figures 3.8, 3.9, 3.10, and 3.11.

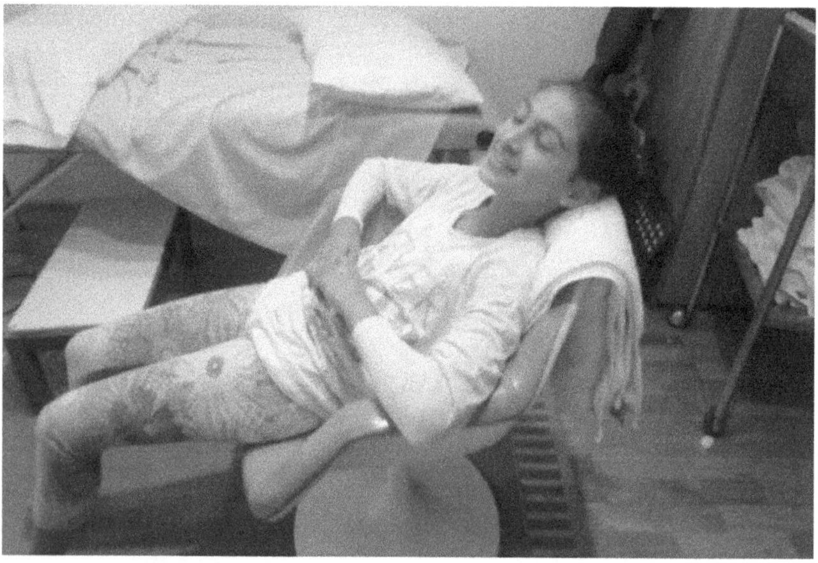

FIGURE 3.8 Sitting at an angle.

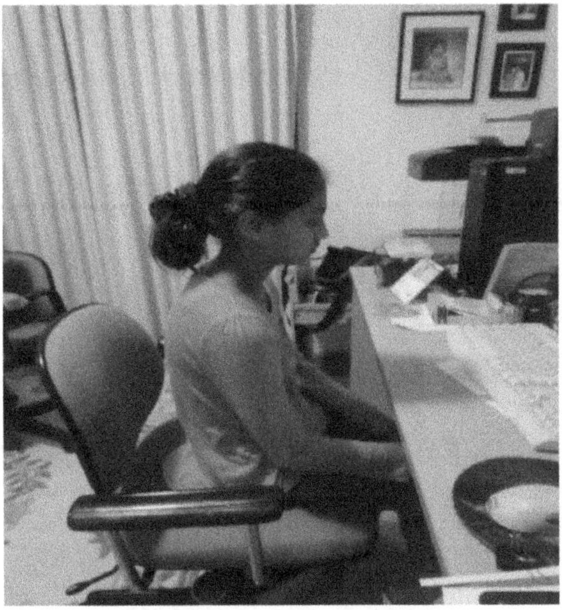

FIGURE 3.9 Sitting at the front of the chair.

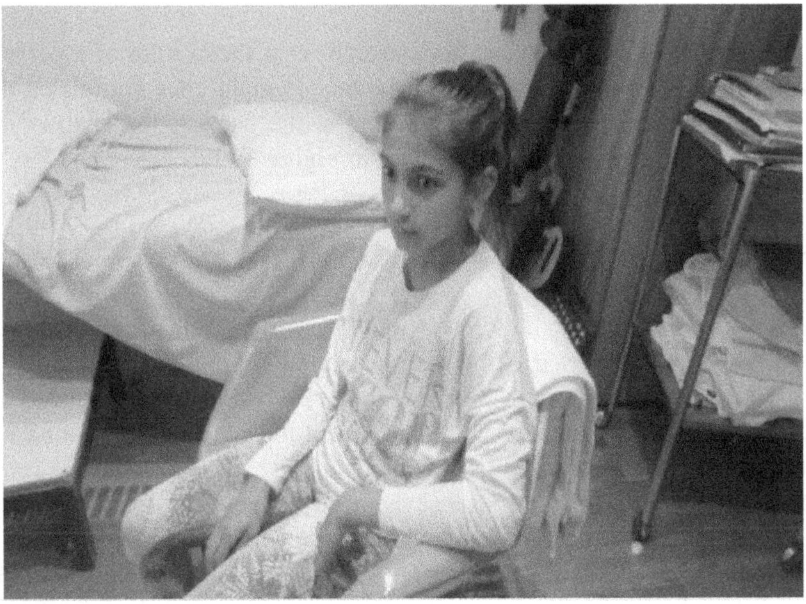

FIGURE 3.10 Sitting at the back of the chair.

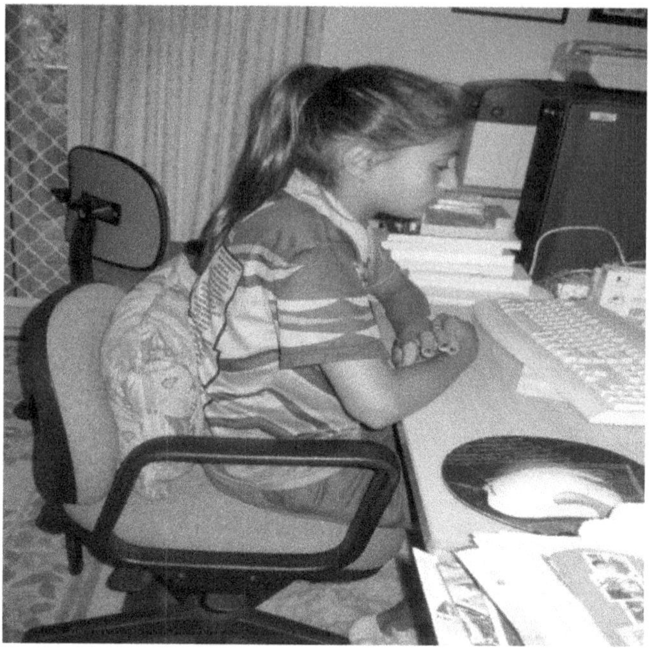

FIGURE 3.11 Sitting with a cushion at the back..

In all sitting positions, the body weight is at the bottom of a person. If the back is supported then all of the body weight does not fall on the bottom. This can be achieved by sitting at the back of the chair or by placing a pillow or a cushion as shown in Figure 3.11.

3.3.1 SITTING IN FRONT OF A COMPUTER

As a rule, the middle of the screen should be at eye level. The back should be straight and supported. This is demonstrated in Figures 3.10 and 3.11.

The arms should be at right angle to the body and be supported. This can be achieved if you place your chair under the table and rest your arms at the table.[5] In case, this is not possible and you have chair with the arms. Raise the level of the chair so that the arms of the chair are at the same level as table. Now place your arms on the arms of the chair. This is shown in Figure 3.12. If you are working with a mouse, then your elbow should be slightly higher than your hand. This can be done by placing a small hand towel under your elbow. This is shown in Figure 3.13.

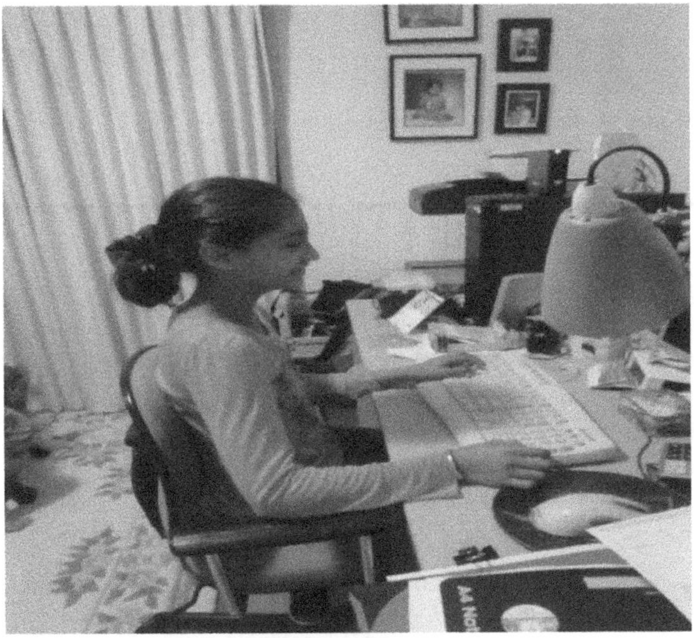

FIGURE 3.12 Sitting in front in front of a computer.

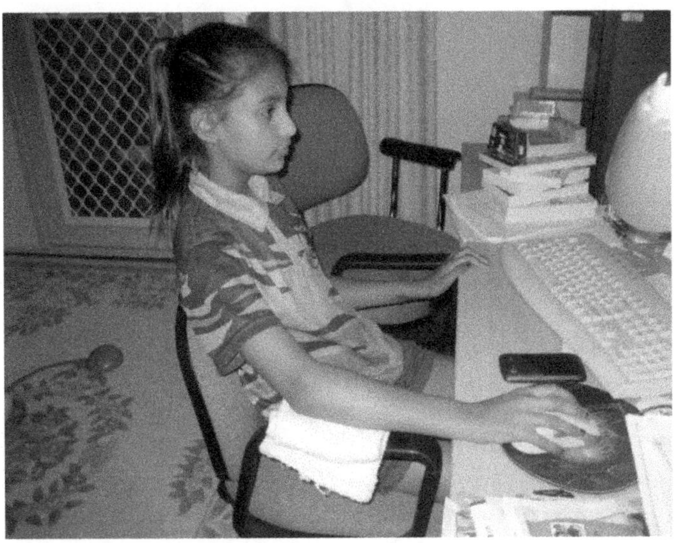

FIGURE 3.13 Sitting in front of computer with elbow raised.

In the sitting position, your upper legs should be almost parallel to the ground. In fact, the angle between the top of your thigh and the knees should be about 10 degrees.

Lower legs should be at right angle to the ground.

3.3.2 GETTING UP FROM A CHAIR

During a typical day, we get up from a chair 50–100 times. The majority of people use their hands to get up. This places the full body weight on the shoulder. This can affect the neck and shoulders overtime. I have treated many patients with shoulder pain. I have noticed that patients who get up from a chair using hands as shown in Figures 3.14 and 3.15, took a long time to recover. It is apparent from the pictures that the person's whole body weight falls on the shoulders.

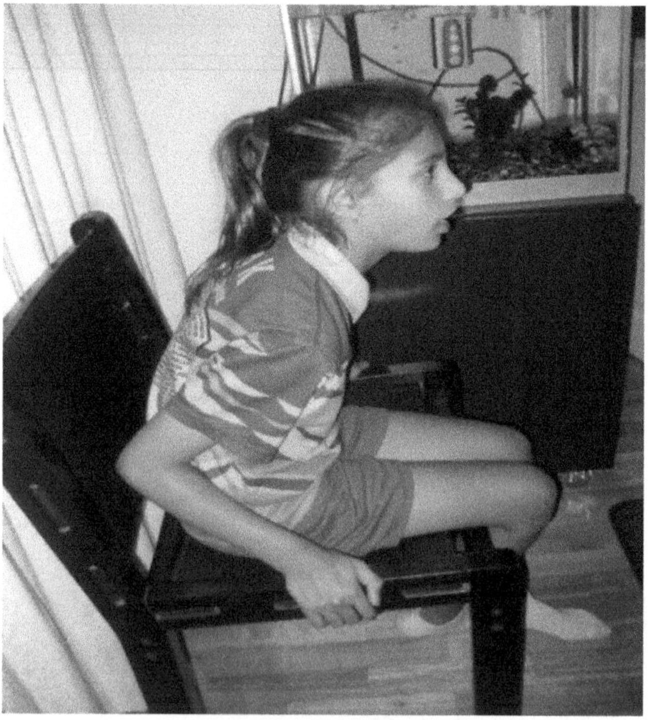

FIGURE 3.14 Getting up from the chair using hands.

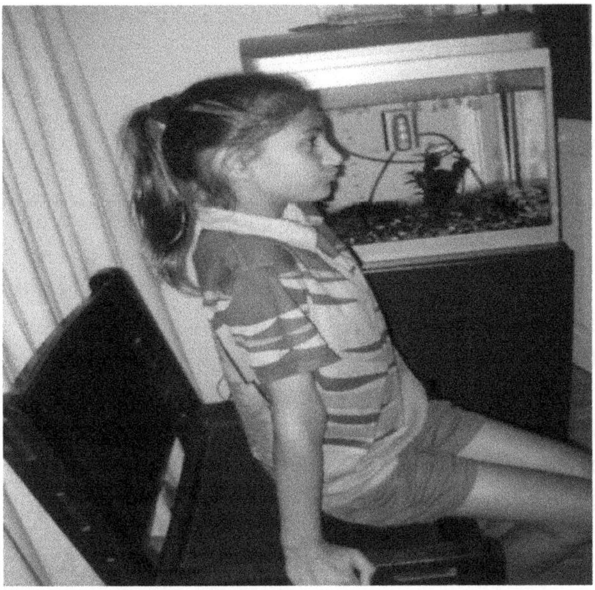

FIGURE 3.15 Getting up from the chair using hands.

The correct way to get up from a chair is to bend forward and use the legs to get up without using hands. This is shown in Figure 3.16.

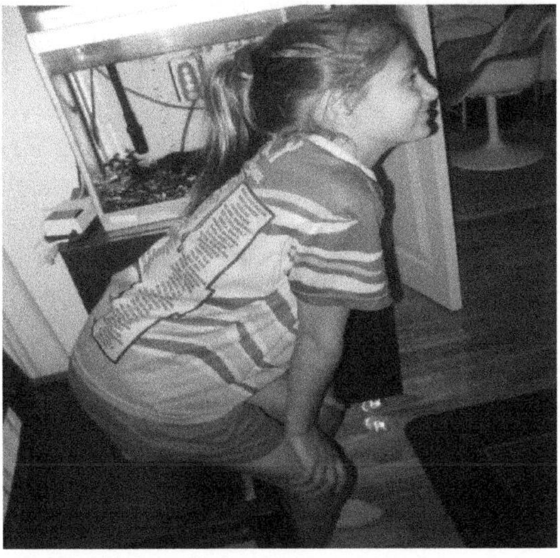

FIGURE 3.16 Getting up from a chair without using hands.

Using the wrong technique to get up can make it very difficult for older persons to get up from chairs without help.

3.4 STANDING POSTURE

A good posture while standing can be stated as "standing tall." Your feet should be approximately shoulder width apart. Knees and hips should be in line with the middle of your feet. Your knees should be slightly bent because looking your knees would restrict blood flow. Your torso should be balanced above the hips keeping the shoulders back. This will keep your body best working position and allowing the lungs to work without any restriction. Your head should be upright while chin slightly leaning downward. Middle of your head should be in line with your shoulders. Your hands can be in your pockets or folded in the lower back.

If you place your place, your hands on your waist you will end up raising your shoulders and it can lead to problems in shoulders if prolonged or done repeatedly.

Standing on hard surfaces, such as concrete over a long period of time can lead to heal spurs.

The majority of people stand correctly. Some who are taller than the average tend to bend their neck and upper thoracic area forward. This can lead to scoliosis in the upper back and pain in your shoulders after a few years. In old age, it can cause breathing problems. These postures are shown in Figures 3.17 and 3.18. However in case, you have developed shoulders going inwards and upper back leaning forward, you can correct it slightly by doing simple exercises. While standing keep your hands at the back instead of front. This will open up your shoulders. In serious cases, you can roll up a small towel and place this in the middle of your back horizontally between C-7 and T-12, and lie on a hard surface as shown in Figure 3.19.

Last piece of advice is for people who tend to keep their head in a particular direction. Invariably they do not know about it. They developed this at some time to relieve pain. This can be corrected if a person sits in front of a mirror and corrects his/her posture. If one does this 2–3 times in a day and after about a week his posture will be corrected.

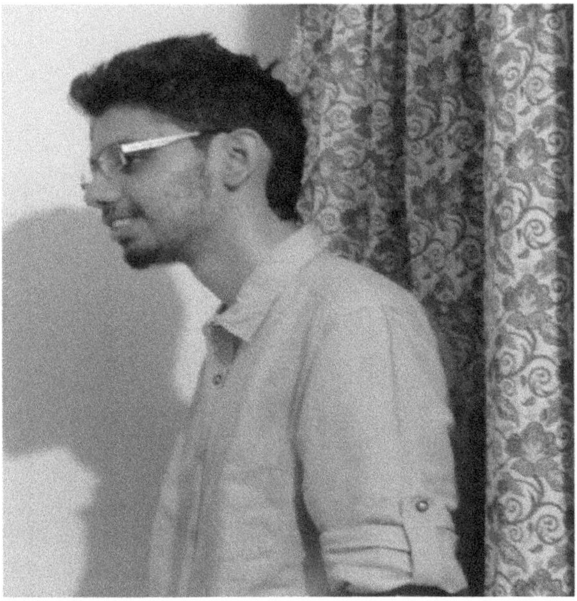

FIGURE 3.17 Standing with neck and upper back bent forward.

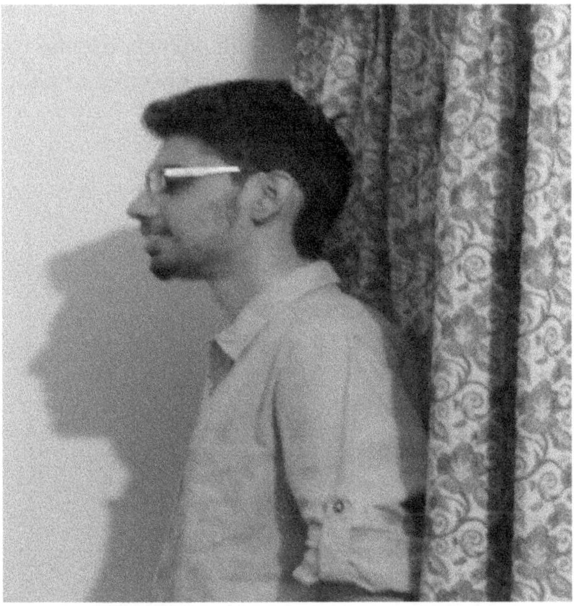

FIGURE 3.18 Correct standing position.

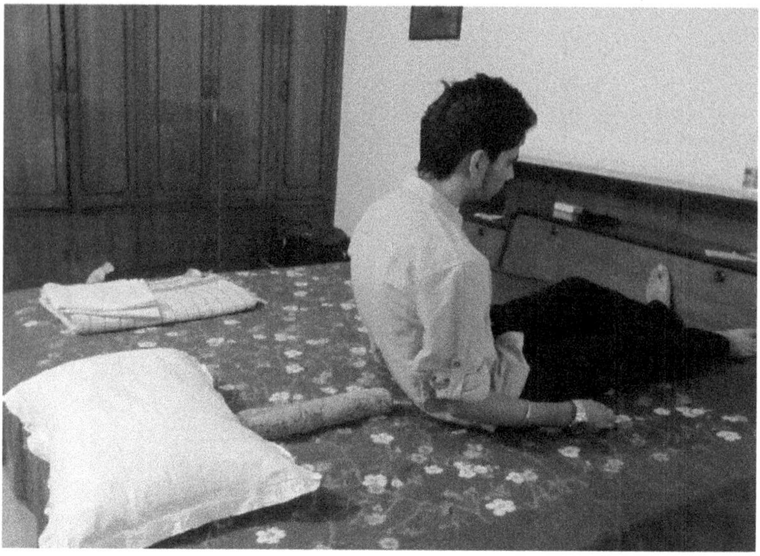

FIGURE 3.19 Exercise to correct hump in the neck and upper back.

3.5 CONCLUSION

Good posture is paramount for good health. Hence, use the guidelines and adjust accordingly. A good posture will keep you free of pain and flexible without any stress on your body.

KEYWORDS

- **Better sleep**
- **breathing problems**
- **headaches**
- **good posture**

REFERENCES

1. Types of Postures by Nancy Clark.
2. *Sleeping Position and Their Effects on Health,* Proceedings of the Singapore PATIENT conference, Singapore, 2014.
3. How to sit with good posture by Anne Asher?
4. What is a good posture by Chris Adams?
5. South African Institute of Vihangam Yoga Health Times. *J. Health.* May **2013,** *1*.

CHAPTER 4

INTEGRATIVE PHARMACOLOGY–INTERCONNECTING THE WORLD OF AYURVEDA (TRADITIONAL INDIAN MEDICINE–TIM), TRADITIONAL CHINESE MEDICINE (TCM), AND CONVENTIONAL MEDICINE (CM)

SUSANA DINIS*

Unus Research Center, Sinestecnopolo ZIL 2, 122 A, 7520-309 Sines, Portugal

**E-mail: susdisa@gmail.com*

CONTENTS

ABSTRACT

Pharmacology studies origin, nature, chemistry, effects, and uses of drugs. It includes pharmacognosy (medicinal drugs from plants), pharmacokinetics (interactions of a drug and the body in terms of its absorption, distribution, metabolism, and excretion), pharmacodynamics (branch concerned with the effect of the drugs on the body), pharmacotherapeutics (branch concerned with the therapeutic use of specific drugs), and toxicology. Even though conventional drugs go through this scientific screening before being in the market, drug-related adverse outcome continues to increase every year. Patients worry about adverse effects and toxicity of many conventional drugs and the inability of conventional medicine (CM) to provide adequate clinical effectiveness for chronic diseases, and are looking for more natural treatments and products over chemical drugs. Traditional Indian medicine (TIM) and traditional Chinese medicine (TCM) are the most ancient yet living traditions, with a strong philosophical basis and can play an important role in new therapies and drug discovery. For this to happen it is crucial not only to give traditional knowledge modern science evidence but also to enlighten modern science with traditional knowledge. The current strategy of drug development of single target–single compound is not suitable for studies on traditional medicines. Pharmacology needs to be reinvented possibly within methods like reverse pharmacology, network pharmacology, genomics, and computational tools, to understand TIM/TCM combinatorial formula rules where each herb plays a different role during treatment. Almost half of TIM/TCM botanical sources have similarities and both medicines have similar philosophies toward individuals, materials, and diseases. Plants are compositional complex mixtures of chemicals and studying them is a challenge. Integrative and interdisciplinary approach may be the key to study them. While herbals well-documented data arises urges the need for new classification, as they have a bigger role than just food supplements. If TIM, TCM, and CM are able to put their egos apart and work together as one we will converge into the medicine of the future with newer, safer, cheaper, and effective therapies, where all the knowledge is integrated in a scientific and holistic view while remembering the importance of individual responsibility for achieving health.

4.1 INTRODUCTION

Since time immemorial people have tested plants for their medicinal properties. Western medicine originated with the Romans and Greeks around 200 A.D. and Western pharmaceuticals only attained their present status in the 1920s with the discovery of penicillin.[1] On the other hand, time-tested Indian and Chinese herbal remedies have helped billions of people for nearly 5000 years and scientists today are still puzzled over their therapeutic effectiveness.[2]

Rigveda (2000 B.C.) is the oldest recorded document regarding use of plants as medicine in India, and this tradition continued in another ancient text, *Atharvaveda* (1500–1000 B.C.), which described more plants and introduced basic concepts. And after that we have the basic scriptures of Ayurveda – *Charaka Samhita* and *Sushruta Samhita.*[3]

According to Chinese medical texts, *Shen Nung* (lived ~3000 B.C.), considered to be the father of Chinese medicine and pharmacology sought out and investigated hundreds of herbs documenting many of them including the poisonous ones.[4] The Yellow Emperor's Internal Classic, considered to be the fundamental doctrinal source of Chinese medicine (*Huang Di Nei Jing*: 475–221 B.C.) systematically documented human structure, physiology, pathology, diagnosis, treatment, and preservation.[5]

Pharmacology is the science of drugs (Greek *pharmakos* – medicine or drug; *logos* – study) and the study of substances that interact with living systems through chemical processes, especially through binding to regulatory molecules and activating or inhibiting normal body processes. Pharmacology's history, knowledge of drugs and their use in disease is as old as the history of mankind, but as a science is quite young.

Dioscorides (40–90 A.D.), a Greek physician, wrote *De Materia Medica*, a reference work on herbs and pharmacy that remained the supreme authority on the subject in western civilization for over 1500 years. Johann Jakob Wepfer (1620–1695 A.D.) was the first to verify through animal experimentation assertions about pharmacological or toxicological actions. But pharmacology just became an independent scientific discipline with Rudolf Buchheim (1820–1879 A.D.), who founded the first institute of pharmacology at the University of Dorpat, and Oswald Schmiedeberg, with his many disciples, helped to establish the high reputation of pharmacology.1 In the second half of the nineteenth century, things changed remarkably as the industrial revolution brought technological development to manufacturing and agriculture inspiring the development of medical technology.

4.2 END OF A PARADIGM

Pharmaceutical industry has been highly successful and has historically seen incredible growth since its beginning. However, for the last decade, this growth process has not led to a corresponding increase in the number and efficacy of new drugs.[6] Despite the fact that conventional drugs go through a major scientific screening before being in the market, drug-related adverse outcomes continues to increase every year.[7] Between 2004 and 2008, there was a 52% increase in side and adverse effects in the inpatient setting, more than half of this increase was due to corticosteroids, anticoagulants, sedatives, and hypnotics.[8] Industry serious innovation deficit, high cost of new drugs, increased toxicity and side effects, lack of clinical effectiveness for chronic diseases, and microbial resistance and emerging diseases are leading public interest to the non conventional medicines.[9]

It is time to change the paradigm; it is time to gather knowledge, not only to give the traditional knowledge modern science evidence but also to enlighten modern science with traditional knowledge. It is extremely difficult to change the health system if we do not change our actual health concept.

CM grew is disease focused, however the increase in life expectancy makes us look to health and see much more than just the absence of disease and illness. Emphasizing similarities rather than differences facilitates the integration of knowledge across cultures and that fusion can conceptualize health also as a dynamic process of adaptation to environmental conditions where it is crucial for the individual to play an active and conscious role to maintain its balance.[10]

4.3 RESEARCH OPPORTUNITIES

With a new concept of health comes a new vision of treatment. TIM and TCM remain the most ancient yet living traditions, with strong philosophical basis and can play an important role in new therapies and drug discovery. Almost half of the botanical sources have similarities and both medicines have similar philosophies toward individuals, materials, and diseases.[11] Despite numerous pharmaceutical drugs being derived from botanicals, when chemical analysis became available (nineteenth century), scientists began to extract and modify the active ingredients from plants and made their own version of plant compounds leading to a declined use of herbal medicines in favor of drugs, a reality that is being reverted again.

Therefore, the interconnection between the conventional and traditional world already occurred it has been controlled by the conventional one. For example, using pharmacological concepts, strategy of drug development of single target – single compound, ephedrine was isolated from *ma huang* (*Ephedra sinica*), a TCM plant, revolutionizing asthma's treatment,[12] likewise, reserpine (*Rauvolfia serpentina*), a TIM plant, revolutionized hypertension treatment.[11,13] But if we want to study traditional formulas with multiple active ingredients or single herbs that have constituents difficult to analyze, pharmacology needs to be reinvented.

4.4 SIMILARITIES

To really understand TIM's and TCM's herbalism, it is crucial to understand the medicinal and medical model of both systems which are based on universal natural law and are considered holistic medicines, which address body, mind, and spirit. Each organ or each physiological part is interrelated, and all are connected to a bigger pattern. Diagnosis and treatment are focused on the patient as a whole person, and less on the symptoms.[14]

When a TIM/TCM formulation is prescribed the treatment should be preferably done with local herbs. Influence of the local seasons and time of the day, different parts of the plants, how they are collected, different tastes (sweet, sour, salty, pungent, bitter, and in TIM also astringent) are taken into account.[15,16]

When several herbs are applied together combined, they will display their superiority over a single herb in the treatment of disease. Herbs of similar action, if used simultaneously, can strengthen the therapeutic effect. Drugs of different actions in combination can expand the therapeutic scope. Noxious herbs may be applied combined with some drugs capable of reducing or removing their side effects or toxicity.[17] The herbs chosen in the prescription not only take into consideration the disease diagnose and its symptoms, but they can also be adapted to an individual's body and emotional constitution, in order to adjust the systems that are out of balance,[2,18] considering each patient has a unique constitution, which can be a very similar concept to what we know as pharmacogenetics in CM.[19]

With all these specific factors, it cannot be expected that after separating all the plants and isolating a unique substance there will be the same controlled effect with no toxicity and adverse effects. No medicine is better than other; it is just a matter of using a different language, a different point of view. It is time to create a global language for better understanding without losing each singularity and specificity.

4.5 NEW APPROACHES

Probably the best method to cross traditional and modern herbalism knowledge has not been developed yet. Plants are complex mixtures of chemicals and studying them is a challenge.[6] Integrative and interdisciplinary approach may be the key to study them.

Drug development, using conventional pharmacology, requires preclinical testing for information on the biological effects of new substances. Clinical testing with Phase I studies on healthy subjects will determine effects on body functions, dose definition, and pharmacokinetics. In Phase II, potential drugs are first tested on selected patients to determine the effects on disease, safety, efficacy, dose, and pharmacokinetics. Phase III involves a larger group of patients to compare the new drug with standard therapy. After being approved and marketed it is possible to gather information on the drug's effect in various populations and any side effects associated with long-term use – Phase IV.[20] All these important data that usually take years to gather after drug is on the market, is available for Chinese and Indian herbal formulas that have been used by thousands of people for thousands of years. Reverse pharmacology is a new discipline that is being used in TIM and it reduces costs, time, and toxicity because it starts with this valuable information that comes after the administration of a known drug. Secondly goes to exploratory studies for tolerability, drug-interactions, dose definition, and paraclinical studies to evaluate target-activity, and on the third phase includes experimental studies.6 It is remarkable the work done to integrate documented clinical observation data and reverse pharmacology may lead to new drug candidates and novel targets,[21] but possibly stays too close to conventional pharmacology and still do not emphasize a more deep understanding of TIM principles and different herbs roles within herbal formulas.[22]

Network pharmacology is being used in TCM exploring interactions between the body and drug, establishing a network for drug-gene-disease association and challenging the traditional one disease-one target-one drug. It has the potential to modernize TCM and TIM, change drug design methods and drug discovery from herbal formulas, but still there is the need to refine computational tools that can gather biological processes, TCM, and TIM knowledge.[23]

4.6 PERSPECTIVES

Increased use of traditional medicines and its phytotherapy demands scientific evidence and it might be done using biomedical sciences advances. Reverse and network pharmacology can be important tools for the process, but there is still lot of work to do. What molecular basis and biological knowledge underlines TIM and TCM and their respective body constitution and syndromes? What are the combination rules of TIM and TCM herbal formulas? Why using some herbs together reduce or eliminate toxicity and adverse effects?

TIM and TCM remain the most ancient yet living medicines, and despite the fact they have grown apart, their principles and life and health vision continuous to have so many similarities. It is time to put differences apart and join resources to get to a major goal.

Being TIM and TCM holistic medicines, they promote human health considering human beings and health in the context of their environment. That is why it is so important not only to understand TIM and TCM active substances and how they work, but also study the parallelism between Chinese and Indian herbs and local herbs from other countries. Using local herbs is a much more respectful way of natural approach, reinforcing human environmental adaptability. Innovative thinking is needed and of course new drug development is important and it will come with TCM and TIM scientific study development but we should focus on what is more urgent right now. It is crucial to reveal scientifically TIM and TCM phytopharmacology in order to make it correctly accessible to thousands of people all over the world that would benefit from it. While herbals well-documented data arises urges the need for new classification, as they have a bigger role than just food supplements. It is crucial to re-examine and adapt legislation to population actual needs. We cannot continue to close our eyes and pretend that traditional phytoformulas do not prevent, cure, and treat diseases just because modern science still has not found an adequate method to prove it. They are real medicines and must be used accordingly.

If TIM, TCM, and CM are able to put their egos apart and work together as one we will converge into the medicine of the future with newer, safer, cheaper, and effective therapies, where all the knowledge is integrated in a scientific and holistic view while remembering the importance of individual responsibility for achieving health.

KEYWORDS

- **CM**
- **conventional drugs**
- **pharmacology**
- **TCM**
- **TIM**

REFERENCES

1. Lüllmann, H. *Color Atlas of Pharmacology;* 2nd Ed., Thieme: New York, 2000.
2. Kwong-Robbins, C. The Art and Science of Chinese Herbal Medicine. *US Pharm,* **2003,** *28*(3).
3. World Health Organization. Benchmarks for Training in Traditional/Complementary and Alternative Medicine: Benchmarks for Training in Ayurveda. 2010. Available at http://www.who.int/medicines/areas/traditionaBenchmarksforTraininginAyurveda.pdf?ua=1.
4. Hinrichs, T. J.; Barnes, L. L. *Chinese Medicine and Healing: An Illustrated History*; 1st Ed., Harvard University Press: Cambridge, 2013.
5. World Health Organisation. Benchmarks for Training in Traditional/Complementary and Alternative Medicine: Benchmarks for Training in Traditional Chinese Medicine. 2010. Available at http://www.who.int/medicines/areas/traditional/Benchmarksfor-TraininginTraditionalChineseMedicine.pdf?ua=1.
6. Patwardhan, B.et al. Reverse Pharmacology and Systems Approaches for Drug Discovery and Development. *Curr. Bioact. Comp.* **2008,** *4*, 201–212.
7. Gandhi, T. K.; Weingart, S. N.; Borus, J. et al. Adverse Drug Events in Ambulatory Care. *N. Engl. J. Med.* **2003,** *348*(16), 1556–1564.

8. Lucado, J.; Paez, K.; Elixhauser, A. *Medication - Related Adverse Outcomes in U.S. Hospitals and Emergency Departments, 2008;* HCUP, Agency for Healthcare Research and Quality: Rockville, MD, April 2011.
9. Humber, J. M. The Role of Complementary and Alternative Medicine: Accommodating Pluralism. *J. Am. Med. Assoc.* **2002,** *288,* 1655–1656.
10. Morandi, A. et al. An Integrated View of Health and Well-Being. In *Cross Cultural Advancements in Positive Psychology;* Springer: Germany, 2013; Vol. 5.
11. Patwardhan, B. et al. Ayurveda and Traditional Chinese Medicine: A Comparative Overview. *Evid. Based Complement. Alternat. Med.* **2005,** *2,* 465–473.
12. Brand, E. When Big Pharma Meets Chinese Medicine. Acupuncture Today. October, 2014, Vol. 15, Issue 10.
13. Lele, R. D. Beyond Reverse Pharmacology: Mechanism-Based Screening of Ayurvedic Drugs. *J. Ayurveda Integr. Med.* **2010,** *1*(4), 257–265.
14. Kwong-Robbins, C. Traditional Chinese Medicine–A Natural and Holistic Approach. *US Pharm.* **2002,** *27*(12), 48–50.
15. Valiathan, M. S. *An Introduction to Ayurveda*; Universities Press: Tamil Nadu, 2013.
16. Zuo, Y. *Science of Chinese Materia Medica*; Publishing House of Shanghai University of Traditional Chinese Medicine: Shanghai, 2003.
17. Zuo, Y. *Science of Prescriptions*; Publishing House of Shanghai University of Traditional Chinese Medicine: Shanghai, 2002.
18. Macioccia, G. *Os Fundamentos da Medicina Chinesa*; Roca: São Paulo, 1992.
19. Patwardhan, B. et al. Classification of Human Population Based on HLA Gene Polymorphism and the Concept of Prakriti in Ayurveda. *J. Altern. Complement. Med.* **2005,** *11*(2), 349–353.
20. *Integrated Pharmacology*; 3rd Ed., Elsevier: New York, 2006.
21. Vaidya, A. D. et al. Current Status of Herbal Drugs in India: An Overview. *J. Clin. Biochem. Nutr.* **2007,** *41,* 1–11.
22. Pathak, N. Reverse Pharmacology of Ayurvedic Drugs Includes Mechanisms of Molecular Actions. *J. Ayurveda Integr. Med.* **2011,** *2*(2), 49–50.
23. Yang, M. et al. Navigating Traditional Chinese Medicine Network Pharmacology and Computational Tools. *Evid. Based Complement. Alternat. Med.* **2013,** *2013,* 731969.

CHAPTER 5

CONCEPT AND PRINCIPLES OF YOGA

GISALA GEORGE*

Department of Physical Education, Mercy College, Palakkad 678006, Kerala, India

**E-mail: srgisala@gmail.com*

CONTENTS

ABSTRACT

Yoga has received remarkable acceptance during past few years and millions of people are practicing yoga on regular basis. Developed over 5000 years ago, yoga has undergone many transformations to develop into a polished form. Yoga is more than practicing certain postures to attain physical stability. Yoga is a group of practices that allows person to be self- disciplined and to attain an unwavering mind. The wealth of a nation is its healthy population. In today's world, where lifestyle disorders have become more prominent due to stress and fast foods, yoga helps to attain a balance between physical and mental states of a human being. This chapter portrays different types of yogic postures and their significance.

5.1 INTRODUCTION

The origin of yoga has been a matter of debate but evidence of yoga can be seen in the early Hindu literatures. The word "Yoga" is derived from the Sanskrit term "Yuj," which means "to join or to unite." People always associate yoga with the physical aspects such as postures. But yoga is more than increasing our physical flexibility and strength. Yoga is an ancient practice that has evolved and changed over time. Yoga is the experience of oneness that is, the experience of union with inner being. Yoga is about the union of jeevatma with paramatma. It is a science by which, the individual approaches truth. It is an ancient art by which one obtains control of one's latent powers and is the means to reach complete self-realization. The continued practice of yoga helps us attain the state of unwavering mind. The primary aim of yoga is to attain harmony between body and mind. Yoga is simply ruling over body and mind.

5.2 TYPES OF YOGA

5.2.1 BHAKTI YOGA OR YOGA OF DEVOTION

It is the one commonly practiced in India. Bhakti yoga is a means of attaining a spiritually liberated state. It focuses on the maintaining a devoted and doubtless relationship with God, thereby achieving "oneness with God." Here man is free from worldly thoughts and spiritual enlightenment is achieved.

5.2.2 KARMA YOGA OR THE YOGA OF ACTION

It helps us to act selflessly without expecting any reward. This thought helps us to remove the evils of ego and thus helps to attain purity of mind and soul.

> *"Karma Yoga is the selfless devotion of all inner as well as the outer activities as a sacrifice to the Lord of all works, offered to the eternal as* Master of all the soul's energies and austerities."—Bhagavad Gita

5.2.3 JNANA YOGA OR THE YOGA OF KNOWLEDGE OR WISDOM

It can be a difficult task requiring a lot of will and patience. It focuses on man's intelligence and considers that gaining knowledge is crucial in knowing the spirit.

5.2.4 HATHA YOGA OR YOGA OF POSTURES

It is the most familiar one. It makes use of asana, pranayama, and meditation to attain mental well-being. Psychic and mental purity are the fruits of hatha yoga. There was a significant increase in muscle strength, flexibility, and cardiorespiratory endurance in individuals after 8 weeks of regular yoga practice.[1]

5.2.5 LAYA YOGA

Laya yoga is the path of total dissolution. Once entered into the state of laya, one loses self consciousness and there is no knowledge of time or individuality. Laya yoga is not as common as other yogas and is taught by very few. It is an ancient form of meditation that helps to prevent fluctuations of mind. Laya yoga helps to eliminate the feeling of "I" and enter into a higher level of consciousness.

5.2.6 RAJA YOGA

It is also known as mental yoga. Through this practice of concentration we learn to calm our mind. Raja yoga is a path of self-discipline and practice.

Raja yoga is divided into eight parts also known as astanga yoga or the eight limbs of yoga.

To secure purify of body, mind, and soul the observation of following is necessary.

- Yama
- Niyama
- Asana
- Pranayama
- Pratyahara
- Dharana
- Dhyana
- Samadhi

5.2.6.1 YAMAS (ABSTENTIONS)

Yamas and Niyamas are set of rules within yoga. It is believed that by following Yamas and Niyamas one can attain peace. They are the fundamental principles that explains how we should interact with other people. The attitude towards ourselves is also important.

The commonly used Yamas include

Ahimsa: do not harm, Satya: truth, Astheya: non-stealing, Aparigraha: non-greediness, Brahmacharya: chastity.

5.2.6.2 NIYAMAS (MORAL OBSERVATIONS)

- Shaucha (internal purity of mind, speech; external purity of body, surroundings)
- Santosha (peace, equilibrium of mind)
- Tapas (internal heat or fire-burns up impurities and ego)
- Svadhyaya (self-study)
- Ishvara Pranidhana (surrender to God through the prayer and meditation)

5.2.6.3 ASANA

It concentrates on physical posture. The idea behind asana is to attain a steady and stable posture. It is a state in which one can remain steady, calm, quiet, and comfortable, both physically and mentally. It increases the flexibility of the body and helps to attain control over emotions. The asana is mainly classified into

a. Meditative asana
b. Cultural asana
c. Relaxation asana

TABLE 5.1 Classification of Asana

a. Meditative asana	b. Cultural asana	c. Relaxation asana
(i) Padmasana	(i) Sirsasana	(i) Savasana
(ii) Vajrasana	(ii) Sarvangasana	(ii) Makarasana
(iii) Sukhasana	(iii) Bhujangasana	(iii) Matsya kridasana
	(iv) Salabhasana	
	(v) Ardha Matsyendrasana	

5.2.6.4 PRANAYAMA

Pranayama is the control or regulation of breath.

> *"For breath is life, and if you breathe well you will live long on earth."*
> *~Sanskrit proverb*

According to BKS Iyengar,[2] one of the foremost yoga teachers in the world, "Prana is the life force which permeates both the individual as well as the universe at all levels." Prana is the vital energy or force that drives life. Correct breathing habit can be established by the regular practice of pranayama. Studies have shown that by regularly practicing pranayama one can control his stress and anxiety. Moreover this also helps to attain a balance of mind and body.

The following procedure can be followed while doing pranayama

- Lie on the back with eyes closed and hands softly resting on the belly, mouth closed.
- Start to notice the quickness of breathing.
- Exhale gently outward.
- As you exhale see the joining of breath in reverse.
- Stay here, deepening the awareness of the breath.

5.2.6.5 PRATYAHARA

Pratyahara is opposite of "Ahara." Whatever we accept is ahara (e.g., O_2, food, etc.). Pratyahara is gaining control over external influences by staying away from wrong choice of food or associations.

By achieving control over senses, we learn to move forward in life with a completely relaxed mind. Pratyahara can be achieved only by constant practice and patience.

5.2.6.6 DHARANA

Dharana deals with the concentration of mind. Our thoughts are fixed on a single object. Through the daily practice of dharana we can do our work more efficiently and effectively. Dharana helps to attain an unwavering mind. In the initial stage we find it very difficult to tame our minds and thoughts. But gradually we realize that concentration becomes easy once we start practicing it.

5.2.6.7 DHYANA

Dhyana and Dharana are mutually linked. The word *dhyana* comes from the Sanskrit word *dhyai*, which means "to think of." Dhyana is usually translated as "meditation." Dhyana helps to differentiate between illusions and reality and finally attain Samadhi. Dhyana has benefits on both mind and body. Some researchers have also tried to study the distinctions between meditation and Dhyana.[3]

5.2.6.8 SAMADHI

This is considered as the final stage in Yoga where union with God is achieved.

5.3 HINTS AND RULES OF YOGASANAS

5.3.1 PLACE

- Ground should be level, clean, and free from noise.
- Should be practiced on a mat on or a carpet.

5.3.2 TIME

Early morning is the ideal time for practicing yoga. You can feel its effects throughout the day.

5.3.3 BEGINNERS

The body will be more flexible in the evening.

5.3.4 CLOTHING

In accordance with the season, any loose and comfortable dress can be selected. The salwar kameez is an ideal dress for women as it is loose yet allowing freedom of movement.

5.3.5 SURROUNDINGS

- One should remain silent while practicing asana.
- Concentration is necessary for the all-round progress of the body and the mind.
- Concentration should be on breathing and on the limbs which may feel stressed.

- Before one begins to practice other asana, one should perform savasana in order to make breathing normal.
- No force or jerk should be exerted which practicing yogasana.
- The time taken to practice yogasanas should be increased gradually as it will help the body to become flexible.
- It is a scientific process which deals with the internal and external parts of the body. One should practice yogasanas under the proper guidance of a yoga expert.
- Before performing yogasana, one should take light food.
- If one is suffering from complicated disorder or severe fever, he/she should not practice asana. There are certain asana that should not be practiced by people suffering from high blood pressure, heart condition, diabetes, spondylitis, eye problems, etc.
- Women should not practice asana during pregnancy and immediately after delivery.
- While doing the asanas, the change from one position to another and vice versa should be done very gently and slowly.
- After practicing yogasanas, savasana should be performed. Savasana is a perfect asana which gives the body speedy relaxation. This in turn helps us to become more energetic.

5.4 BENEFITS OF YOGASANA

- Gives sufficient exercise to the internal organs—with this, an individual can maintain good health and longevity of life.
- A small airy place and very little equipment are required for yogasana practice.
- It is a solo-practice, whereas two or more individuals are required in other games.
- It helps to develop physical and mental powers to calm the mind and control the senses.
- Not expensive.
- Keeps the body free of diseases.
- The body becomes more flexible.
- One looks younger and lives longer.
- Blood in the blood vessels is purified.
- Concentration is improved.

- Yogasana helps to improve the flexibility of the spine.
- Yogasana is a non-violent activity which keeps a person to become morally good.
- Stimulates different glands of the body which helps the body to acquire a balanced growth.
- Constipation, gas-trouble, diabetes, blood-pressure, headache, etc. can be overcome.
- Intellectual and spiritual development is achieved along with physical and mental development.
- There is no restriction of age or sex for yogasana and one can enjoy sound health for a long time.
- Reduce fatigue and soothe the nerves.

5.5 MEDITATION AS ANTI-AGING MEDICINE

Meditation is our most potent form of natural, anti-aging medicine. Meditation is easy to learn. We need a quiet environment along with meditative tools such as mantra and a meditative attitude. Go to a private place by yourself or with another mediator where you will not be interrupted. Allow 10–20 minutes for meditation, and stick with it.

Sit down on a comfortable mat, cushion, or chair and try to relax every muscle in your body from bottom to top. Close your eyes and breathe deeply. Silently repeat a word or mantra. It can be religious or philosophical as long as it makes you feel good. When thoughts intrude, just say, "Oh well" to yourself, and start all over. Adopt a calm passive attitude, a mental state in which you do not judge yourself or others. After you finish, sit quickly for a couple of minutes and try to carry your calm, anti-aging, meditative attitude into your daily activities.

Meditation has also been shown to produce the following general medical benefits:-

- Reduction of anxiety
- Reduction of chronic pain
- Lowered level of cortisone
- Increase in cognitive function
- Lowered blood pressure
- Improvement in post traumatic stress syndrome

5.6 STRESS MANAGEMENT

Ashtanga yoga (yama, niyama, asana, pranayama, prathyahara, dharana, dhyana, samadhi) will help us to achieve totally stress free life. Yoga nidra and Savasana are the most effective methods of stress release. Regular practice of pranayama (breathing exercises) will help to control our feelings.

Most anxieties are related to a specific fear, like performance anxiety or social anxiety. These anxieties are usually rooted to a negative experience in the past. Anxiety usually results in the excitation of various organs of the body.

5.7 HEALTH BENEFITS

The body consists of various systems and organs, which are related and coordinated with each other, to give the best possible health and efficiency. When this system is interrupted, it results in disease and lack of vitality. Yoga brings these systems into balance with one another, thereby helping to prevent and cure disease.

The aim of Yoga is to attain better mental, physical, and spiritual health.

The fundamental difference between the yogic exercises and ordinary physical exercises is that physical exercises emphasize harsh movements and they produce large quantities of lactic acid in the muscle fibers, thus causing fatigue. Healing power of yoga is great for the physical, mental and spiritual health and for our total well-being.

The daily practice of yogasana will help in physical, mental, and spiritual progress. And thus one attains equilibrium between self, nature, and God. Similarly, harmony between all the members of a society leads to social happiness. It will lead an individual to find out meaning for the past and fills the future with hope. The blessing of yoga is precisely that it teaches us to live in the present. Thus practicing yogasana will help in our integral development.

5.8 SELECTED YOGIC POSTURES WITH PICTURES, THEIR SIGNIFICANCE, AND ACTION

5.8.1 SURYANAMASKARA

Suryanamaskara which comes under yogasanas includes different postures. By practicing various bodily postures, some of the dormant psychological systems of the body are activated. Activities energy centers of the body, promotes general health, since it involves the movement of all parts of the body (Fig. 5.1).

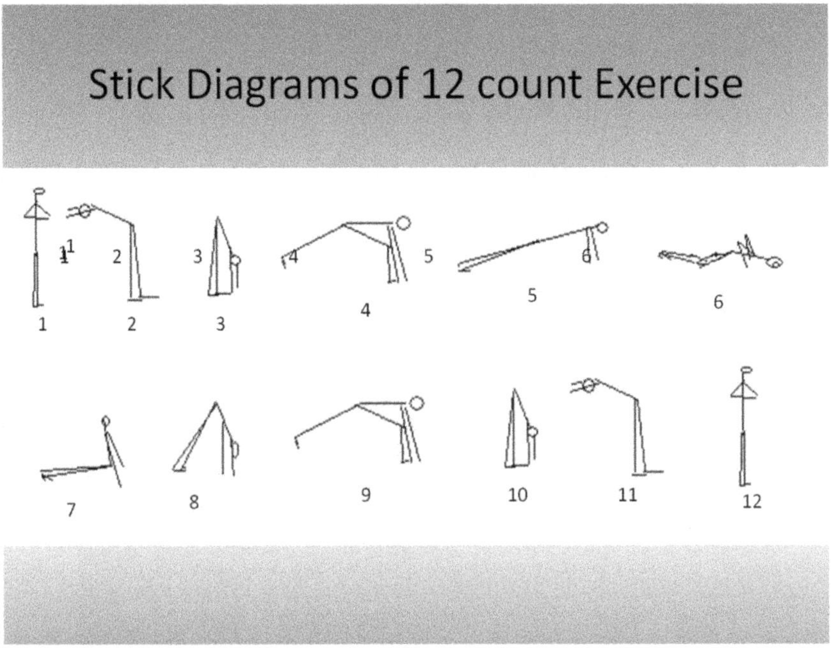

FIGURE 5.1

5.8.2 PRANAYAMA

Activate respiratory and nervous system, good for anxiety and stress management (Fig. 5.2).

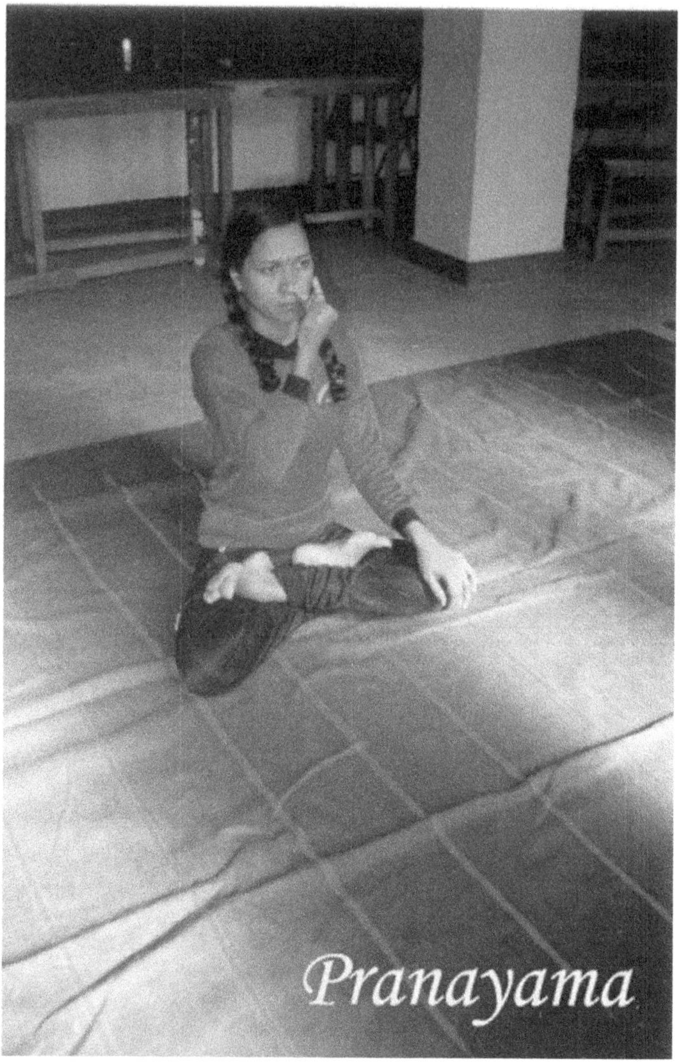

FIGURE 5.2

5.8.3 HALASANA

Halasana activates the entire spine, stretches the spinal muscles and tones the nerves of both inside out side of spine (Fig. 5.3).

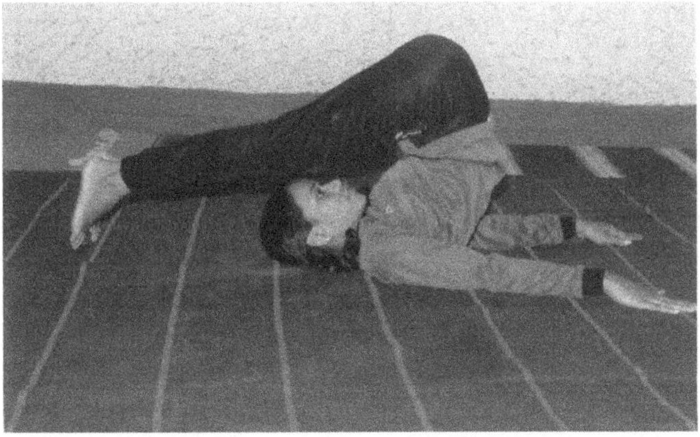

FIGURE 5.3

5.8.4 PADANGUSTHASANA

Acts on the back and lower stomach, curves indigestion (Fig. 5.4).

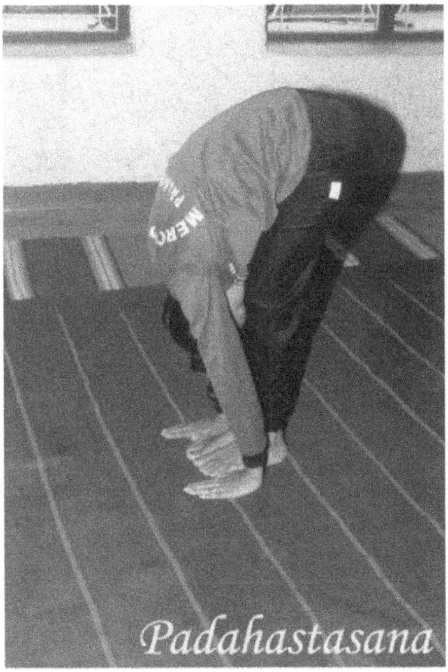

FIGURE 5.4

5.8.5 PAVANAMUKTHASANA

Acts at the central back portion, relievers back and hip pairs, regulates blood pressure (Fig. 5.5)

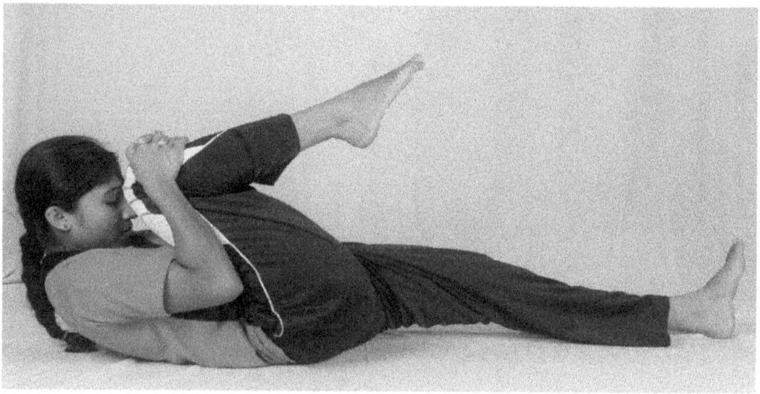

FIGURE 5.5

5.8.6 SALABASANA

Acts at stomach region, stimulating intestine, liver, spleen, and pancreas (Fig. 5.6).

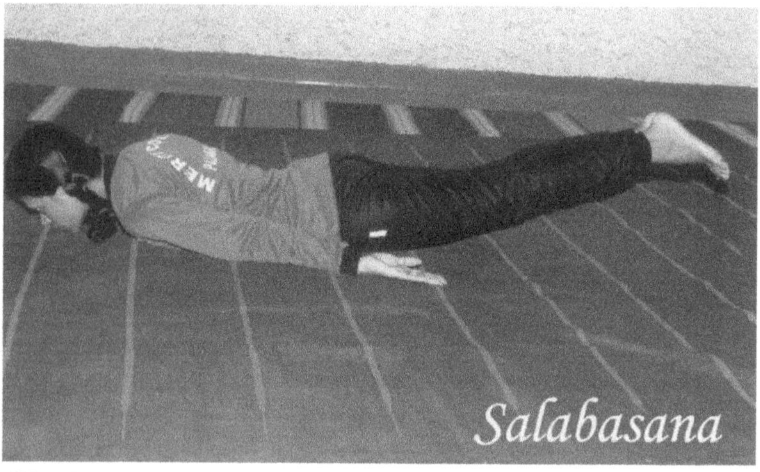

FIGURE 5.6

5.8.7 YOGAMUDHRA

Acts on lower back, right back and activates back muscles and digestion (Fig. 5.7).

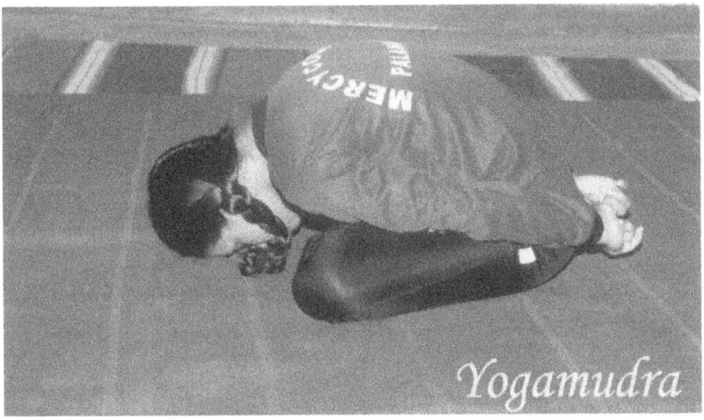

FIGURE 5.7

5.8.8 BHUJANGASANA

Acts on chest, activates respiratory system, cures asthma, spondylitis, and stomach ache (Fig. 5.8).

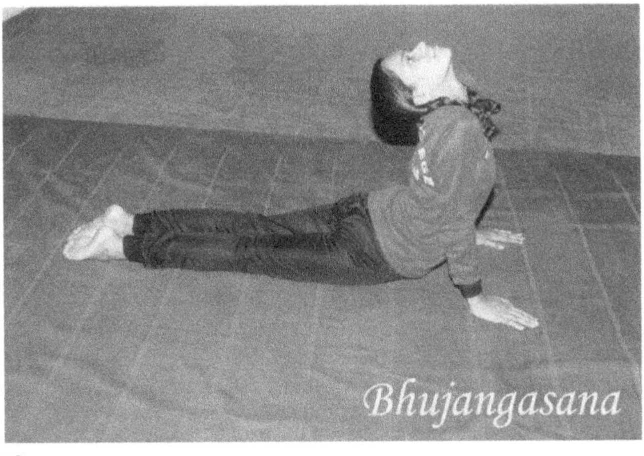

FIGURE 5.8

5.8.9 DHANURASANA

Acts on back region and stomach, cures intestinal disorders and diabetes (Fig. 5.9).

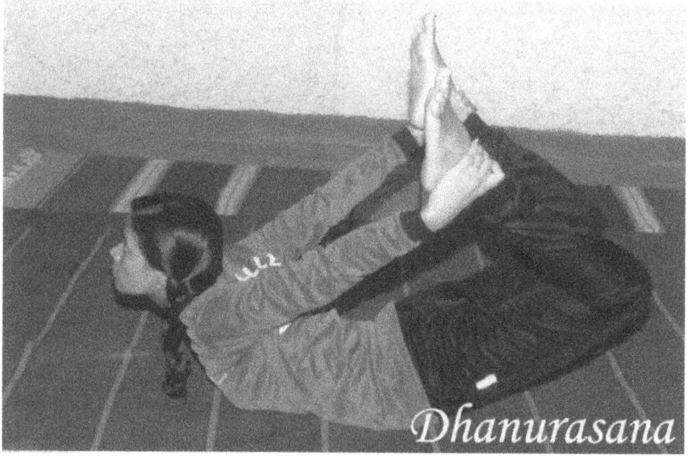

FIGURE 5.9

5.8.10 PASCHIMOTTANASANA

Activates stomach, liver, spleen, and kidney, increases appetite, reduces stomach and back pains, cures diabetes (Fig. 5.10).

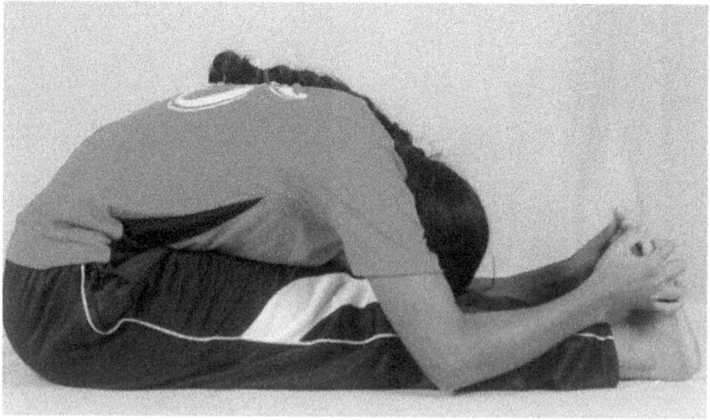

FIGURE 5.10

5.8.11 CHAKRASANA

Acts on stomach, chest, and spinal cord, activates respiratory system. The final position looks like wheel and hence the name (Fig. 5.11).

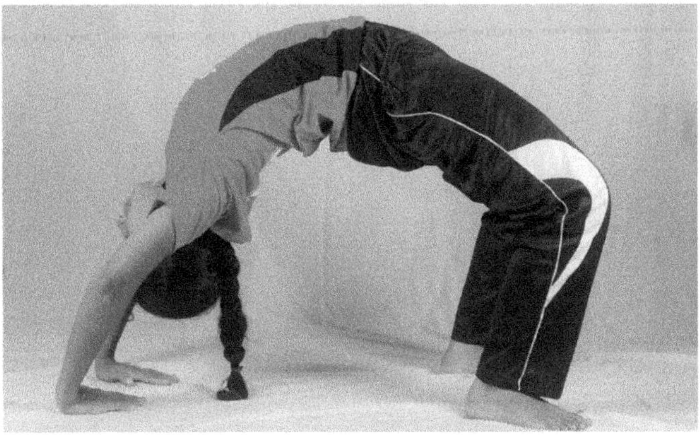

FIGURE 5.11

5.8.12 TRIKONASANA

Acts on back muscles, activates lungs, and relieves back and hip pains (Fig. 5.12).

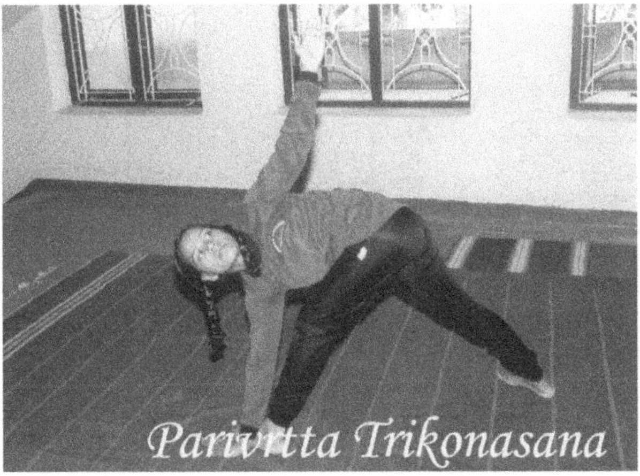

FIGURE 5.12

5.8.13 SARVANGASANA

Acts in neck region and on thyroid and parathyroid gland (Fig. 5.13).

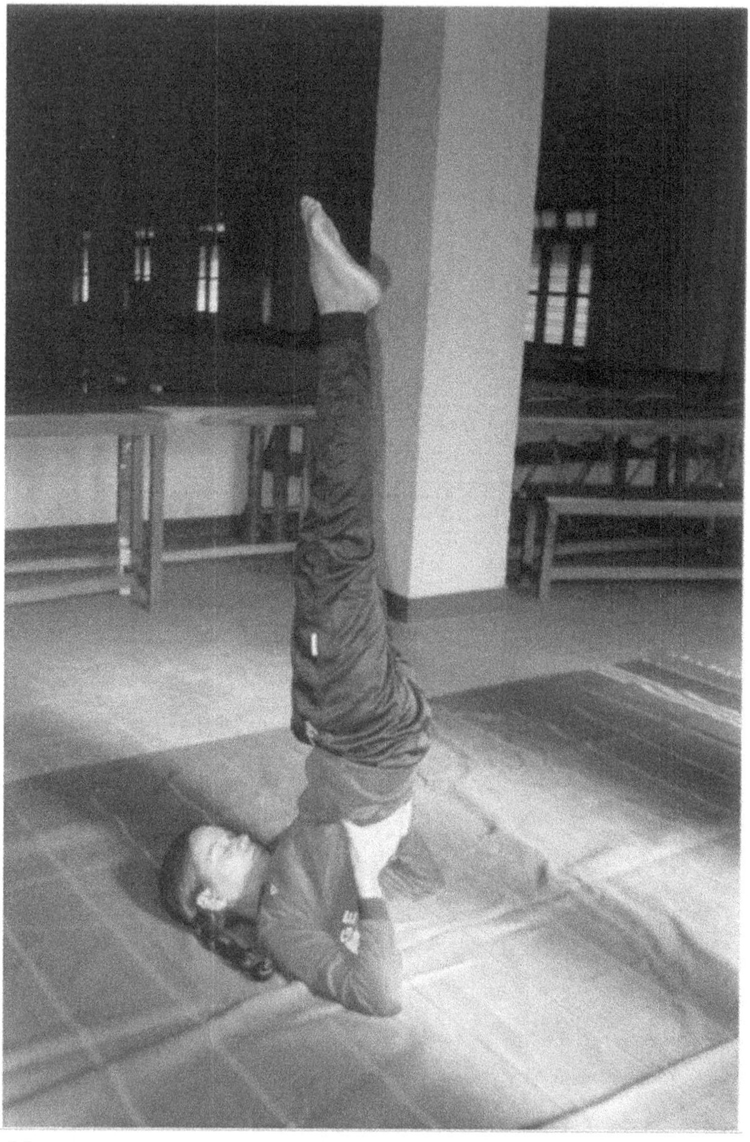

FIGURE 5.13

5.8.14 PADMASANA

Acts on stomach and muscles, a typical asana for meditation bestows peace of mind, a good posture for meditation and pranayama (Fig. 5.14).

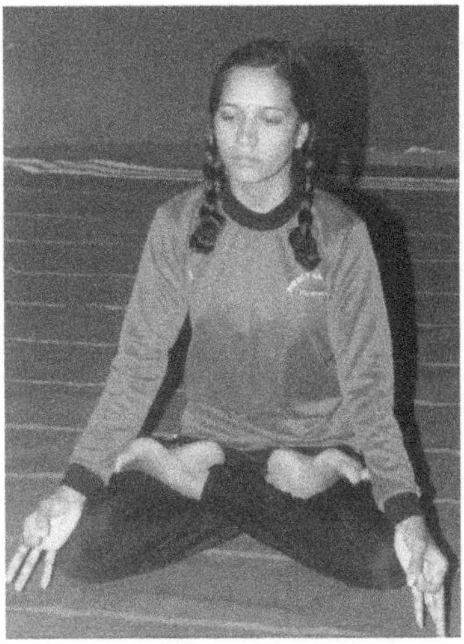

FIGURE 5.14

5.8.15 SIDDHASANA

Increases will power and the duration of meditation (Fig. 5.15).

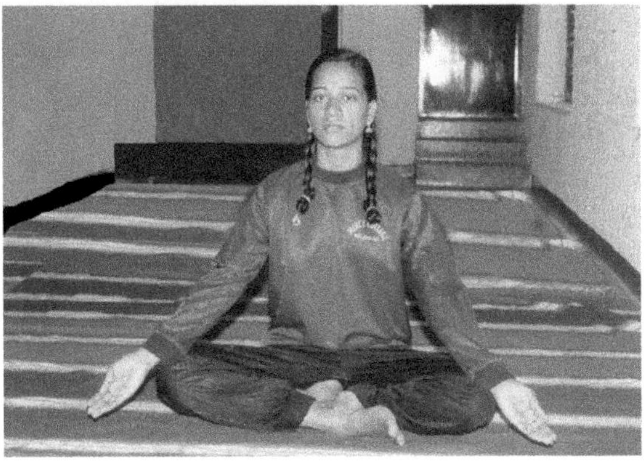

FIGURE 5.15

5.8.16 VAJRASANA

Acts on anal region, strengthens muscles, bestows the power of concentration, good posture for meditation, and pranayama (Fig. 5.16).

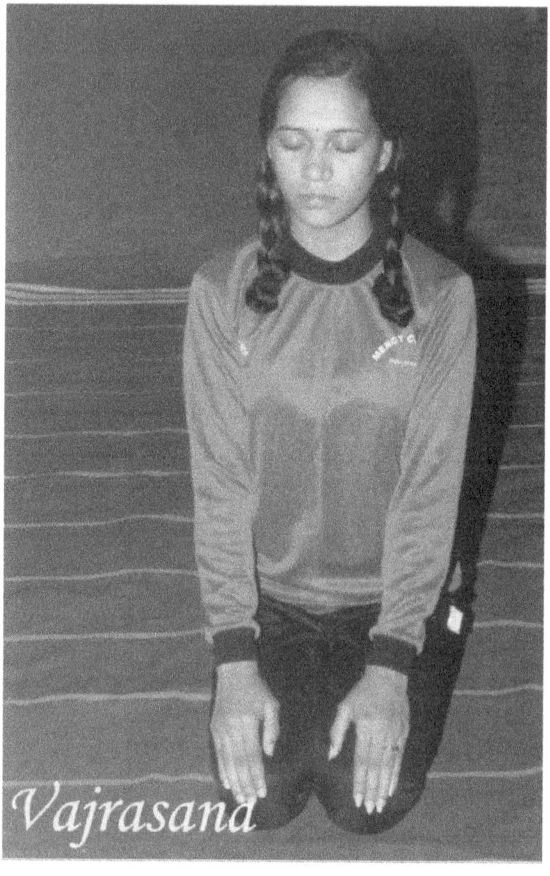

FIGURE 5.16

5.8.17 SUKHASANA

Comfortable asana for suffering long time, regulates inhalation and exhalation, gives peace of mind, related to meditation (Fig. 5.17).

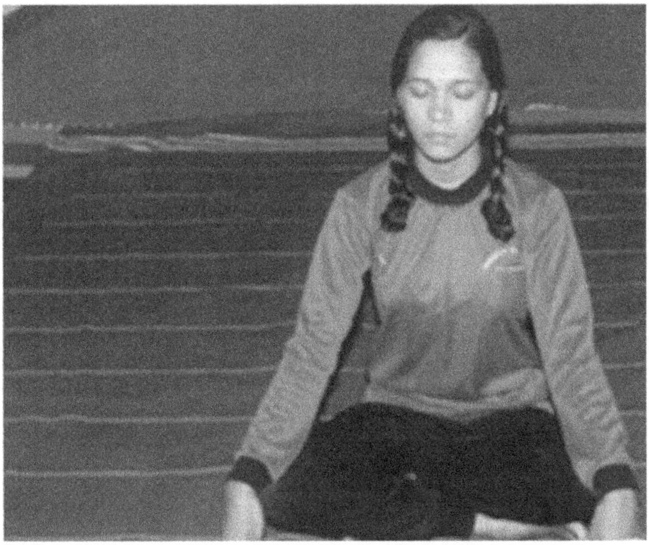

FIGURE 5.17

5.9 CONCLUSION

Yoga has been proved to be effective for those who have incorporated yoga practice in their daily lives. Regular practice of yoga provides physical benefits in addition to the rejuvenation of mind. Yoga helps to develop a positive attitude toward life. June 21 was declared as the International day of yoga by United Nations General Assembly on December 11, 2014. This shows the world wide acceptance of yoga. Yoga is not just an exercise but it is a journey toward healthy living.

KEYWORDS

- **pranayama**
- **jnana yoga**
- **yamas**
- **jeevatma**
- **paramatma**

REFERENCES

1. Tran, M. D.; Holly, R. G.; Lashbrook, J.; Amsterdam, E. A. Effects of Hatha Yoga Practice on the Health-related Aspects of Physical Fitness. *Prevent. Cardiol.* **2001,** *4*(4), 165–170.
2. Iyengar, B. K. S. *Light on Yoga: The Classic Guide to Yoga by the World's Foremost Authority*; Thorsons: Hammersmith, London. ISBN-13: 978-8172235017.
3. Srinivasan, T. M. (2013). From Meditation to Dhyana. *Int. J. Yoga*. **2013,** *6*(1), 1.

CHAPTER 6

THE POTENTIAL BACTERICIDAL PROPERTIES OF SOME PLANTS COMMONLY USED IN AYURVEDIC MEDICINAL PRACTICES OF SOUTH INDIA

INDU M. NAIR[1] and A. A. MOHAMED HATHA[2*]

[1]*School of Environmental Sciences, Mahatma Gandhi University, P.D. Hills, Kottayam 686562, Kerala, India*

[2]*Department of Marine Biology, Microbiology and Biochemistry, School of Marine Sciences, Cochin University of Science and Technology, Cochin 682016, Kerala, India*

[*]*Corresponding author. E-mail: mohamedhatha@gmail.com, mohamedhatha@cusat.ac.in*

CONTENTS

ABSTRACT

The antibacterial potential of crude extracts of 15 plants, which were traditionally used in Indian medicinal practices have been tested against both gram-negative and gram-positive strains using Agar well method. On the basis of the medicinal aspects of different parts of the plants, 24 extracts were prepared. Nine plants extracts were found to have excellent antibacterial property and eight extracts shows moderate activity. The study points to the possibility of the plant, such as *E. hirta, L. inermis, C. dactylon, C. roseus*, and *S. asoca* for further discovery of new metabolites with active antibacterial properties.

6.1 INTRODUCTION

Ayurveda is a Sanskrit term, made up of the words "*ayus*" and "*veda*." "*Ayus*" means life and "*Veda*" means knowledge or science. It is the science of life and longevity, which is the oldest healthcare system in the world, sprouted in the pristine land of India 5000 years ago, and it combines the profound thoughts of medicine and philosophy. It is a complete naturalistic system that depends on the diagnosis of body's humors like vata, pitta, and kapha. *Charaka Samhita* was written around 900 BC and contains 341 plant-based medications, which is considered as the first treatise with respect to Indian Ayurveda. About 395 medicinal plants and 57 animal-derived products were described in *Sushruta Samhita*.[1] Ayurveda also has treatments for specific health problems. The ideas from Hinduism and ancient Persian beliefs had laid the foundation of ayurveda. The aim is to protect health and prolong life ("*Swasthyas swasthya rakshanam*") and to eliminate diseases and dysfunctions of the body ("*Aturasya vikar prashamanamcha*").[2] "Food be our Medicine" is an important concept in ayurveda, which can prevent and eradicates the diseases.

Plant-based medicines, which are the most eco-friendly system of health care, get its roots too deep in the Indian culture. Native plants have served as a key source of drugs for centuries. The Indian subcontinent is an enormous storehouse of medicinal plants that are used in traditional medical treatments.[3] For the development of new novel drugs, plants have provided potential insight as they were used conventionally for the well-being of human beings.[5] Natural products as a mean for both medicinal and health purposes were noticed throughout the course of evolution.

Based on the ancient belief, which says that plants are created to supply man with food and proper health, man relied on the curative properties of medicinal plant, prior to the introduction of chemical medicines.[6,7] Traditional medicine and therapies are the main root of developing new novel compounds with therapeutic values, though the accepted modern medicine has gradually evolved by the scientific and observational hard works of many scientists.[8]

Secondary metabolites (also referred to as natural products, phytochemicals, or specialized metabolites) are the products of metabolism, which are not essential for normal growth, development, or reproduction, which serve to meet the secondary requirements of the producing organisms. They also make the organisms potent to overcome interspecies competition, provide defensive mechanisms, and facilitate reproductive processes.[9] Plants which are immobile autotrophs, have to tackle a number of ruthless situations, which includes their own pollination and seed dispersal, fluctuations in the availability of the simple nutrients for the survival and the coexistence of herbivores, and pathogens in their micro environment.[10] To withstand the biotic and abiotic stresses, plants have adapted by diverse ways, which is reflected at the phytochemical level results in the production of numerous specialized secondary metabolites,[11] like saponins, tannins, alkaloids, alkenyl phenols, glycol-alkaloids, flavonoids, sesquiterpenes lactones, terpenoids, and phorbol esters provides the valuable medicinal properties to the plants, which help to withstand the biotic and abiotic stresses.[12,13] At the time of infection, the host response of plants activates various secondary metabolite pathways results in the production of compounds with antimicrobial properties.[14] Secondary metabolites play protective roles like antioxidant, free radical-scavenging, UV light-absorbing, and antiproliferative agents and defend the plant against microorganisms, and also be active as allelopathic defenders.[15,16,17] Feeding deterrence also results in the synthesis of phytochemicals, which are bitter and/or toxic to herbivores.[18]

The antibiotic resistance in bacteria is a serious universal threat in healthcare today and can occur in a significant minority of infected patients and predominantly for the one who have other basic health conditions, regular hospitalizations, or frequent exposures to antibiotics.[19] "Antimicrobial resistance: no action today, no cure tomorrow," which is the theme of World Health Day 2011 point out toward the severity of antibiotic resistance. The treatment of bacterial infections is increasingly complicated by the ability of bacteria to develop resistance to antimicrobial agents.[20] Multidrug resistance due to the expression by bacteria of an efflux pump is a rising clinical problem. Gram-negative bacteria have inherent multidrug resistance to several antimicrobial compounds due to the presence of efflux pumps.[21] Frequent and improper use of antibiotics in the treatment of human as well as animal production system has resulted in the selection of drug resistant mutants. Drug resistance among bacteria is of concern among health practitioners as the infection caused by them are difficult to treat. Since the discovery of new antibiotics is not keeping pace with the emergence of drug resistant mutants, alternative options are, being sought to reduce the selection pressure for drug resistant mutants in the environment. While prudent use of antibiotics is one important step, other step being the screening of plant based alternatives that have antibacterial activity. In this regard, the antibacterial activity of some medicinal plants commonly used in Ayurvedic medicinal practices was evaluated against some pathogenic bacteria.

6.2 MATERIALS AND METHODS

6.2.1 PLANT MATERIAL AND PREPARATION OF EXTRACTS

The aqueous extracts of 15 plants, which were used in Ayurvedic formulations, were selected for evaluating the antibacterial properties. Based on the therapeutic uses of different parts of the plant, in some cases more than one part of the same plant viz. roots, stem, leaves, flowers, fruits, etc were used. Details of the plant with figures (Fig.6.1–6.15) analyzed are represented in the Table 6.1.

TABLE 6.1 Details of Plants.[55]

1. *Catharanthus roseus* (L.) G. Don.

   Synonym: *Vinca rosea* L., *Lochnera rosea* (L.) Reichub.

   Family: *Apocynaceae.*

   English: Madagascar Periwinkle

   Folk: Sadaabahaar, Nayantaaraa, Nityakalyaani.

   Vernacular name (Malayalam): Kashithetti

   Officinal parts used: Leaf

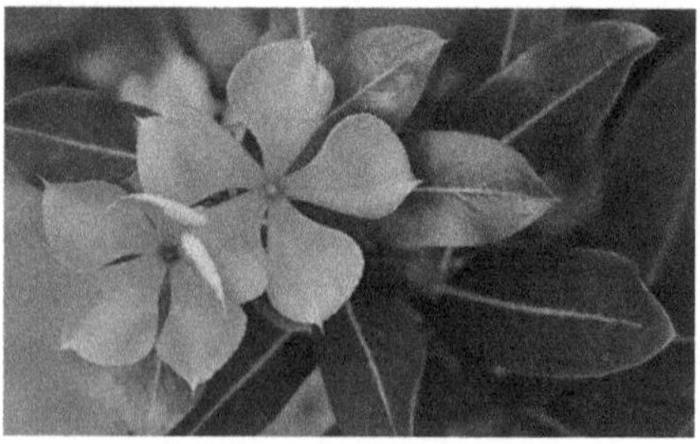

FIGURE 6.1 *Catharanthus roseus.*

TABLE 6.1 *(Continued)*

2. *Tabernaemontana divaricata* L.

   Synonym: *E. divaricata* (L.) Alston., *Tabernaemontana coronaria* R. Br.

   Family: *Apocynaceae.*

   English: East Indian Rosebay.

   Ayurvedic: Nandivrksha, Tagar.

   Siddha/Tamil: Nandiyaavattam.

   Vernacular name (Malayalam): Nandyarvattam

   Officinal parts used: Leaf and flower

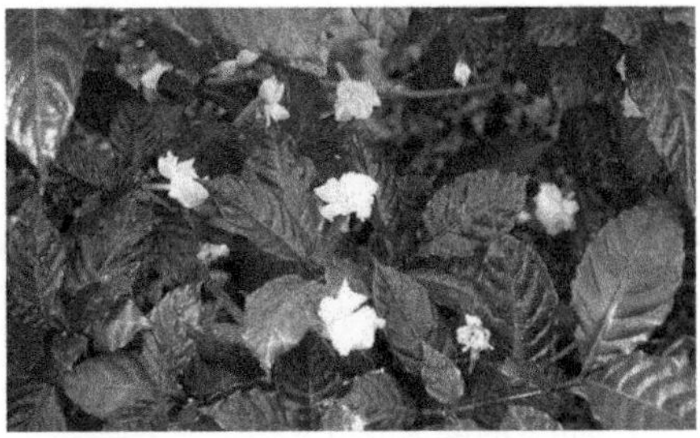

FIGURE 6.2 *Tabernaemontana divaricata.*

3. *Eclipta alba* (Linn.) Hassk.

   Synonym: *E. prostrata* Roxb.

   Family: *Compositae; Asteraceae.*

   English: Trailing Eclipta Plant.

   Ayurvedic: Bhringaraaja, Bhringa, Bhringaja, Bhrngaaraka, Bhrngaara, Maarkava, Kesharaaja

   Unani: Bhangraa.

   Siddha/Tamil: Karisalaankanni

   Vernacular name (Malayalam): Kaiyonni

   Officinal parts used: Leaf

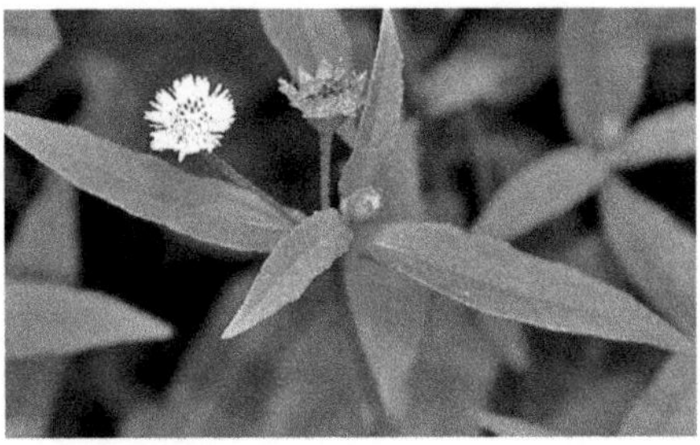

FIGURE 6.3 *Eclipta alba.*

4. *Sida rhombifolia* Linn.

   Family: *Malvaceae.*

   English: Common Bala.

   Ayurvedic: Mahaabalaa, Mahaasamangaa, Sahadevaa, Kshetrabalaa.

   Unani: Bariyaara

   Siddha/Tamil: Athi Bala-chedi, Chitrmutti, Tennacham.

   Vernacular name (Malayalam): Kurumthotti

   Officinal parts used: Leaf and root

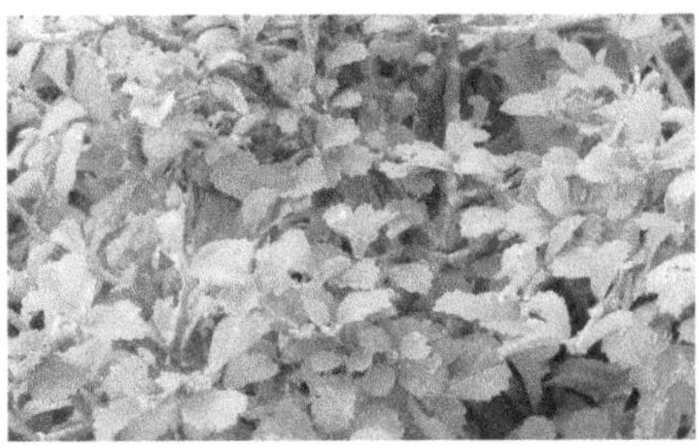

FIGURE 6.4 *Sida rhombifolia.*

TABLE 6.1 *(Continued)*

5. *Euphorbia hirta* Linn.

   Synonym: *E. pilulifera* auct. non Linn.

   Family: *Euphorbiaceae.*

   English: *Euphorbia*, Australian Asthma Weed, Pill-bearing Spurge.

   Ayurvedic: Dudhi, Dudhikaa, Naagaarjuni, Vikshirini.

   Unani: Dudhi Khurd.

   Siddha/Tamil: Amman pachharisi.

   Vernacular name (Malayalam): Chithirapala

   Officinal parts used: Leaf

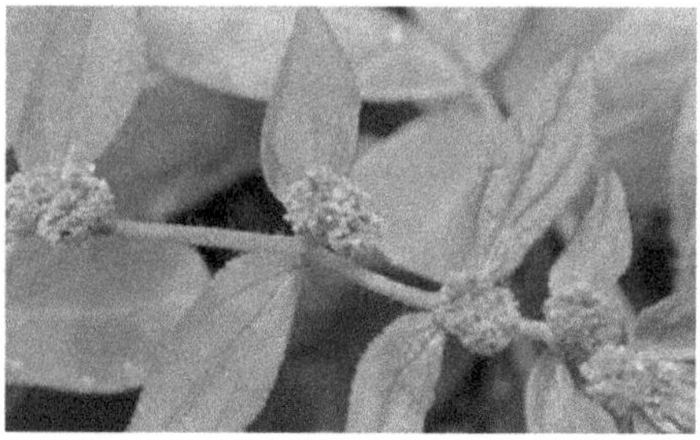

FIGURE 6.5 *Euphorbia hirta.*

6. *Ficus benghalensis* Linn.

   Family: *Moraceae.*

   English: Banyan tree.

   Ayurvedic: Vata, Nyagrodha, Bahupaada, Dhruv.

   Unani: Bargad, Darakht-e-Reesh.

   Siddha/Tamil: Aalamaram.

   Vernacular name (Malayalam): Peral

   Officinal parts used: Leaf and fruit

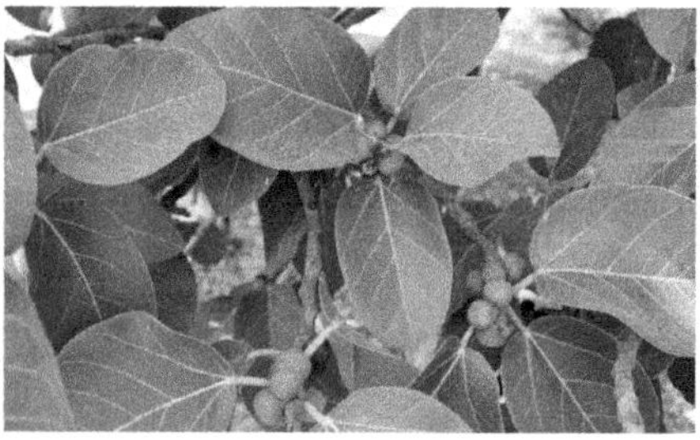

FIGURE 6.6 *Ficus benghalensis.*

7. *Biophytum sensitivum* (Linn.) DC.

   Synonym: *Oxalis sensitiva* Linn.

   Family: *Oxalidaceae.*

   Ayurvedic: Lajjaalu (var.) Vipareet Lajjaalu (non-classical), Alambushaa

   Folk: Lajoni, Jhalai, Lakajana.

   Vernacular name (malayalam): Mukkutti

   Officinal parts used: Leaf

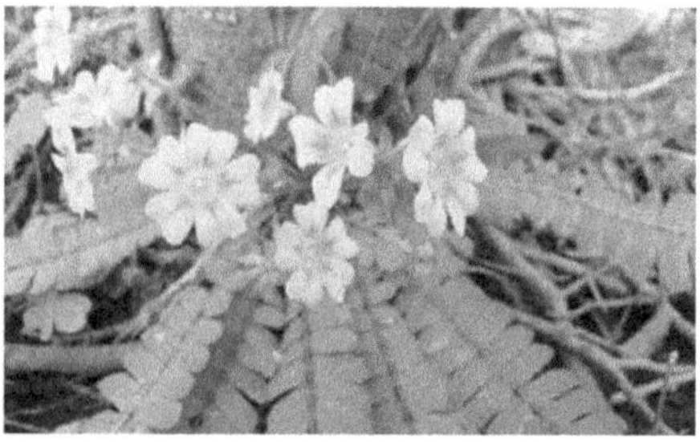

FIGURE 6.7 *Biophytum sensitivum.*

TABLE 6.1 *(Continued)*

8. *Saraca asoca* (Roxb.) DeWilde.

Synonym: *S. indica* auct. non L.

Family: *Caesalpiniaceae.*

English: Ashoka tree.

Ayurvedic: Ashoka, Ashoku, Hempushpa, Taamrapallava, Pindapushpa, Gandhapushpa.

Unani: Ashoka.

Siddha/Tamil: Asogam.

Vernacular name (Malayalam): Ashokam

Officinal parts used: Leaf and flower

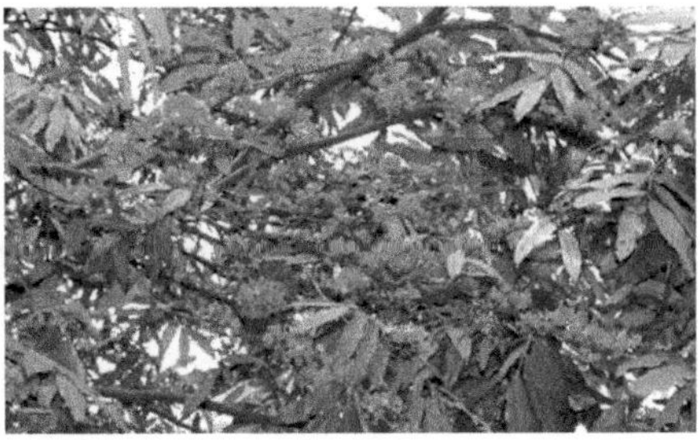

FIGURE 6.8 *Saraca asoca.*

9. *Plectranthus amboinicus* Lour.

Synonym: *C. aromaticus* Benth.

Family: *Lamiaceae.*

English: Indian Borage.

Ayurvedic: Parna-yavaani.

Siddha/Tamil: Karpoorvalli.

Folk: Pattaa Ajawaayin. Pattharachuur (Bengal)

Vernacular name (Malayalam): Panikkoorkka

Officinal parts used: Leaf

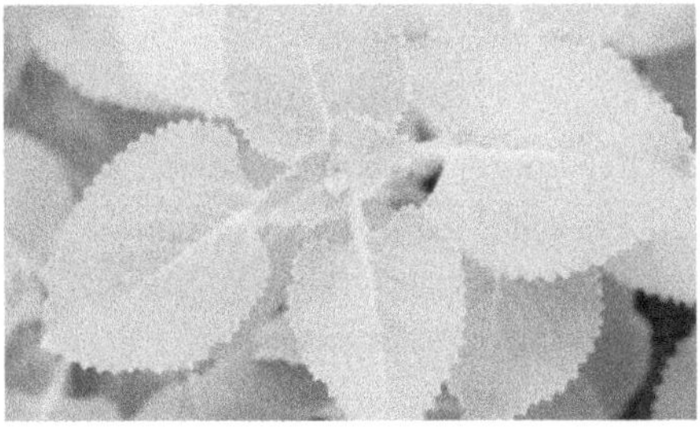

FIGURE 6.9 *Plectranthus amboinicus.*

10. *Andrographis paniculata* Wall. ex Nees

Family: *Acanthaceae.*

English: Creat.

Ayurvedic: Kaalmegha, Bhuunimba, Vishwambharaa, Yavtikta, Kalpanaatha, Kiraata-tikta (var.).

Unani: Kiryaat.

Siddha/Tamil: Nilavembu.

Vernacular name (Malayalam): Neelaveepu

Officinal parts used: Leaf and root

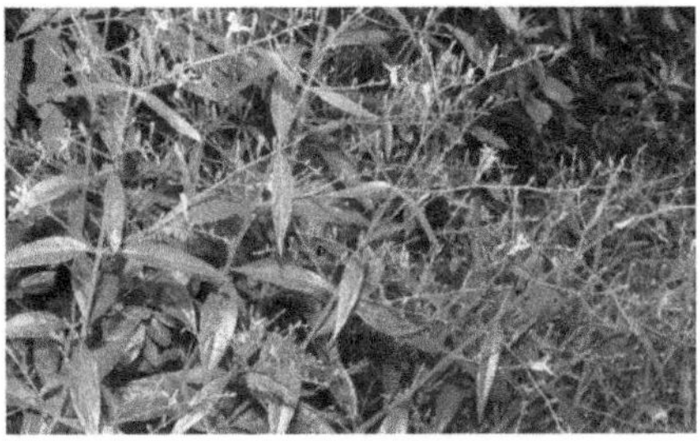

FIGURE 6.10 *Andrographis paniculata.*

TABLE 6.1 *(Continued)*

11. *Lawsonia inermis* Linn.

Family: *Lythraceae.*

English: Henna.

Ayurvedic: Madayanti, Madayantikaa, Mendika, Ranjaka.

Unani: Hinaa, Mehndi.

Siddha/Tamil: Marithondi, Marudum.

Vernacular name (Malayalam): Mailanchi

Officinal parts used: Leaf and flower

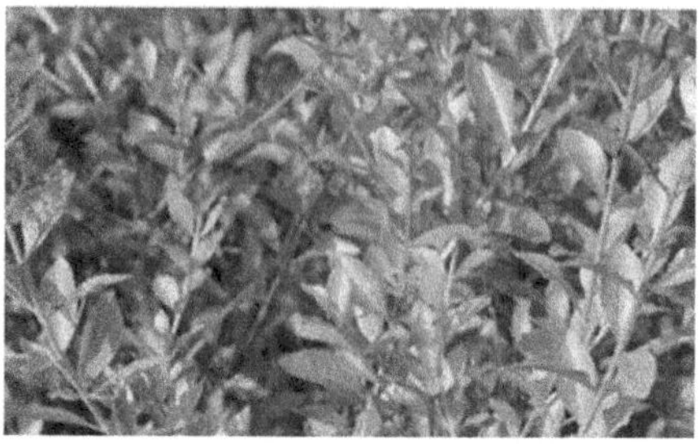

FIGURE 6.11 *Lawsonia inermis.*

12. *Boerhavia diffusa* Linn.

Synonym: *B. repens* Linn., *B. procumbens* Roxb.

Family: *Nyctaginaceae.*

English: Horse-purslane, Hogweed.

Ayurvedic: Punarnavaa, Katthilla, Shophaghni, Shothaghni. Varshaabhu

Unani: Itsit, Bishkhaparaa.

Siddha/Tamil: Mookkirattai.

Vernacular name (Malayalam): Punarnava

Officinal parts used: Leaf and stem

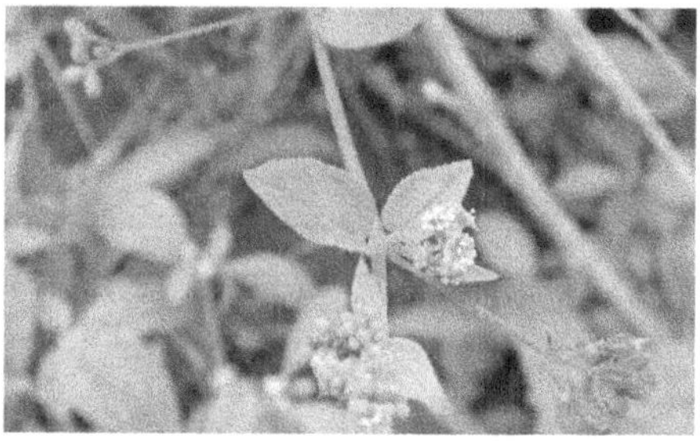

FIGURE 6.12 *Boerhavia diffusa.*

13. *Cynodon dactylon* Pers.

Family: *Gramineae; Poaceae.*

Ayurvedic: Duurvaa, Bhaargavi, Shatvalli, Shatparvaa, Tiktaparvaa, Shatviryaa, Sahastravirya, Shitaa.

Unani: Duub.

Siddha/Tamil: Arugampallu.

Vernacular name (Malayalam): Karuka

Officinal parts used: Leaf

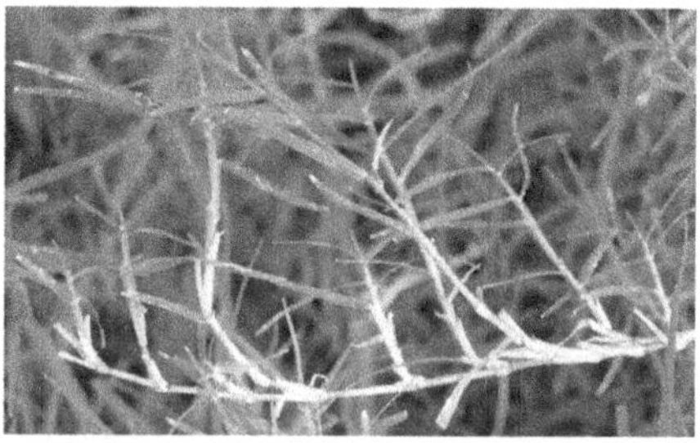

FIGURE 6.13 *Cynodon dactylon.*

TABLE 6.1 *(Continued)*

14. *Ixora coccinea* Linn.

    Family: *Rubiaceae.*

    English: Jungleflame Ixora.

    Ayurvedic: Bandhuka, Paaranti.

    Siddha/Tamil: Vetchi, Thechii.

    Folk: Rukmini, Rangan.

    Vernacular name (Malayalam): Nandyarvattam

    Officinal parts used: Leaf and flower

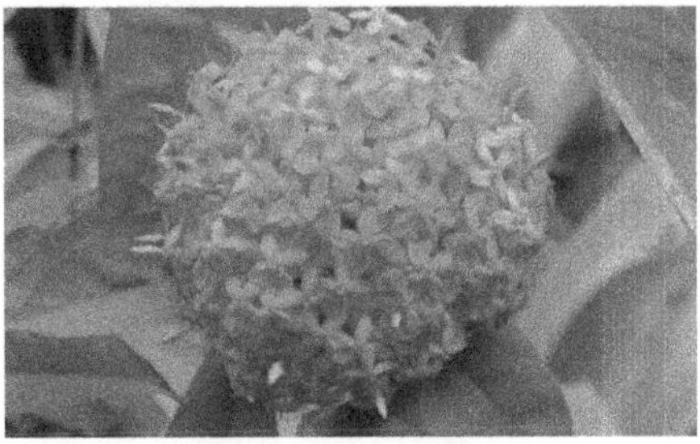

FIGURE 6.14 *Ixora coccinea.*

15. *Centella asiatica* (Linn.) Urban.

    Synonym: Hydrocotyle asiatica Linn.

    Family: Umbelliferae; Apiaceae.

    English: Asiatic Pennywort, Indian Pennywort.

    Ayurvedic: Manduukaparnikaa, Maanduuki, Saraswati, Brahma-manduuki, Manduukaparni,

    Siddha/Tamil: Vallaarai.

    Vernacular name (Malayalam): Nandyarvattam

    Officinal parts used: Leaf and flower

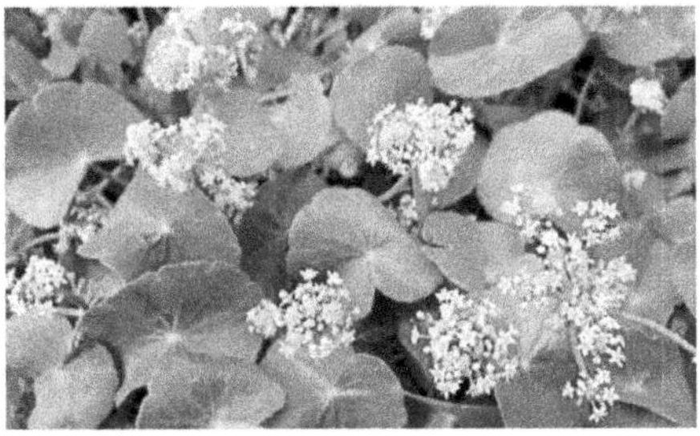

FIGURE 6.15 *Centella asiatica.*

The fresh plants were collected randomly from the local areas and were cleaned, and washed in sterile distilled water. In order to obtain the plant extracts, about 100 g of each washed plant parts were crushed with mortar and pestle (Fig. 6.16). The extracts were sieved through a fine mesh cloth were centrifuged at 1500 rpm for 20 min and sterilized using a membrane filter (0.45-micron sterile filter). Garlic extract was made in a different way due to the difficulty to filter the crushed material. One hundred grams of the descaled and cleaned garlic were taken, and surface sterilized using ethanol.[22] The ethanol was allowed to evaporate in a sterile laminar flow chamber and the garlic was homogenized aseptically using a sterile mortar, and pestle. The aqueous extract was aseptically squeezed out using sterile cheesecloth.

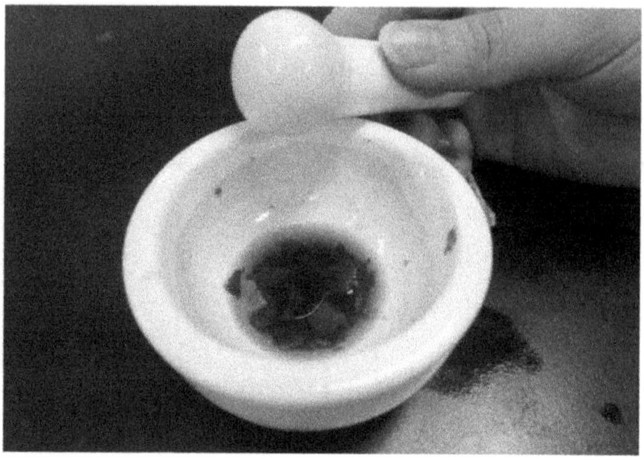

FIGURE 6.16 Preparation of plant extracts.

6.2.2 BACTERIAL STRAINS AND INOCULUMS PREPARATION

Both gram-positive and gram-negative bacterial strains were used in this study to find out the broad-spectrum activity of the medicinal plants. The gram-positive strains used in this study were *Staphylococcus aureus* (*S. aureus*) and *Bacillus subtilis* (*B. subtilis*). The gram-negative strains used includes eight serotypes of *Salmonella*, two serotypes of *Vibrio,* three serotypes of *Escherichia coli* (*E. coli)* and *Aeromonas hydrophila (A. hydrophila)*, and are mentioned in Table 6.2.

TABLE 6.2 List of Bacterial Strains.

No.	Bacterial strains
I	Gram-positive
1.	*Staphylococcus aureus*
2.	*Bacillus subtilis*
II	Gram negative
1.	*Salmonella paratyphi, Salmonella mgulani, Salmonella bareilly* *Salmonella enteritidis, Salmonella senftenberg, Salmonella bovis* *Salmonella typhimurium, Salmonella weltevreden* *Salmonella worthington*
2.	*Aeromonas hydrophila*
3.	*Vibrio cholera, Vibrio vulnificus*
4.	*Escherichia coli* O25, *Escherichia coli* O86, *Escherichia coli* O63

6.2.3 ANTIBACTERIAL ACTIVITY TESTING USING AGAR WELL METHOD (CUP-PLATE METHOD)

Using a sterile cotton swab, the nutrient broth cultures were swabbed on the surface of sterile Mueller–Hinton agar (MHA) plates. Agar wells were prepared with the help of sterilized cork borer (Fig. 6.17) with 10 mm diameter.[23] Using a micropipette, 100 μl of plant extracts were added to different wells in the plate. The plates were incubated in an upright position at 37 °C for 24 h. The diameter of inhibition zones was measured in millimeters (Figs. 6.18 and 6.19) and the results were recorded. Inhibition zones with diameter less than 12 mm were considered as having no antibacterial activity. Diameters between 12 and 16 mm were considered as moderately active, and greater than 16 mm were considered as highly active.[24]

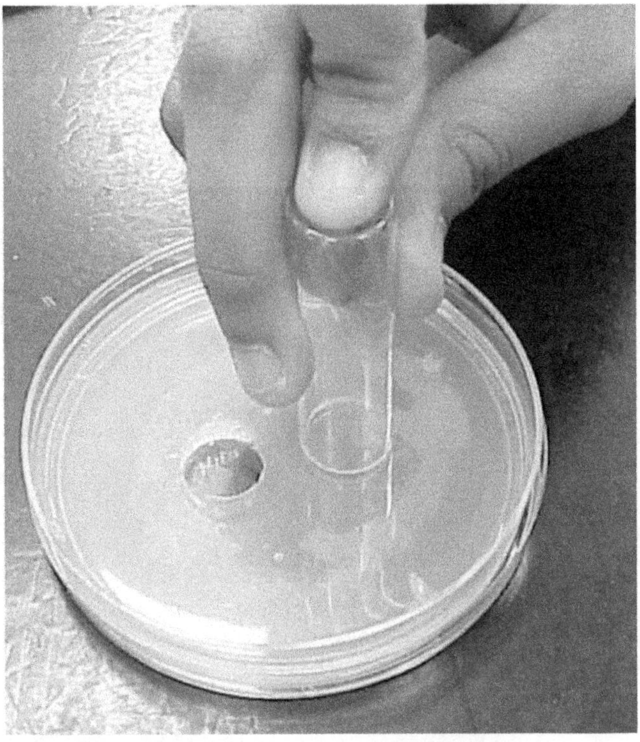

FIGURE 6.17 Preparation of well on Mueller–Hintonagar plates.

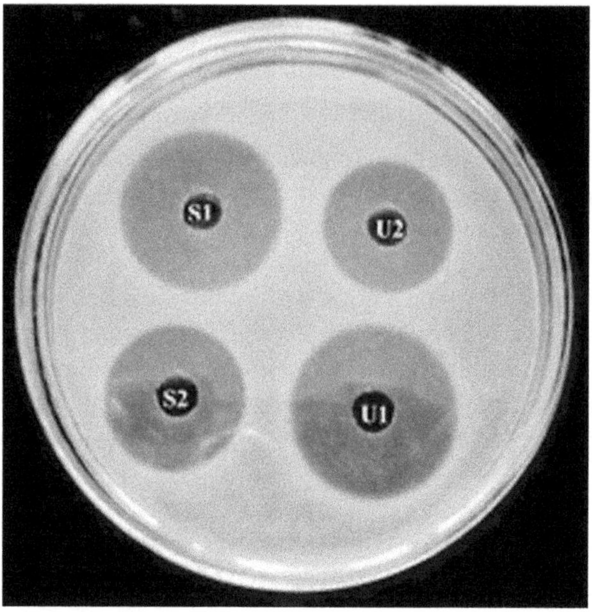

FIGURE 6.18 Antibacterial activity testing using agar well method (cup-plate method) diameter of zone of inhibition.

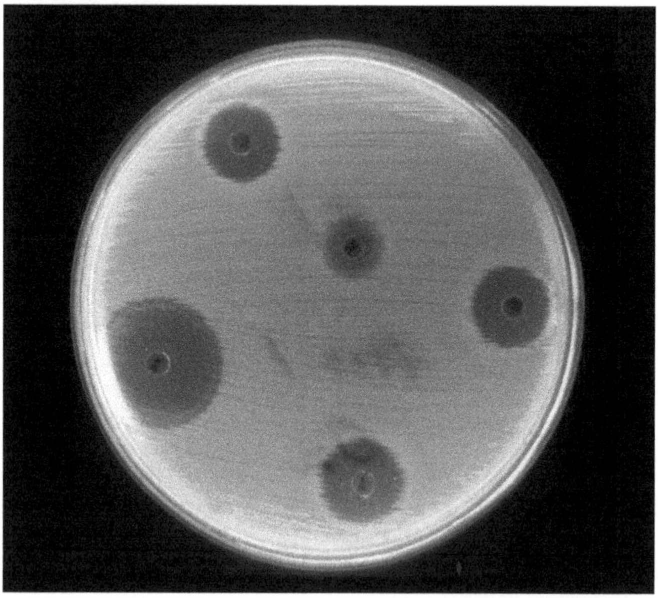

FIGURE 6.19 Antibacterial activity testing using agar well method (cup-plate method).

6.2.4 ANTIBIOTIC SENSITIVITY TESTING

The test microorganisms were also tested for their sensitivity against the antibiotics, such as penicillin, ampicillin, chloramphenicol, ciprofloxacin, kanamycin, erythromycin, lincomycin, gentamycin, vancomycin, amikacin, nitrofurantoin, novobiocin, nalidixic acid, streptomycin, and tetracycline by the disk diffusion method.[24] The cultures were enriched in sterile nutrient broth for 6–8 h at 37 °C. The cultures were aseptically swabbed on the surface of sterile MHA plates. The antibiotic discs were aseptically placed over the seeded MHA plates and were incubated at 37 °C for 24 h, and the diameter of the inhibition zones (Fig. 6.20) was measured in millimeters. Based on the interpretation chart, the inhibition zone size were categorized as susceptible (S), intermediate (I), or resistant (R).

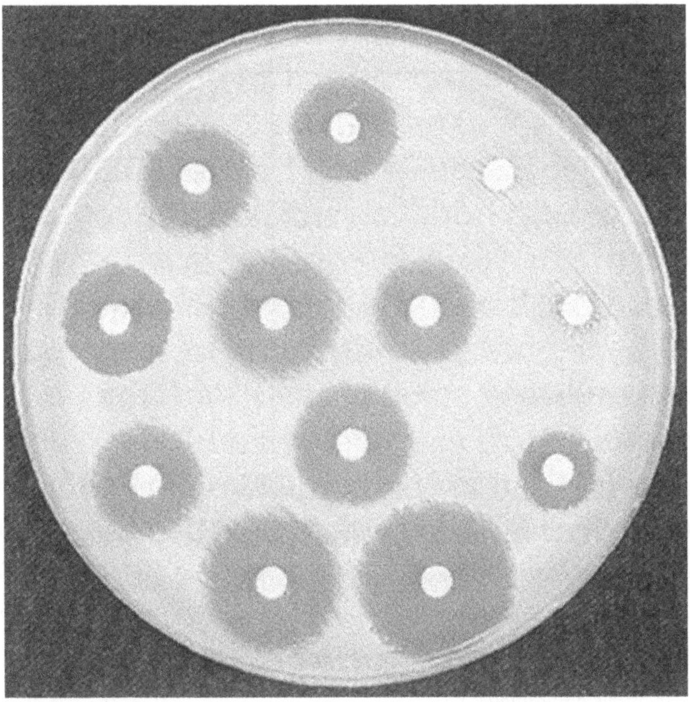

FIGURE 6.20 Antibiotic sensitivity testing using disc-diffusion method.

6.3 RESULT AND DISCUSSION

6.3.1 ANTIBACTERIAL ACTIVITY OF PLANT EXTRACTS

In this study crude extracts of 15 plants, which were traditionally used in Indian medicinal practices have been tested against both gram-negative and gram-positive strains. On the basis of the medicinal aspects of different parts of the plants, 24 extracts were prepared. Nine plants were found to have excellent antibacterial property and eight extracts shows moderate activity. The diameters of inhibition zones of plant extracts against different serotypes of *Salmonella, Vibrio, A. hydrophila, E. coli, B. subtilis*, and *S. aureus* by agar well method are represented in Tables 6.3 and 6.4.

TABLE 6.3 Diameters of Inhibition Zones of Plant Extracts against Different Serotypes of *Salmonella* by Agar Well Method.

No.	Plants	Zone of inhibition (mm)								
		SP	**SM**	**SBa**	**SE**	**SS**	**SB**	**ST**	**SWe**	**SW**
1.	*Catharanthus roseus* (L)	16	0	16	19	12	0	15	0	20
2.	*Lawsonia inermis* (L)	12	13	12	12	14	0	0	0	0
	(Fl)	12	14	15	12	0	20	20	12	26
3.	*Saraca asoca* (L)	0	0	17	16	14	14	14	18	12
	(Fl)	0	0	12	12	14	16	12	0	12
4.	*Ficus benghalensis* (Fr)	12	12	0	0	0	0	0	14	12
5.	*Eclipta alba* (L)	0	0	0	16	0	0	0	0	0
6.	*Cynadon dactylon* (L)	0	0	0	0	15	0	0	18	12
7.	*Euphorbia hirta* (L)	20	20	14	15	20	20	12	16	16
8.	*Biophytum sensitivum* (L)	0	0	0	18	12	0	0	0	12
9.	*Tabernemondana divaricata* (Fl)	0	0	0	0	0	0	14	20	0
10.	*Ixora coccinea* (Fl)	0	0	0	0	0	20	0	0	0
11.	*Plectranthus amboinicus* (L)	0	0	13	0	0	0	0	0	0

SP Salmonella paratyphi, SM Salmonella mgulani, SBa Salmonella bareilly, SE Salmonella enteritidis, SS Salmonella senftenberg, SB Salmonella bovis, ST Salmonella typhimurium, SWe Salmonella weltevreden, SW Salmonella worthington.

L Leaf, S Stem, Fl Flower, Fr Fruit.

TABLE 6.4 Diameters of Inhibition Zones of Plant Extracts against *A. Hydrophila*, Two Serotypes of *Vibrio*, Three Serotypes of *E. coli*, *B. subtilis*, and *S. aureus*.

No.	Plants	Zone of inhibition (mm)							
		AH	VC	VV	EC O25	EC O86	EC O63	BS G^{+ve}	SA G^{+ve}
1.	*Catharanthus roseus* (L)	0	0	0	0	0	0	0	13
2.	*Boerhavia diffusa* (L)	0	0	0	0	0	0	21	15
3.	*Lawsonia inermis* (Fl)	0	0	12	0	0	0	0	20
4.	*Saraca asoca* (L)	0	0	0	0	0	0	0	13
	(Fl)	0	0	0	12	0	0	0	13
5.	*Cynadon dactylon* (L)	16	0	0	0	0	0	28	19
6.	*Sida rhombifolia* (L)	12	0	0	0	0	0	0	0
7.	*Tabernemondana divaricata* (Fl)	0	0	0	0	0	0	0	13
	(L)	0	0	0	0	0	0	0	12
8.	*Ixora coccinea* (Fl)	0	0	0	0	0	0	0	12
9.	*Centella asiatica* (L)	0	0	0	0	0	0	0	12
10.	*Plectranthus amboinicus* (L)	0	0	0	0	0	0	0	0

AH *Aeromonas hydrophila*, VC *Vibrio cholerae*, VV *Vibrio vulnificus*, EC *Escherichia coli*, SA *Staphylococcus aureus*, BS *Bacillus subtilis*, G^{+ve} Gram-positive.

L Leaf, S Stem, Fl Flower, Fr Fruit.

6.3.1.1 INHIBITORY EFFECT OF INHIBITORY EFFECT OF SIDA RHOMBIFOLIA (S. RHOMBIFOLIA, FAMILY: MALVACEAE)

Root and leaf extract of *S. rhombifolia* was tested for their potency in controlling the growth of both gram-positive and gram-negative strains. The root extract do not owes any antibacterial property while the leaf extract of *S. rhombifolia* shows moderate activity (inhibition zone of 12 mm) in checking the growth of *A. hydrophila.* But the plants do not control the gram-positive strains used in this study. The results are not consistent with preceding reports unfolding the antibacterial activities of root extract of *S. rhombifolia*[25] and the activity of the methanol extract against *E. coli* and *Salmonella typhimurium* (*S. typhimurium*).[26]

6.3.1.2 INHIBITORY EFFECT OF ECLIPTA PROSTRATA (E. PROSTRATA, FAMILY: ASTERACEAE)

Officinal part such as leaf and stem of *E. prostrata*was examined for their antibacterial activities. The stem extracts of the plant do not show any bactericidal properties. *E. prostrata* leaf extracts suppress the growth of *Salmonella enteritidis* (*S. enteritidis*) with an inhibition zone of 16 mm. But based on the observations by Pandey *et al.*[4], hexane extract of *Eclipta alba* possess high antibacterial activity against *S. aureus, E. coli* whereas acetone, ethanol, methanol, and aqueous extracts showed intermediate activity against *S. aureus* and *E. coli*.

6.3.1.3 INHIBITORY EFFECT OF TABERNAEMONTANA DIVARICATA (T. DIVARICATA) AND CATHARANTHUS ROSEUS (C. ROSEUS, FAMILY: APOCYNACEAE)

The leaf extracts of *C. roseus* reveals its potential in controlling the growth of both gram-positive and negative strains. Among the gram-negative strains this plant target the serotypes of *Salmonella* with a maximum zone of inhibition as 20 mm. Show *et al.*[27] also reported some potentially active antibacterial agents from leaf extract of *C. roseus* against *S. aureus*. Similarly, Govindasamy *et al.*[28] reports the bactericidal property of the leaf extract against *S. aureus*.

The leaf and flower extract of *T. divaricata* also possess bactericidal properties, but the leaf extract is found to be effective only in controlling the growth of *S. aureus*. Bijeshmon *et al.*[29] reported the bactericidal activity of the flower extract by inhibiting the growth of *S. aureus* and *E. coli*. But this study reveals that the growth of *E. coli* is not controlled but the growth of *S. aureus* can be checked. Three novel compounds ethyl-4-n-octyl benzoate 1 and ethyl-4- n-decyl benzoate 2 from the flowers of *T. divaricata* and digalactosyl deconate three from the latex of *T. divaricata* have been isolated by Venkatachalapathi *et al.*[30] with antibacterial activity.

6.3.1.4 INHIBITORY EFFECT OF EUPHORBIA HIRTA (E. HIRTA, FAMILY: EUPHORBIACEAE)

In checking the growth of serotypes of *Salmonella*, the leaf extract of *E. hirta* is found to be very effective with a maximum inhibition zone of 20 mm and were ineffective in controlling the growth of other gram- negative and positive strains. The antimicrobial activities of the methanolic extracts of *E. hirta* L leaves were evaluated by Rajeh *et al.*,[31] revealed the potential in controlling the growth of both gram-positive and negative strains. However, in this study, the gram-positive strains were found to be resistant. Moderate antimicrobial activity of leaves extracts in controlling the growth of *S. typhi* was reported by Perumal *et al.*[32] which supports with the current investigation. However, this study revealed the impotency of the extract in controlling the growth of *S. aureus*. Hussain *et al.*[33] had reported the efficiency of extract in controlling the growth of *S. aureus*.

6.3.1.5 INHIBITORY EFFECT OF FICUS BENGHALENSIS (F. BENGHALENSIS, FAMILY: MORACEAE)

The leaf extract of *F. benghalensis* do not possess any antiseptic properties against the tested bacterial strains though the fruit extract of *F. benghalensis* shows moderate activity in controlling *Salmonella* strains only. The antibacterial activity of the plant was recorded by Murti *et al.*[34] in controlling the survival of *S. aureus*. Koona *et al.*[35] reported that *B. subtilis* and *E. coli* were effectively controlled by the methanolic extract of leafs, but the present evaluation do not support their findings.

6.3.1.6 INHIBITORY EFFECT OF BIOPHYTUM SENSITIVUM (B. SENSITIVUM, FAMILY: OXALIDACEAE)

Gram-positive strains were found as resistant to the leaf extracts of *B. sensitivum*, but have checked the growth of *Salmonella* serotypes. The leaf extract of *B. sensitivum* shows its potency in controlling the growth of with an inhibition zone of 18 mm. Natarajan *et al.*[36] revealed the potency of leaf extract in controlling the proliferation of *B. subtilis*, *S. aureus*, *E. coli,* and *S. typhimurium*. Their findings disagree with this study, but in controlling the growth of other serotypes of *Salmonella* the leaf extract were found to be efficient. The finding of Gangadharan *et al.*[37] reveals the resistance of *B. subtilis*, *S. aureus*, *E. coli*, and *S. typhimurium,* which supports this study. Namboodiri *et al.*[38] also reports the bactericidal property of leaf extract against *S. aureus* and *E. coli.*

6.3.1.7 INHIBITORY EFFECT OF SARACA ASOCA (S. ASOCA, FAMILY: FABACEAE)

The proliferation of *Salmonella* strains, *E. coli* and gram-positive *S. aureus* can be efficiently tackled by the use of *S. asoca* flower extracts but the leaf extract controls *Salmonella* serotypes and *S. aureus*.

6.3.1.8 INHIBITORY EFFECT OF LAWSONIA INERMIS (L. INERMIS, FAMILY: LYTHRACEAE)

The flower extract of *L. inermis* was found to be promising in controlling the growth of both gram-positive and negative test organisms with a maximum inhibition zone of 26 mm, inhibiting *Salmonella worthington* (*S. worthington*), and 20 mm for *S. aureus.* Moderate bactericidal activities were observed for the leaf extract, which checks only the growth of gram-negative *Salmonella* strains. Habbal *et al.*[39] and Rahmoun *et al.*[40] evaluate the antibacterial potential of the leaf extract and reported that the extract can control both gram-positive and negative strains. While the present work, disagree with the finding, which records the efficiency of extract in controlling the growth of gram-positive strains. But according to Sukanya *et al.*[41] *S. aureus* and *E. coli* have resistance toward the activity of leaf extract, which agrees with the current investigation.

6.3.1.9 INHIBITORY EFFECT OF PLECTRANTHUS AMBOINICUS (P. AMBOINICUS, FAMILY: LAMIACEAE)

The leaf extract of *P. amboinicus* controls only the growth of gram-negative *S. bareily* with an inhibition zone of 13 mm. However, Oliveira *et al.*[42] reported the potential of this plant in controlling the growth of Methicillin Resistant *S. aureus.*

6.3.1.10 INHIBITORY EFFECT OF ANDROGRAPHIS PANICULATA (A. PANICULATA, FAMILY: ACANTHACEAE)

The leaf extracts of *A. paniculata* were found to be inefficient in controlling the growth of both gram- positive and negative test organisms. The finding of Leelarasamee *et al.*[43] agrees with the present investigation. But Mishra *et al.*[44] reports bactericidal property of methanolic extract of *A. paniculata* in controlling the growth of *S. aureus*.

6.3.1.11 INHIBITORY EFFECT OF BOERHAVIA DIFFUSA (B. DIFFUSA, FAMILY:NYCTAGINACEAE)

The root and leaf extract of *B. diffusa* were analyzed for their efficiency in controlling the growth of gram-positive and negative strains. The results revealed that the root extract do not have the potential to control the growth of the test organisms. But the leaf extract can inhibit the growth of gram-positive stains used in this study. An inhibition zone of diameter 21 mm and 15 mm were observed for *B. subtilis* and *S. aureus*, respectively. The gram-negative strains were resistant to the action of leaf extract. Akinnibosun *et al.*[45] reported that the aqueous and ethanolic extracts of *B. diffusa* had antibacterial activity on *E. coli*, *S. aureus*, and *P. aeruginosa*. But in the present investigation, *E. coli* were not controlled by the extract.

6.3.1.12 INHIBITORY EFFECT OF CYNODON DACTYLON (C. DACTYLON, FAMILY: POACEAE)

E. coli and serotypes of *Vibrio* were resistant to the bactericidal activity of the leaf extract of *C. dactylon. A. hydrophila, Salmonella* serotypes and gram-positive strains were effectively controlled by the leaf extract with a zone of inhibition 28 mm for *B. subtilis* and 19 mm for *S. aureus*. Kumar *et al.*[46], and Jazani *et al.*[47] also observed the antibacterial activity of *C. dactylon* extract in controlling the growth of gram-positive strains.

6.3.1.13 INHIBITORY EFFECT OF IXORA COCCINEA (I. COCCINEA, FAMILY: RUBIACEAE)

The flower extract of *I. coccinea* inhibits the growth of one-gram- positive and negative strains. The diameter of zone of inhibition for *Salmonella bovis* (*S. bovis*) and gram-positive *S. aureus* was 20 mm and 12 mm, respectively. The rest of the test organisms were resistant toward the action of flower extract. According to Sukanya *et al.*[41] *I. coccinea* extract were found to be ineffective or showed poor inhibition on bacteria like *E. coli* and *S. aureus*.

6.3.1.14 INHIBITORY EFFECT OF CENTELLA ASIATICA (C. ASIATICA, FAMILY: UMBELLIFERAE)

The leaf, stem and root extract of *C. asiatica* were evaluated for their bactericidal activities. Gram-positive *S. aureus* was the only strain susceptible to the bactericidal activity of leaf extract of *C. asiatica* with 12 mm zone of inhibition. Other officinal parts evaluated were found to have no antiseptic properties with regard to the test organisms. Dash *et al.* and Arumugam *et al.*[48,49] evaluated the bactericidal potential of Petroleum Ether, Ethanol, Chloroform, n-Hexane and Aqueous extracts of *C. asiatica*, and reveals that those extracts were effective in controlling the growth of *S. aureus*, *B. subtilis*, and *E. coli*.

Based on the diameter of inhibition zones obtained from the agar well method, the plant extracts were classified as no activity, moderate, and highly active. Inhibition zones with diameter less than 12 mm were considered as having no antibacterial activity. Diameters between 12 and 16 mm were considered as moderately active, and greater than 16 mm were considered as highly active out of the 24 aqueous extracts prepared from the officinal parts of 15 plants, seven extracts do not possess any bactericidal activity against the test organisms. Nine plants were found to have excellent antibacterial property and eight extracts shows moderate activity (Table 6.5).

The plant extracts which control the growth of both positive and negative strains were categorized to be having broad-spectrum activity and those, which control any one of the strains were categorized as narrow spectrum. Based on the range of the activity, the plant extracts were classified as broad and narrow spectrum. Of the 18 plants extract with bactericidal activity, eight possess broad spectrum and 10 with narrow spectrum activity, and are represented in Table 6.6. In controlling the growth of gram-positive test organisms, nine plants extracts were found to be effective and 14 plants extract controls the growth of gram-negative strains (Table 6.7). The results also revealed that gram-negative strains were more vulnerable to the bactericidal activity of plant extracts than gram-positive ones. Janakiraman *et al.*[50] and Pitchamuthu *et al.*[51] also reported that gram-positive bacteria were more prone to the action of antibacterial compounds. However, gram-negative bacteria were found to be more resistant to the action of bactericidal compounds[52] than gram-positive strains. This is attributed to the presence of hydrophilic outer membrane rich in lipopolysacchride molecules and enzymes coupled with periplasmic space, which is capable of breaking down the foreign molecules.[53] In case of gram-positive bacteria such outer membranes and cell wall structures were lacking.[54] Generally, it was observed from this study that serotypes of *Salmonella* were extremely susceptible to the action of plant extracts. Serotypes of *E. coli* were resistant to the bactericidal properties of the extracts of plant officinal parts. The resistance is in the order *E. coli* > *Vibrio* > *B. subtilis* > *A. hydrophila* > *S. aureus* > *Salmonella.*

TABLE 6.5 Classification Based on Antibacterial Activity, Based on Inhibition Zone Diameter in Millimeters.

No.	Plants with officinal parts		
	No activity < 12 mm	**Moderate between 12 and 16 mm**	**High > 16 mm**
1.	*Boerhavia diffusa* (R)	*Lawsonia inermis* (L)	*Catharanthus roseus* (L)
2.	*Andrographis paniculata* (L)	*Saraca asoca* (L)	*Boerhavia diffusa* (L)
3.	*Ficus benghalensis* (L)	*Ficus benghalensis* (Fr)	*Lawsonia inermis* (Fl)
4.	*Eclipta prostrata* (S)	*Eclipta prostrata* (L)	*Saraca asoca* (L)
5.	*Sida rhombifolia* (R)	*Sida rhombifolia* (L)	*Cynadon dactylon* (L)
6.	*Centella asiatica* (S)	*Tabernemondana divaricata* (L)	*Euphorbia hirta* (L)
7.	*Centella asiatica* (R)	*Centella asiatica* (L)	*Biophytum sensitivum* (L)
8.		*Plectranthus amboinicus* (L)	*Tabernemondana divaricata* (Fl)
9.			*Ixora coccinea* (Fl)

L Leaf, S Stem, Fl Flower, Fr Fruit, R Root, Rh Rhizome, B Bulb.

TABLE 6.6 Classification Based on the Specificity of Action, Based on Inhibition Zone Diameter in Millimeters.

No.	Activity	
	Broad spectrum	**Narrow spectrum**
1.	*Catharanthus roseus* (L)	*Boerhavia diffusa* (L)
2.	*Lawsonia inermis* (Fl)	*Lawsonia inermis* (L)
3.	*Saraca asoca* (L)	*Ficus benghalensis* (Fr)
4.	*Saraca asoca* (Fl)	*Eclipta prostrata* (L)
5.	*Cynadon dactylon* (L)	*Euphorbia hirta* (L)
6.	*Tabernemondana divaricata* (Fl)	*Biophytum sensitivum* (L)
7.	*Tabernemondana divaricata* (L)	*Sida rhombifolia* (L)
8.	*Ixora coccinea* (Fl)	*Centella asiatica* (L)
9.		*Plectranthus amboinicus* (L)
10.		*Tabernemondana divaricata* (L)

L Leaf, S Stem, Fl Flower, Fr Fruit, R Root, Rh Rhizome, B Bulb.

TABLE 6.7 Classification Based on Controlling Gram-Negative and Gram-Positive Strains, Based on Inhibition Zone Diameter in Millimeters.

Sl. No.	Gram-negative	Gram-positive
1.	*Catharanthus roseus* (L)	*Catharanthus roseus* (L)
2.	*Lawsonia inermis* (Fl)	*Lawsonia inermis* (Fl)
3.	*Saraca asoca* (L)	*Saraca asoca* (L)
4.	*Saraca asoca* (Fl)	*Saraca asoca* (Fl)
5.	*Cynadon dactylon* (L)	*Cynadon dactylon* (L)
6.	*Tabernemondana divaricata* (Fl)	*Tabernemondana divaricata* (Fl)
7.	*Lawsonia inermis* (L)	*Tabernemondana divaricata* (L)
8.	*Ixora coccinea* (Fl)	*Ixora coccinea* (Fl)
9.	*Ficus benghalensis* (Fr)	*Boerhavia diffusa* (L)
10.	*Eclipta prostrata* (L)	
11.	*Euphorbia hirta* (L)	
12.	*Biophytum sensitivum* (L)	
13.	*Sida rhombifolia* (L)	
14.	*Plectranthus amboinicus* (L)	

L Leaf, S Stem, Fl Flower, Fr Fruit, R Root, Rh Rhizome, B Bulb.

6.3.2 ANTIBIOTIC SENSITIVITY TESTING

The diameter of the inhibition zone obtained against various plant extract by agar well method was compared to those obtained against commonly prescribed antibiotics (Tables 6.8 and 6.9).

TABLE 6.8 Diameters of Inhibition Zones of Antibiotics against Different Serotypes of *Salmonella.*

No.	Antibiotics	Zone of inhibition (mm)								
		SP	SM	SBa	SE	SS	SB	ST	SWe	SW
1.	Penicillin (P)	12	12	12	14	14	17	0	12	0
2.	Ampicillin (A)	0	12	0	12	13	14	0	0	0
3.	Nalidixic acid (Na)	0	20	24	26	24	0	24	24	0
4.	Chloramphenicol (C)	21	25	28	28	26	20	31	28	20
5.	Ciprofloxacin (Cf)	23	26	27	29	28	20	28	27	21
6.	Kanamycin (K)	17	14	15	15	15	0	0	15	14
7.	Erythromycin (E)	0	0	0	0	0	14	0	0	0
8.	Lincomycin (L)	0	0	0	0	0	0	0	0	0
9.	Gentamycin (G)	15	15	16	15	16	0	10	16	16
10.	Vancomycin (Va)	0	0	0	0	0	14	0	0	0
11.	Amikacin (Ak)	16	15	19	17	18	0	16	19	16
12.	Tetracycline (T)	14	14	16	18	18	24	23	16	13
13.	Streptomycin (S)	14	14	16	15	15	0	16	16	13
14.	Nitrofurantoin (Nf)	0	15	12	15	15	17	12	12	16
15.	Novobiocin (Nv)	0	14	0	0	0	12	0	0	0

SP Salmonella paratyphi, SM Salmonella mgulani, SBa Salmonella bareilly, SE Salmonella enteritidis, SS Salmonella senftenberg, SB Salmonella bovis, ST Salmonella typhimurium, SWe Salmonella weltevreden, SW Salmonella worthington.

TABLE 6.9 Diameters of Inhibition Zones of Antibiotics against *A. Hydrophila*, Two Serotypes of *Vibrio*, Three Serotypes of *E. coli*, *B. subtilis*, and *S. aureus*.

No.	Antibiotics	Zone of inhibition (mm)							
		AH	VC	VV	EC O25	EC O86	EC O63	BS G^{+ve}	SA G^{+ve}
1.	Penicillin (P)	0	0	0	0	0	0	0	33
2.	Ampicillin (A)	0	0	0	0	0	0	0	27
3.	Nalidixic acid (Na)	20	18	0	22	21	0	0	0
4.	Chloramphenicol (C)	26	18	0	25	28	28	0	29
5.	Ciprofloxacin (Cf)	25	30	25	25	27	0	23	31
6.	Kanamycin (K)	12	18	17	12	12	0	15	16
7.	Erythromycin (E)	0	0	15	0	0	15	0	20
8.	Lincomycin (L)	0	0	0	0	0	18	0	22
9.	Gentamycin (G)	11	20	17	13	13	20	12	16
10.	Vancomycin (Va)	0	0	0	0	0	0	0	0
11.	Amikacin (Ak)	12	17	21	14	12	13	18	22
12.	Tetracycline (T)	19	19	12	16	16	0	0	25
13.	Streptomycin (S)	15	0	0	13	15	13	12	12
14.	Nitrofurantoin (Nf)	12	0	0	13	0	13	0	16
15.	Novobiocin (Nv)	0	13	18	0	0	0	0	16

AH *Aeromonas hydrophila*, VC *Vibrio cholerae*, VV *Vibrio vulnificus*, EC *Escherichia coli*, SA *Staphylococcus aureus*, BS *Bacillus subtilis*, G^{+ve} Gram-positive.

6.3.2.1 ANTIBIOTICS V/S PLANT EXTRACTS AGAINST SALMONELLA PARATYPHI (S. PARATYPHI)

Five extracts were found to be effective in controlling the growth of *S. paratyphi*. Of which the leaf extract of *E. hirta* presented higher diameter of inhibition zones, which can compete with the reference antibiotics expect Chloramphenicol and ciprofloxacin. The leaf extract of *C. roseus* with 16 mm inhibition zone can also be used as an alternative to Amikacin, which gives diameter of inhibition 16 mm. Extracts from the leaf and flower of *L. inermis*, *F. benghalensis* gives the same range of antibacterial property with respect to Penicillin. Seven of the antibiotics do not show any bactericidal property.

6.3.2.2 ANTIBIOTICS V/S PLANT EXTRACTS AGAINST SALMONELLA MGULANI (S. MGULANI)

In controlling the growth of *S. mgulani*, four plant extracts were found to be potent. The leaf extract of *E. hirta* and Nalidixic acid shows a maximum inhibition zone of 20 mm. Twelve of the antibiotics could not check the growth. Antibiotics like tetracycline, kanamycin, streptomycin, and novobiocin having the same inhibition zone of diameter (14 mm), which was comparable to the activity of flower extract of *L. inermis*. The fruit extract of *F. benghalensis* with 12 mm inhibition zone can also used as substitutes to Pencillin and ampicillin.

6.3.2.3 ANTIBIOTICS V/S PLANT EXTRACTS AGAINST SALMONELLA BAREILLY (S. BAREILLY)

The growth of *S. bareily* was controlled by six extracts. gentamycin, tetracycline, and streptomycin can be replaced with the leaf extract of *C. roseus* as both antibiotics and plant extract gives 16 mm zone of diameter. The leaves and flower extract of *L. inermis* with inhibition zone of 12 mm and 15 mm and flower extract of *S. asoca* (12 mm) were comparable with penicillin, nitrofurantoin and kanamycin. The inhibition zone of leaf extract of *E. hirta* and *P. amboinicus* were also comparable with the activity of antibiotics. Five of the antibiotics do not owe the potency to control the bacteria.

6.3.2.4 ANTIBIOTICS V/S PLANT EXTRACTS AGAINST S. ENTERITIDIS

S. enteritidis growth was effectively controlled by eight extracts, which is comparable to the reference antibiotics like ampicillin and tetracycline. The bacteria have resistance toward erythromycin, lincomycin, vancomycin, and novobiocin.

6.3.2.5 ANTIBIOTICS V/S PLANT EXTRACTS AGAINST *SALMONELLA SENFTENBERG* (*S. SENFTENBERG*)

The bactericidal activity of streptomycin, nitrofurantoin, and kanamycin is similar to the activity of *C. dactylon* and Penicillin to the flower and leaf extract of *S. asoca*, and *L. inermis*, against *S. senftenberg*.

6.3.2.6 ANTIBIOTICS V/S PLANT EXTRACTS AGAINST *S. BOVIS*

Flower extract of *L. inermis*, *I. coccinea*, and leaf extract of *E. hirta* shows the equal range of antibacterial property with respect to chloramphenicol and ciprofloxacin in suppressing the growth of *S. bovis*. The leaf extract of *S. asoca* and antibiotics like ampicillin, erythromycin, and vancomycin possess the same range of activity in inhibiting the growth of *S. bovis*.

6.3.2.7 ANTIBIOTICS V/S PLANT EXTRACTS AGAINST *SALMONELLA WELTEVREDEN* (*S. WELTEVREDEN*)

The survival of *S. weltevreden* has been efficiently controlled by six extracts, of which flower extracts of *L. inermis* and leaf extract of *E. hirta* can compete with the activity of Penicillin, nitrofurantoin and gentamycin, tetracycline, streptomycin, respectively. In controlling the growth of *S. typhimurium*, six extracts were found to be effective, in comparison with some of the reference antibiotics. But eight of the antibiotics do not possess the ability to control *S. typhimurium*.

6.3.2.8 ANTIBIOTICS V/S PLANT EXTRACTS AGAINST *S. WORTHINGTON*

The flower extract of *L. inermis* shows excellent zone of inhibition with 26 mm diameter in controlling the growth of *S. worthington*. No antibiotics used in the study exceed the value set by *L. inermis*. Ciprofloxacin is the only antibiotic, which suppresses the growth when compared to the leaf extract of *C. roseus*. The leaf extract of *E. hirta* can also used instead of gentamycin, amikacin, and nitrofurantoin, which show equal zone of diameter.

6.3.2.9 ANTIBIOTICS V/S PLANT EXTRACTS AGAINST A. HYDROPHILA

The growth of *A. hydrophila* was suppressed by the leaf extract of *C. dactylon* and *S. rhombifolia* with zone of inhibition 16 mm and 12 mm, respectively. The leaf extract of *S. rhombifolia* can be used an alternative to kanamycin and nitrofurantoin, as the diameter of inhibition zones were alike (12 mm). Six of the antibiotics do not owe any bactericidal property.

6.3.2.10 ANTIBIOTICS V/S PLANT EXTRACTS AGAINST SEROTYPES OF VIBRIO

Vibrio vulnificus (*V. vulnificus*) was controlled by the flower extract of *L. inermis* and comparable with the results of Tetracycline.

6.3.2.11 ANTIBIOTICS V/S PLANT EXTRACTS AGAINST SEROTYPES OF E. COLI

E. coli O25 was the only serotype of *E. coli* used in the study, which was controlled by the flower extract of *S. asoca*, comparable with kanamycin.

6.3.2.12 ANTIBIOTICS V/S PLANT EXTRACTS AGAINST B. SUBTILIS

B. subtilis, a gram-positive bacterium was controlled by the leaf extract of *B. diffusa* and *C. dactylon*. The comparison with antibiotics reveals that no antibiotics used in the study could control this bacterium when compared to the activity of *C. dactylon*, which shows an inhibition zone of 28 mm. Except ciprofloxacin, all other antibiotics can be substituted with the leaf extract of *B. diffusa*, as the zone of inhibition was 21 mm.

6.3.2.13 ANTIBIOTICS V/S PLANT EXTRACTS AGAINST S. AUREUS

In controlling the growth of *S. aureus*, ten of the extracts were found to be effective, of which the flower extract of *L. inermis* gives an inhibition zone of 20 mm, which can be used as an alternative to erythromycin. Even though their antibacterial activities were moderately lower than that of the reference compounds (antibiotics), the crude extracts of most of the plants showed bactericidal activity.

The results regarding the comparison with antibiotics and plant extracts suggesting its possible use in the treatment of infections caused by the test pathogenic bacteria.

6.4 CONCLUSION

Multidrug resistance among bacteria is an immense threat to successful treatment of infective microbial diseases. The advance of effective plant-based products for improving health care needs is constrained by a number of issues, which includes the recognition of significant active secondary metabolites. Thousands of phytochemicals with *in vitro* microbicidal activities were reported factually, but animal and human studies have to be done for determining their effectiveness including toxicological studies as well as an examination of their effects on useful natural micro biota. The use of different plant natural compounds as antibacterial agents is an interesting strategy for developing bioactive products. The increasing consumer demand for effective, safe, natural products, calls for the research interest among scientists from divergent fields in the study of phytochemicals and ingenious screening programs are required to discover the plant based antimicrobials. This study-evaluated potency of plant extracts used in traditional medicine in controlling the growth of both gram- positive and negative strains. Of the 18-plant extract with bactericidal activity, eight possess broad spectrum and 10 with narrow spectrum activity, while many of the extracts showed activity against *Salmonella* and *S. aureus*. The results points to the possibility of the plant, such as *E. hirta, L. inermis, C. dactylon, C. roseus*, and *S. asoca* for further discovery of new metabolites with active antibacterial properties. These studies raises an intriguing idea in selecting particular plants, which may help the future research in the evolution of a novel plant based natural antimicrobials.

KEYWORDS

- **ayurveda**
- **medicine**
- **bacterial strains**
- **antibiotic resistance**

REFERENCES

1. Dev, S. Ancient–Modern Concordance in Ayurvedic Plants: Some Examples. *Environ. Health Perspect.* **1999,** *107,* 783–789.
2. Thakar, V. J. Historical development of basic concepts of Ayurveda from *Veda* up to Samhita. *Ayu.* **2010,** *31*(4), 400–402.
3. Pandey, M. M.; Rastogi, S.; Rawat, A. K. S. Indian Traditional Ayurvedic System of Medicine and Nutritional Supplementation. *Evid. Based Complement. Alternat. Med.* **2013,** Article ID 376327.
4. Pandey, M. K.; Singh, G. N.; Sharma, K. R.; Lata, S. Antibacterial Activity of *Eclipta Alba* (L.) Hassk. *J. Appl. Pharm. Sci.* **2011,** *1*(7), 104–107.
5. Maurice, M. I.; Angela, R. D.; Okunji, O. C. New Antimicrobials of Plant Origin. *Perspectives on New Crops and New Uses;* Janick, J., Ed.; ASHS Press: Aiexandria, 1999.
6. Hong-Fang, J.; Xue-Juan, L.; Hong-Yu, Z. Natural Products and Drug Discovery: Can Thousands of Years of Ancient Medical Knowledge Lead Us to New and Powerful Drug Combinations in the Fight against Cancer and Dementia? *EMBO rep.* **2009,** *10,* 3.
7. Ahvazia, M.; Khalighi-Sigaroodi, F.; Charkhchiyan, M. M.; Mojab, F.; Mozaffarian, V. A.; Zakeri, H. Introduction of Medicinal Plants Species with the Most Traditional Usage in Alamut Region. *Iran. J. Pharm. Res.* **2012,** *11*(1), 185–194.
8. Bhushan, P.; Vaidya, A. D. B.; Mukund, C. Ayurveda and Natural Products Drug Discovery. *Curr. Sci.* **2004,** *86,* 6–25.
9. Vaishnav, P.; Demain, A. L. Unexpected Applications of Secondary Metabolites. *Biotech. Adv.* **2010,** *29,* 223–229.
10. Kennedy, D. O.; Wightman, E. L. Extracts and Phytochemicals: Plant Secondary Metabolites and the Enhancement of Human Brain Function. *Adv. Nutr.* **2011,** *2,* 32–50.
11. Cox, P.; Balick, M. The Ethnobotanical Approach to Drug Discovery. *Sci. Am.* **1994,** *270,* 80.
12. Kliebenstein, D. J.; Osbourn, A. Making New Molecules – Evolution of Pathways for Novel Metabolites in Plants. *Curr. Opin. Plant. Biol.* **2012,** *15,* 415–423.
13. Tiwari, S.; Singh, A. Toxic and Sub-Lethal Effects of Oleadrin on Biochemical Parameters of Freshwater Air Breathing Murrel, *Chant Punctatus (Bloch). Indian J. Exp. Biol.* **2004,** *42,* 413–418.

14. Bednarek, P. Chemical Warfare or Modulators of Defence Responses – The Function of Secondary Metabolites in Plant Immunity. *Curr. Opin. Plant. Biol.* **2012,** *15,* 407–414.
15. Harborne, J. R. *Introduction to Ecological Biochemistry,* 4th Ed., Elsevier: London, 1993.
16. Wink, M. Evolution of Secondary Metabolites from an Ecological and Molecular Phylogenetic Perspective. *Phytochemistry.* **2003,** *64,* 3–19.
17. Tahara, S. A Journey of Twenty-Five Years through the Ecological Biochemistry of Flavonoids. *Biosci. Biotechnol. Biochem.* **2007,** *71,* 1387–1404.
18. Rattan, R. S. Mechanism of Action of Insecticidal Secondary Metabolites of Plant Origin. *Crop Prot.* **2010,** *29,* 913–920.
19. Hooper, D. C.; Demaria, A.; Limbago, B. M.; O'Brien, T. F.; Mccaughey, B. Antibiotic Resistance: How Serious is the Problem, and What Can e Done? *Clin. Chem.* **2012,** *58*(8), 1182–1186.
20. Tenover, F. C. Mechanisms of Antimicrobial Resistance in Bacteria. *Am. J. Med.* **2006,** *119,* 3–10.
21. Piddock, L. J. V. Clinically Relevant Chromosomally Encoded Multidrug Resistance Efflux Pumps in Bacteria. *Clin. Microbiol. Rev.* **2006,** *19,* 382–402.
22. Indu, M. N.; Hatha, A. A. M.; Abirosh, C.; Harsha, U.; Vivekanandan, G. Antimicrobial Activity of Some of the South-Indian Spices against Serotypes of *Escherichia Coli, Salmonella, Listeria Monocytogenes* and *Aeromonas Hydrophila. Braz. J. Microbiol.* **2006,** *37,* 153–158.
23. Srinivasan, D.; Sangeetha, N.; Suresh, T.; Lakshmanaperumalsamy, P. Antibacterial Activity of Neem and Tamarind Leaves. *Asian J. Microbiol. Enviorn. Sci.* **2001,** *3,* 67–73.
24. Bauer, A. W.; Kirby, W. M. M.; Sherris, J. C.; Turck, M. Antibiotic Susceptibility Testing by Standardized Single Disk Method. *Am. J. Clin. Pathol.* **1996,** *45,* 493–496.
25. Ranjan, S. R.; Shankar, M. U.; Kumar, P. S.; Saiprasanna, B. Evaluation of Antidiarrhoeal Activity of *Sida Rhombifolia* Linn. Root. *Int. Res. J. Pharm.* **2011,** *2,* 157–160.
26. Woldeyes, S.; Adane, L.; Tariku1, Y.; Muleta, D.; Begashaw, T. Evaluation of Antibacterial Activities of Compounds Isolated From *Sida Rhombifolia* Linn. (Malvaceae). *Nat. Prod. Chem. Res.* **2012,** *1,* 1.
27. Show, S.; Banerjee, S.; Chakraborty, I.; Sikdar, M. *In Vitro* Comparison between Antibacterial Activity of *Catharanthus Roseus* and *Nyctanthes Arbour Tristis* on Antibiotic Resistant *Staphylococcus Aureus* Strain. *Indo Am. J. Pharm. Res.* **2014,** *4,* 3.
28. Govindasamy, C.; Srinivasan, R. *In Vitro* Antibacterial Activity and Phytochemical Analysis of *Catharanthus Roseus* (Linn.) G. Don. *Asian Pac. J. Trop. Biomed.* **2012,** *2,* 155–158.
29. Bijeshmon, P. P.; George, S. Antimicrobial Activity and Powder Microscopy of the Flowers of *Tabernaemontana Divaricata* R. Br. *Indo Am. J. Pharm. Res.* **2014,** *4,* 3.
30. Venkatachalapathi, S.; Saranya, C.; Ravi, S. Isolation and Characterization of Bio Active Compounds from *Tabernaemontana Divaricata* and a Study of its Antioxidant and Antibacterial Activity. *Indo Am. J. Pharm. Res.* **2014,** *4* (5), 2401–2406.
31. Rajeh, M. A. B.; Zuraini, Z.; Sasidharan, S.; Latha, L. Y.; Amutha, S. Assessment of *Euphorbia Hirta* L. Leaf, Flower, Stem and Root Extracts for their Antibacterial and Antifungal Activity and Brine Shrimp Lethality. *Molecules.* **2010,** *15,* 6008–6018.

32. Perumal, S.; Pillai, S.; Cai, L. W.; Mahmud, R.; Ramanathan, S. Determination of Minimum Inhibitory Concentration of *Euphorbiahirta* (L.) Extracts by Tetrazolium Microplate Assay. *J. Nat. Prod.* **2012,** *5,* 68–76.
33. Hussain, M.; Farooq, U.; Rashid, M.; Bakhsh, H.; Majeed, A.; Khan, I. A.; Ranal, S. L.; Shafeeq-Ur-Rahman, M.; Aziz, A. Antimicrobial Activity of Fresh Latex, Juice and Extract of *Euphorbia Hirta* and *Euphorbia Thymifolia*–An *in Vitro* Comparative Study. *Int. J. Pharma Sci.* **2014,** *4*(3), 546–553.
34. Murti, K.; Kumar, U. Antimicrobial Activity of *Ficus Benghalensis* and *Ficus Racemosa* Roots *L. Am. J. Microbiol.* **2011,** *2*(1), 21–24.
35. Koona, S. J.; Rao, B. S. *In Vitro* Evaluation of Antibacterial Activity of Crude Extracts of *Ficus Benghalensis* Linn, the Banyan Tree Leaves. *Ind. J. Nat. Prod.* **2012,** *3*(2), 281–284.
36. Natarajan, D.; Shivakumar, M. S.; Srinivasan, R. Antibacterial Activity of Leaf Extracts of *Biophytum Sensitivum* (L.) DC. *J. Pharm. Sci. Res.* **2010,** *2*(11), 717–720.
37. Gangadharan, A.; Jacob, E.; Jose, D. Phytochemical Analysis, Antibacterial and Antihyaluronidase Activity of Three Indigenous Medicinal Plants. *World J. Pharm. Pharma. Sci.* **2014,** *3*(6), 751–761.
38. Namboodiri, A. G.; Parameswaran, R. Fibro-Porous Polycaprolactone Membrane Containing Extracts of *Biophytum Sensitivum*: A Prospective Antibacterial Wound Dressing. *J. Appl. Polym. Sci.* **2013,** *129,* 2280–2286.
39. Habbal, O.; Hasson, S. S.; El-Hag, A. H.; Al-Mahrooqi, Z.; Al-Hashmi, N.; Al-Bimani, Z.; Al-Balushi, M. S.; Al-Jabri, A. A. Antibacterial Activity of *Lawsonia Inermis* Linn (Henna) against *Pseudomonas Aeruginosa*. *Asian Pac. J. Trop. Biomed.* **2011,** *1,* 173–176.
40. Rahmoun, M. N.; Benabdallah, M.; Villemin, D.; Boucherit, K.; Mostefa-Kara, B.; Ziani-Cherif, C.; Choukchou-Braham, N. Antimicrobial Screening of the Algerian *Lawsonia Inermis* (Henna). *Der Pharma Chemica.* **2010,** *2*(6), 320–326.
41. Sukanya, S. L.; Sudisha, J.; Hariprasad, P.; Niranjana, S. R.; Prakash.; Fathima, S. K.. Antimicrobial Activity of Leaf Extracts of Indian Medicinal Plants against Clinical and Phytopathogenic Bacteria. *Afr. J. Biotechnol.* **2009,** *8*(23), 6677–6682.
42. Oliveira, F. F. M.; Torres, A. F.; Gonçalves, T. B.; Santiago, G. M. P.; Carvalho, C. B. M.; Aguiar, M. B.; Camara, L. M. C.; Rabenhorst, S. H.; Martins, A. M. S.; Junior, J. T. V.; Nagao-Dias, A. T. Efficacy of *Plectranthus Amboinicus* (Lour.) Spreng in a Murine Model of Methicillin-Resistant *Staphylococcus Aureus* Skin Abscesses. *Evid. Based Complement. Alternat. Med.* **2013,** *2013,* 291–592.
43. Leelarasamee, A.; Trakulsomboon, S.; Sittisomwong, N. Undetectable Anti-Bacterial Activity of *Andrographis Paniculata* (Burma) Wall. ex ness. *J. Med. Assoc. Thai.* **1990,** *73,* 299–304.
44. Mishra, P. K.; Singh, K. R.; Gupta, A.; Chaturvedi, A.; Pandey, R.; Tiwari, S. P.; Mohapatra, T. M. Antibacterial Activity of *Andrographis Paniculata* (Burm. F.) Wall. ex ness Leaves against Clinical Pathogens. *J. Pharm. Res.* **2013,** *7,* 459–462.
45. Akinnibosun, F. I.; Akinnibosun, H. A.; Ogedegbe, D. Investigation on the Antibacterial Activity of the Aqueous and Ethanolic Extracts of The Leaves of *Boerhavia Diffusa L. Sci. World J.* **2009,** *4,* 2.
46. Kumar, A.; Kashyap, P.; Sawarkar, H.; Muley, B.; Pandey, A. Evaluation of Antibacterial Activity of *Cynodon Dactylon* (L.) Pers. *Int. J. Herbal Drug Res.* **2011,** *1*(2), 31–35.

47. Jazani, N. H.; Mikaili, P.; Shayegh, J.; Haghighi, N.; Aghamohammadi, N.; Zartoshti, M. Evaluation of Antibacterial Activities of *Cynadon Dactylon*on Multi Drug Resistant Bacterial Isolates in Comparing with Ciprofloxacin. *J. Am. Sci.* **2011,** *7,* 6.
48. Dash, B. K.; Faruquee, H. M.; Biswas, S. K.; Alam, M. K.; Sisir, S. M.; Prodhan, U. K. Antibacterial and Antifungal Activities of Several Extracts of *Centella Asiatica L.* against Some Human Pathogenic Microbes. *Life Sci. Med. Res.* **2011,** *2011,* 35.
49. Arumugam, T.; Ayyanar, M.; Pillai, Y. J. K.; Sekar, T. Phytochemical Screening and Antibacterial Activity of Leaf and Callus Extracts of *Centella Asiatica. Bangladesh J. Pharmacol.* **2011,** *6,* 55–60.
50. Janakiraman, N.; Sahaya, S.; Johnson, M. Anti-Bacterial Studies on *Peristrophe Bicalyculata (Retz.) Nees. Asian Pac. J. Trop. Biomed.* **2012,** *2,* 147–150.
51. Pitchamuthu, A.; Muthiah, G.; Rajaram, P. Preliminary Study on the Antimicrobial Activity of *Enicostemma Littorale* Using Different Solvents. *Asian Pac. J. Trop. Med.* **2012,** *5,* 552–555.
52. Okwu, D. E.; Josaiah, C. Evaluation of the Chemical Composition of Two Nigerian Medicinal Plants. *Afr. J. Biotechnol.* **2006,** *5,* 357–361.
53. Shan, B.; Cai, Y. Z.; Brooks, J. D.; Corke, H. The *in Vitro* Antibacterial Activity of Dietary Spice and Medicinal Herb Extract. *Int. J. Food Microbiol.* **2007,** *117,* 112–119.
54. Chowdhury, A. A.; Islam, M. S. Antibacterial Activity of *Trema Orientalis. Dhaka Univ. J. Pharam. Sci.* **2004,** *3*(1–2), 115–117.
55. Khare, C. P. *Indian Medicinal Plants, an Illustrated Dictionary;* Springer-Verlag: New York, 2007.

CHAPTER 7

ANTIBACTERIAL EFFECT OF GREEN TEA AND BLACK TEA EXTRACT AGAINST SELECTED GENERA OF BACTERIA

K. A. TREASA NIMY[1], VINCENT TERRENCE REBELLO[1*], and T. K. MUKUNDAN[2]

[1]PG Department of Zoology and Aquaculture, St. Albert's College, Banerji Road, Ernakulam-682018, Kerala, India.

[2]PG Department of Zoology, S.N.M. College, Maliankara, Kerala, India

[*]Corresponding author. E-mail: drterencerebello2012@gmail.com

CONTENTS

ABSTRACT

Green tea has been used for thousands of years as a beverage and therapeutic agent. In countries such as Japan and China, drinking of tea has remained is very common. Most traditional uses of green tea is focused on ritual, but it has also been used as a whole body tonic, used to rejuvenate mind and to provide vitality for life. Over the last few decades green tea has been subjected to many scientific and medical studies to determine the extent of its long-purported health benefits, with some evidence suggesting that regular green tea drinkers may have a lower risk of developing heart disease and certain types of cancer. Although green tea does not raise the metabolic rate enough to produce immediate weight loss, a green tea extract containing polyphenols and caffeine has been shown to induce thermogenesis and stimulate fat oxidation, boosting the metabolic rate 4% without increasing the heart rate.

7.1 INTRODUCTION

The history of antimicrobials begins with the observations of Pasteur and Joubert, who discovered that one type of bacteria could prevent the growth of another. An antimicrobial agent that destroys microbes, inhibits their growth or prevents or counteracts their pathogenic action. Disinfectants are antimicrobial substances used on non-living objects or outside the body. They did not know at that time that the reason one bacterium failed to grow was that the other bacterium was producing an antibiotic. Technically, antibiotics are only those substances that are produced by one microorganism that kill, or prevent the growth, of another microorganism. Of course, in today's common usage, the term antibiotic is used to refer to almost any drug that attempts to rid your body of a bacterial infection. Antimicrobials include not just antibiotics, but synthetically formed compounds as well. The discovery of antimicrobials paved the way for better wellbeing for millions around the world. Before penicillin became a viable medical treatment in the early 1940s, no true cure for gonorrhea, strep throat, or pneumonia existed. Patients with infected wounds often had to have a wounded limb removed, or face death from infection. Now, most of these infections can be cured easily with a short course of antimicrobials. However, with the development of antimicrobials, microorganisms have adapted and become resistant to previous antimicrobial agents. The old antimicrobial technology was based either on poisons or heavy metals, which may not have killed the microbe completely, allowing the microbe to survive, change, and become resistant to the poisons and/or heavy metals.

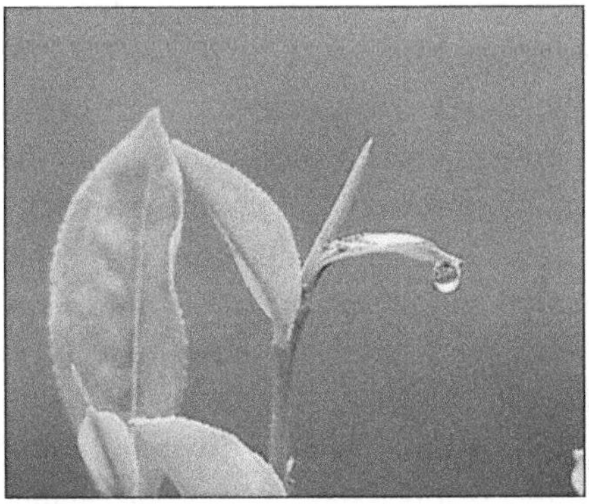

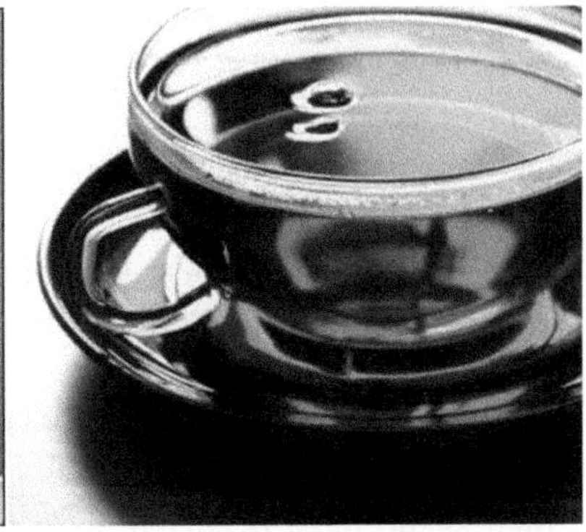

Black tea is nothing more than the leaves of the *C. sinensis* that have been processed a certain way. It is one of the four types of teas [white, green, oolong (partially oxidized) and black]. Black tea is the most consumed of the four types of teas. They are the highest in caffeine, but still have antioxidant properties, just not quite as much as others. The tea leaves are allowed to completely oxidize. Black tea is first withered to induce protein breakdown and reduce water content (68–77% of original). The leaves then undergo a process known in the industry is disruption or leaf maceration, which through bruising or cutting disrupts leaf cell structures, releasing the leaf juices and enzymes that activate oxidation. The oxidation process takes between 45–90 min. to 3 hr. and is done at high humidity between 20-30°C, transforming much of the catechins of the leaves into complex tannin. Orthodox processed black teas are further graded according to the post-production leaf quality by the Orange Pekoe system, while *Crush, Tear, Curl* (CTC; or Cut, tear, curl) teas use a different grading system. Orthodox tea leaves are heavily rolled either by hand or mechanically on a cylindrical rolling table or a rotovane. The rolling table consists of a ridged table-top moving in an eccentric manner to a large hopper of tea leaves, of which the leaves are pressed down onto the table-top. The process produces a mixture of whole and broken leaves, and particles which are then sorted, oxidized, and dried. The rotovane consisted of an auger pushing withered tea leaves through a vane cylinder which crushes and evenly cuts the leaves. CTC black teas is a production method developed by William Mc Kercher and consist of machines with contra-rotation rotors with surfaces patterning that cut and tear the leaves producing a product popular for use in tea bags. The rotovane to often use to precut the withered tea prior to the CTC and to create broken orthodox processed black tea.

It is medically approved that drinking black tea can tremendously relive you from several health disorders including prevention of cancer growth, the most deadly disease in the world. Black tea contains several health benefits which are described in the following lines respectively. One of the first black tea benefits is prevention of life-threatening clogging of arteries thereby by preventing onset of cardiovascular diseases like heart attack and strokes. The medical specialist from Boston University School found out in its test that drinking four cups of black tea in a day has amazing result in improving the condition of cardiovascular syndromes in the heart patient. One of the other black tea benefits is that it inhibits the growth of cancer which is the most deadly disease in the world today. Recent lab studies show that drinking black tea regularly can bring down the cancer growth because the black tea chemical has certain property that acts strongly in decreasing the cancer growth in the body. It has recently been found that black tea contains TF-2 anti-cancer compound that surprisingly suppresses Cox-2 gene which is responsible for inflammation and other medical disorders in the body. You will be quite surprised to know that many viruses can be neutralized by drinking black tea. Various germs in the body are responsible for disorders such as diarrhoea, pneumonia, cystitis and skin infections. Black tea contains such strong property that can be used to terminate these germs and save body from diseases brought forth by the germs. Medicinal properties of tea were known to mankind since antiquity. Antibacterial property of tea was first reported from Japan by using Japanese tea against various diarrhoeal pathogens. Subsequent studies with four kinds of Japanese green tea and 24 bacterial isolates from infected root canals provided enough evidences to support the bactericidal activity of tea. Extracts of tea have shown significant bactericidal activity against methicillin resistant *Staphylococcus aureus* (MRSA) even at concentrations available in ordinarily brewed tea. There have been studies conducted in the past to evaluate the antibacterial activity of tea against *Salmonella serotypes* primarily associated with diarrhoeal illness. However there is paucity in the information available, regarding the antibacterial activity of black tea extracts against serotypes of *Salmonella* causing enteric fever. The phytochemical screening of tea revealed the presence of alkaloids, saponins, tannins, catechin and polyphenols and also showed that moderate daily consumption of green tea killed *S. aureus* and other harmful bacteria (Toda *et al.* 1991).[1] Green tea and black tea showed marked bactericidal activity at their concentration in beverage and they might act as a prophylachic agent against pertussis infection. (Horiuchi *et al.* 1992).[2]

Green tea has been used for thousands of years as a beverage and therapeutic agent. In countries such as Japan and China, the drinking of teas has remained a commonality among the people of these countries. Most traditional uses of Green tea is focused on ritual, but has been used as a whole body tonic; used to rejuvenate one mind and to provide vitality for life. Over the last few decades green tea has been subjected to many scientific and medical studies to determine the extent of its long-purported health benefits, with some evidence suggesting that regular green tea drinkers may have a lower risk of developing heart disease and certain types of cancer. Although green tea does not raise the metabolic rate enough to produce immediate weight loss, a green tea extract containing polyphenols and caffeine has been shown to induce thermogenesis and stimulate fat oxidation, boosting the metabolic rate 4% without increasing the heart rate. According to a survey released by the United States Department of Agriculture (USDA, 2007), the mean content of flavonoids in a cup of green tea is higher than that in the same volume of other food and drink items that are traditionally considered of health contributing nature, including fresh fruits, vegetable juices or wine. Flavonoids are a group of phytochemicals in most plant products that are responsible for such health effects as anti-oxidative and anti carcinogenic functions. However, based on the same USDA survey, the content of flavanoids may vary dramatically amongst different tea products. Today, Green tea is prized because of its high antioxidant activity and harnesses the potential to treat and prevent many diseases, especially cancer. The primary constituents of Green tea that lend to its high antioxidant activity are the polyphenols. The most well-known polyphenols are catechins and gallocatechins. Polyphenols are one sub grouping of a larger classification of molecules known as flavonoids. Flavonoids are well known for their antioxidant potential. Green tea also contains several other constituents, such as tannins, that allow it to be a useful remedy for diarrhea. It also contains caffeine, vitamins, and minerals. Although not as high as amounts the amount found in coffee, the caffeine in Green tea has been shown to stimulate the central nervous system.

Green tea benefits oral health and reduces cavities in at least five ways. It kills the bacteria that cause cavities. Research from the past decade has identified a number of substances in green tea that can weaken the cavity-causing effects of bacteria, including *Streptococcus mutans*. It blocks the attachment of the bacteria associated with dental caries to the teeth. It inhibits the collagenase activity of the bacteria that live below the gum line. The polyphenols in green tea are anti-inflammatory, so they reduce gum disease (gingivitis). Finally, it increases the resistance of tooth enamel to acid induced erosion. The antibacterial effects of green tea against oral bacteria and several pathogenic strains common in the GI tract also have been well documented. Green tea polyphenols completely inhibited the growth and adherence of *Porphyromonas gingivalis* in a concentration of 250–500 mcg/mL. After 5 min. of contact, green tea polyphenol solution (1mg/mL) inhibited the proliferation of *S. mutans*. In general, green tea extracts proved to be bactericidal. They inhibited the growth of diarrhea-causing *S. aureus*, *S. epidermidis*, *V. parahaemolyticus*, *C. jejuni* and *V. cholerae*. The extracts also proved effective against pathogenic and to some extent, against penicillin-resistant, *S. aureus*. In vitro tests also showed that green tea was effective against some pathogenic fungi. Green tea appears to be of great benefit to the skin. The active polyphenols, which are found in both black and green tea, may protect against sunburn. Green and black tea extracts were rubbed on areas of the skin of human volunteers, to test the ability to protect against sun damage from relatively low levels of ultraviolet (UV) radiation aimed at the subjects forearms. The subjects had less acute redness formation after exposure to UV light than untreated areas.

7.2 REVIEW OF LITERATURE

Several studies have been made on the antibacterial activity of tea against different bacterial genera. Some of the works are those of a study by Mbata *et al.*[3] was undertaken to determine the antibacterial activity of the crude Extract of Chinese Green tea on *L. monocytogenes* were investigated using Agar-gel diffusion, Paper disc diffusion and micro broth dilution techniques. The results obtained showed that methanol and water extract exhibit antibacterial activity against *L. monocytogenes*. The leave extract produced inhibition zone ranging from 10.0 to 20.1 mm against the text bacteria. The methanol extract produce larger zone of inhibition against the text bacteria. He also conducted investigation on the antibacterial activities of processed Kenyan and Nigerian Tea, against six organisms, *P. aeruginosa*,

S. aureus, *V. cholerea*, *Salmonella* sp, *Proteus* spp. and *Escherichia coli* using agar gel diffusion method. The result obtained showed that 20% extract of both teas showed antibacterial activities against *S. aureus*, *E. coli*, *Proteus* spp. and *V. cholerea* 01. *Salmonella* spp. and *Pseudomonas* were resisted.

Tiwari *et al.*[4] attempted to describe the synergistic antimicrobial activity of tea and antibiotics against enteropathogenes. Both green tea or black tea extract effectively inhibited the growth of *S. typhimurium* 1402/84 *S. typhi*, *S. typhi* Ty2a, *S. dysenteria*, *Y. enterocolittica* C770 and *E. coli* (EPEC P_2 1265). The growth inhibitory concentration of tea extract was lower for green tea as compared to black tea extract. Tea extract showed synergistic activity with Chloramphenicol and other antibiotics like Gentamycin, Methicillin and Nalidixic and against text strains. Antibacterial activity of *C. sinensis* extracts against dental caries was studied by Rasheed and Haider.[5] It block the attachment of the bacteria associated with dental caries to the teeth. It was also determined the antimicrobial activity of the fermented tea kombucha using an absorbent disc method against *A. tumefaciens*, *B. cereus*, *S. cholerasuis*, *S. aureus* and *E. coli*. Antimicrobial activity was observed in the fermented samples containing 33g/L total and (7g/L acetic acid). *C. albicans* was not inhibited by kombucha.

Shetty *et al.*[6] reported that the green tea extracts inhibited the growths of diarrhea causing *S. aureus*, *S. epidermidis*, *V. parahaemolyticus*, *C. jejuni* and *V. cholera*. Antibacterial activity of tea polyphenols against *C. botulinum* was studied by Yokihiko and Watanabe.[7] They found *C. botulinum* spores were killed when inoculated into tea drinks. Horiuchi *et al*[2] examined the bactericidal activity of tea and catechins against *B. pertussis*. Green tea, black tea and coffee showed marked bactericidal activity at their concentrations in beverages, while puerh tea killed the bacteria in a moderate way. This study suggest that green tea, black tea, epigallocatechin gallate (EGCG) and theaflavin digallate (TF3) might act as prophylactic against pertussis infection.

Chosa, H. *et al.*[8] reported the antimicrobial and microcidal activities of tea and catechins against *Mycoplasma*. At a concentration of 0.2% green tea and black tea showed microbial activities against *M. pneumoniae* and *M. orale* but not against *M. Salivarium*. Extracts of puerh tea showed a slight microbial activity against *M. pneumoniae* and *M. orale*. These result suggest that tea and catechins can be used as prophylactic agent against *M. pneumoniae* infection.

Diker *et al.*[9,10] showed that black and green tea extracts (50 times the usual level of tea used for consumption) had bactericidal activity against *C. jejuni*, *C. coli* and *Helicobacter pylori*. Horiba *et al.*[11] carried out investigation on the antibacterial and bactericidal effect of Japanese green tea. The result obtained show that the tea inhibit the growth of various bacterial strains isolated from patients with infected root canal. Antibacterial and bactericidal activity of Japanese green tea has been studied by Toda *et al.*[12]. They found that extracts of Japanese green tea leaves inhibited the growth of various bacteria causing diarrheal disease. All tea samples tested showed antibacterial activity against *S. aureus*, *S. epidermidis*, *V. cholera* 01, *V. cholerae non 01*, *V. parahaemolyticus*, *V. mimicus*, *Campylobacter jejuni* and *Pl. shigelloides*. *Salmonella* and *Shigella* showed susceptibilities different depending on the kind of Japanese green tea. The bactericidal activity was shown even at the drinking concentration in daily life.

Kawanamura and Takeo[13] reported, the catechin fraction of black tea, at about 0.4 mg/ml, was shown to be antimicrobial against *S. mutans*, related to dental carrier found in human teeth. Stagg and Millin[14] was undertaken to determine the nutritional and therapeutic values of tea. They found that green tea has much higher catechin content than black tea. As a result, green tea may have more antibacterial activity than black tea.

7.3 MATERIALS AND METHODS

7.3.1 COLLECTION OF SAMPLE

Two types of tea were used for this study – green tea and black tea. The samples were collected from Tata Tea Ltd.

7.3.2 SAMPLE PREPARATION

7.3.2.1 AQUEOUS EXTRACT

The aqueous extraction of the water soluble ingredients was carried out. 100 ml of boiling water was added to 2 g of tea and mixture was concentrated to one-fifth volume. Then it was filtered after standing for 10 min. The resulting 2% tea extract was labeled and used further for diffusion studies. The same procedure was repeated for the preparation of 5 and 10% W/V concentrations of tea.

7.3.3 TEST ORGANISM

The organisms used in this work were 2–3 h broth cultures of *S. aureus*, *E. coli*, *Pseudomonas* spp. and *Proteus* spp.

7.4 METHODS

7.4.1 ANTIBACTERIAL SUSCEPTIBILITY TESTING

Antibacterial test of the tea extracts were tested on the test organisms using the agar-gel diffusion test and paper disc diffusion test.

7.4.2 AGAR GEL DIFFUSION SUSCEPTIBILITY TEST

In the agar gel diffusion test as described by Opara and Anasa.[15]

- Five wells of about 6 mm diameter were aseptically punched on Mueller-Hinton Agar (MHA) plates using a sterile cork borer allowing at least 25 mm between adjacent wells and between peripheral wells and the edge of the Petri dish.
- Sterile cotton swabs were used to inoculate the surface of the sterile MHA plate with the test organisms.
- Fixed volumes (0.1 ml) of the tea extract were then introduced into the wells in the plates.
- A control well was in the centre with 0.01 ml of the extracting solvent.
- The plates incubated at 37°C for 24 h.
- Antibacterial activity was indicated by growth-free "zone of inhibition" near the well.

7.5 RESULT

The aqueous extract of the green tea and black tea showed various levels of antibacterial activity when tested by Agar gel diffusion method. The extract showed greater antibacterial activity on *S. aureus*, moderate effect against *P. aeruginosa* and least effect on *E. coli* and *Proteus* spp. Antibacterial activity of aqueous extract of green tea and black tea on test organism and zone of inhibition are given in the following tables (Tables 7.1–7.3).

TABLE 7.1. The Antibacterial Activity of 10% Aqueous Extract of Green Tea and Black Tea on Test Organisms.

Sl. No.	Microorganisms	Zone of Inhibition (mm)	
		Green Tea	Black Tea
1	*Staphylococcus aureus*	32 mm	23 mm
2	*Pseudomonas aeruginosa*	16 mm	12 mm
3	*Escherichia coli*	10 mm	9 mm
4	*Proteus* spp.	9 mm	-

TABLE 7.2 The Antibacterial Effect of 5% Aqueous Extract of Green Tea and Black Tea Against Test Organisms.

Sl. No.	Microorganisms	Zone of Inhibition (mm)	
		Green Tea	Black Tea
1	*Staphylococcus aureus*	20 mm	13 mm
2	*Pseudomonas aeruginosa*	18 mm	-
3	*Escherichia coli*	-	-
4	*Proteus* spp.	-	-

TABLE 7.3 The Antibacterial Effect of 2% Aqueous Extract of Green Tea and Black Tea Against Test Organisms.

Sl. No.	Microorganisms	Zone of Inhibition (mm)	
		Green Tea	Black Tea
1	*Staphylococcus aureus*	15 mm	11 mm
2	*Pseudomonas aeruginosa*	-	-
3	*Escherichia coli*	-	-
4	*Proteus* spp.	-	-

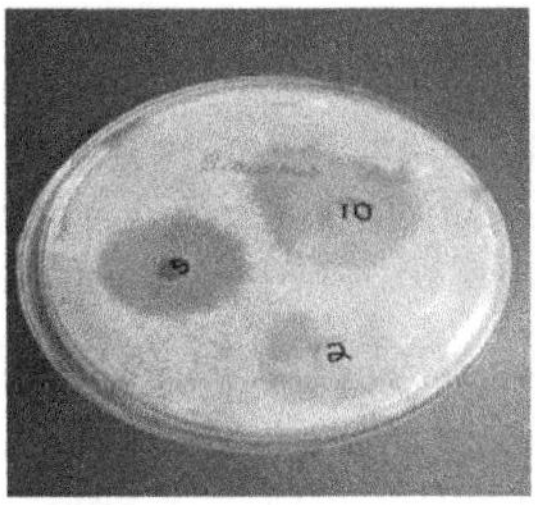

1

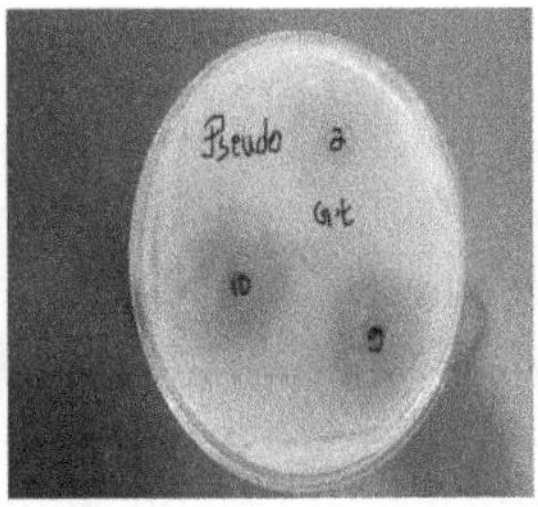

2

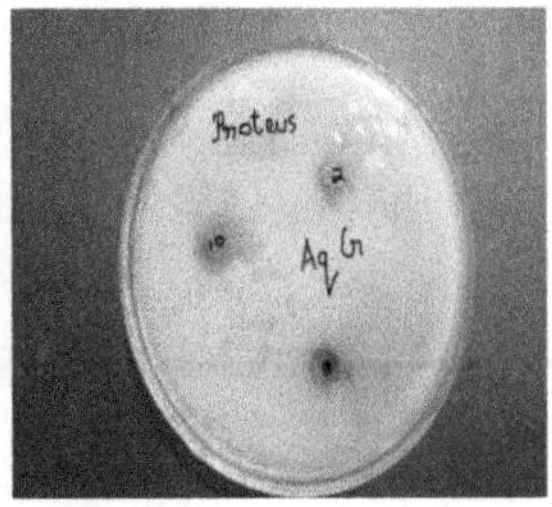

3

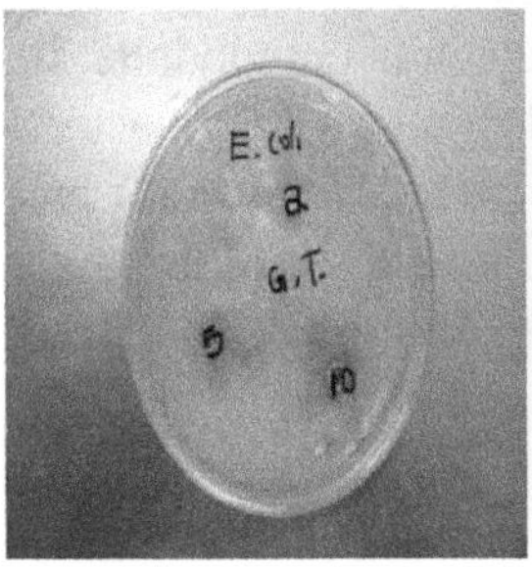

4

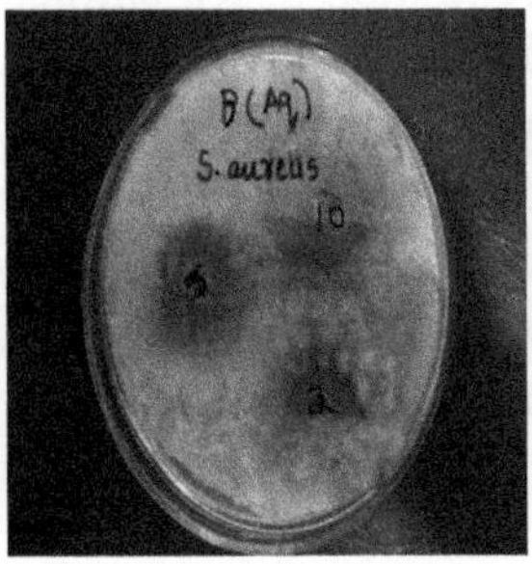

5

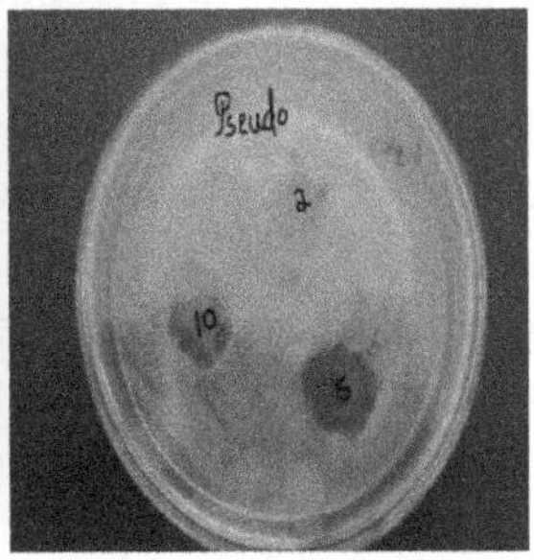

6

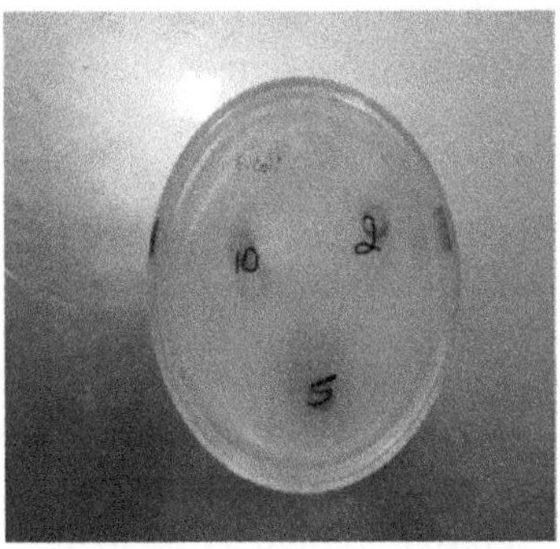

7

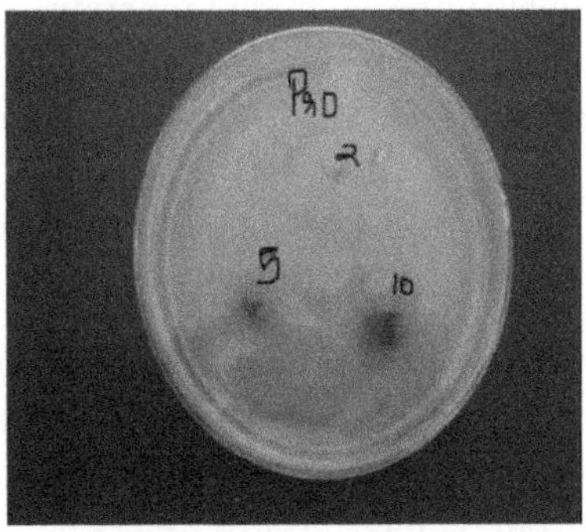

8

FIGURES 1–4 represent the antimicrobial effect of different concentrations of green tea against *S. aureus*, *Pseudomonas* sp., *Proteus* sp. and *E. coli* respectively.

FIGURES 5–8 represent the antimicrobial effect of black tea extracts on *S. aureus, Pseudomonas* sp., *E. coli* and *Proteus* sp.

7.6 DISCUSSION

The results of this study showed that the leaves extract of *C. sinensis* indicates the presence of potent antibacterial activity, which confirms its use against infection. The fresh green tea aqueous extract was found to have high antimicrobial activity than black tea extracts. All the test microorganisms found to be sensitive to aqueous green tea extracts at high concentration (10% w/v). Black tea extract also exhibit antibacterial property except for *Proteus* sp. It was also found that antimicrobial property increases with increase in the concentration of tea extract (2% <5% <10%). These observations may be attributed to green tea catechin compounds and polyphenols. These compounds have been found to possess antibacterial action. The catechin and polyphenols have been found to possess antibacterial and antiviral action as well as anticarcinogenic and antimutagenic properties. It is hoped that this may help to avoid the side effects of antibiotics. In future, the combined use of tea and antibiotics could be also useful in fighting emerging drug-resistant problem especially among enteropathogens.

Green tea is the healthiest beverage on the planet. It is loaded with antioxidants and nutrients that have powerful effects on the body. This includes improved brain function, fat loss, a lower risk of cancer and many other incredible benefits**.** The 10 health benefits of green tea that have been confirmed in human research studies.

1. **Green tea contains various bioactive compounds that can improve health**

   It is loaded with polyphenols like flavonoids and catechins, which function as powerful antioxidants. These substances can reduce the formation of free radicals in the body, protecting cells and molecules from damage. These free radicals are known to play a role in aging and all sorts of diseases. One of the more powerful compounds in green tea is the antioxidant Epigallocatechin Gallate (EGCG), which has been studied to treat various diseases and may be one of the main reasons green tea has such powerful medicinal properties. Green tea also has small amounts of minerals that are important for health. Try to choose a higher quality brand of green tea, because some of the lower quality brands can contain excessive levels of fluoride.

2. **Compounds in green tea can improve brain function and make you smarter**

   It contains less caffeine than coffee, but enough to produce an effect. It also contains the amino acid L-theanine, which can work synergistically with caffeine to improve brain function.

3. **Green tea increases fat burning and improves physical performance**

   It has been shown to boost the metabolic rate and increase fat burning in the short term, although not all studies agree.

4. **Antioxidants in green tea may lower your risk of various types of cancer**

   Green tea has powerful antioxidants that may protect against cancer. Multiple studies show that green tea drinkers have a lower risk of various types of cancer.

   - **Breast cancer:** A meta-analysis of observational studies found that women who drank the most green tea had a 22% lower risk of developing breast cancer, the most common cancer in women.
   - **Prostate cancer:** One study found that men drinking green tea had a 48% lower risk of developing prostate cancer, which is the most common cancer in men.
   - **Colorectal cancer:** A study of 69,710 Chinese women found that green tea drinkers had a 57% lower risk of colorectal cancer.

   Multiple other observational studies show that green tea drinkers are significantly less likely to get various types of cancer. It is important to keep in mind that it may be a bad idea to put milk in your tea, because it can reduce the antioxidant value.

5. **Green tea may protect your brain in old age, lowering your risk of Alzheimer's and Parkinson's**

   The bioactive compounds in green tea can have various protective effects on neurons and may reduce the risk of both Alzheimer's and Parkinson's, the two most common neurodegenerative disorders.

6. **Green tea can kill bacteria, which improves dental health and lowers your risk of infection**

   The catechins in green tea may inhibit the growth of bacteria and some viruses. This can lower the risk of infections and lead to improvements in dental health, a lower risk of caries and reduced bad breath.

7. **Green tea may lower your risk of Type II Diabetes**

   According to a review of 7 studies with a total of 286,701 individuals, green tea drinkers had an 18% lower risk of becoming diabetic. Some controlled trials show that green tea can cause mild reductions in blood sugar levels. It may also lower the risk of developing type II diabetes in the long term.

8. **Green tea may reduce your risk of cardiovascular disease**

   It has been shown to lower total and LDL cholesterol, as well as protect the LDL particles from oxidation. Observational studies show that green tea drinkers have a lower risk of cardiovascular disease.

9. **Green tea can help you lose weight and lower your risk of becoming obese**

   Some studies show that green tea leads to increased weight loss. It is particularly effective at reducing the dangerous abdominal fat.

10. **Green tea may decrease your risk of dying and help you live longer**

    Of course, we all have to die eventually. That is inevitable. However, given that green tea drinkers are at a lower risk of cardiovascular disease and cancer, it makes sense that it could help you live longer. In a study of 40,530 Japanese adults, those who drank the most green tea (5 or more cups per day) were significantly less likely to die during an 11 year period:

    - **Death of all causes:** 23% lower in women, 12% lower in men.
    - **Death from heart disease:** 31% lower in women, 22% lower in men.
    - **Death from stroke:** 42% lower in women, 35% lower in men.

KEYWORDS

- **green tea**
- **black tea**
- **caffeine**
- **microorganism**
- **polyphenols**

REFERENCES

1. Toda, M.; Okubo, S.; Iklgai, H.; Susuki, T.; Shimammura, T. The Protective Activity of the Tea against Infection by *Vibrio Cholerae* 01. *J. Appl. Bacteriol.* **1991,** *70,* 109–112.
2. Horiuchi, Y.; Toda, M.; Okubo, S. Protective Activity of Tea and Catechins against *Bordetella Pertussis. Kansenshogaku Zasshi.* **1992,** *66,* 599–605.
3. Mbata, T. I.; Lu Debiao, A.; Saikia. Antibacterial Activity of the Crude Extract of Chinese Green Tea (*Camellia Sinesis*) on *Listeria Monocytogenes. Internet J. Microbiol.* **2008,** *2*(2), 1571–1573.
4. Tiwari, R. P.; Bharti, S. K.; Kaur, H. D.; Dikshit, R. P.; Hoondal, G. S. Synergistic Antimicrobial Activity of Tea & Antibiotics. *Indian J. Med. Res.* **2005,** *122,* 80–84.
5. Rasheed, A.; Haider, M. Antibacterial Activity of *Camellia Sinensis* Extracts against Dental Caries. *Arch. Pharm Res.* **1998,** *21*(3), 348–352.
6. Shetty, M. et al. Antibacterial Activity of Tea (*Camellia Sinensis*) and Coffee (*Coffia Arabica*) with Special Reference to *Salmonella Typhimurium*. *J. Commun. Dis.* **1994,** *26,* 147–150.
7. Yokihiko, H.; Watanbe, M. Antibacterial Activity of Tea Polyphenols against *Clostridium Botulinum. J. Jpn. Soc. Food Sci. Technol.* **1989,** *36*(12), 951–955.
8. Chosa, H.; Toda, M.; Okubo, S. Antimicrobial and Microbicidal Activities of Tea and Catechins against Mycoplasma. *Kansenshogaku Zasshi.* **1992,** *66,* 606–611.
9. Diker, K. S.; Akan, M.; Hascelik, G.; Yuradakok, M. The Bactericidal Activity of Tea against *Campylobacter Jejuni* and *Campylobacter Coli. Lett. Appl. Microbiol.* **1991,** *12,* 34–35.
10. Diker, K. S.; Hascelik, G. The Bactericidal Activity of Tea against *Helicobacter Pylori. Lett. Appl. Microbiol.* **1994,** *19,* 299–300.
11. Horiba, N.; Maekawa, Y.; Ito, M.; Yamamoto, T. A Pilot Study of Japanese Green Tea as a Medicament, Antibacterial and Bactericidal Effects. *J. Endod.* **1991,** *17,* 122–124.
12. Toda, M.; Okubo, S.; Hiyoshi, R.; Shimamura, T. Antibacterial and Bactericidal Activities of Japanese Green Tea. *Jpn. J. Bacteriol.* **1989,** *44*(4), 669–672.

13. Kawanamura, J.; Takeo, T. Antibacterial Activity of Tea Catechin to *Streptococcus Mutans*. *J. Jpn. Soc. Food Sci. Technol.* **1989,** *36,* 463–467.
14. Stagg, G. V.; Millin, D. J. The Nutritional and Therapeutics Value of Tea – A Review. *J. Sci. Food Agric.* **1975,** *26,* 1439–1459.
15. Opara, A. A.; Anasa, M. A. The Antibacterial Activity of Tea and Coffee on Selected Organisms. *J. Medi. Lab. Sci.* **1993,** *3,* 45–48.

CHAPTER 8

IN VITRO ANTI-PLATELET AGGREGATION PROPERTY OF *HERACLEUM CANDOLLEANUM* (WIGHT ET ARN.) GAMBLE, A PROMISING TRIBAL MEDICINAL PLANT FROM WESTERN GHATS

HEMAND ARAVIND*

Department of Biotechnology, Navajyothi Sree Karunakara Guru Research Centre for Ayurveda and Siddha, Uzhavoor, Kottayam 686634, Kerala, India

**E-mail:hemandaravind@gmail.com*

CONTENTS

ABSTRACT

Heracleum candolleanum (*Apiaceae*) is a plant used by Kani tribes of Western Ghat region for inflammatory relief. The plant is commonly known as "Vatamparathi" and in siddha it is termed as chittelam. The plant is an aromatic, perennial, and rhizomatous herb mostly found in 6000 feet above sea level. The anti-platelet activity of methanol extract of root, leaf, and seed was studied using platelet-rich plasma (PRP) in different concentrations (50–500 µg/ml). Among them methanol extract of root showed dose-dependent anti-platelet activity with maximum activity 89.54% at 500 µg/ml concentration compared with that of standard drug aspirin. In conclusion, these observations suggested that root extract of *H. candolleanum* exhibits excellent levels of inhibitory action on platelets *in vitro* (secretion and platelet aggregation suppression) and may be due to the presence of phytochemical contents of plant.

8.1 INTRODUCTION

Heracleum candolleanum (Wight et Arn.) Gamble, *Apiaceae* a tribal medicinal plant endemic to Western Ghats, locally known as "Vathamparathi." In siddha medicine, it is mentioned as chittelam. The plant found in the Western Ghats region of peninsular India at an altitude above 6000 feet and is used by tribes of the region for various ailments such as nervous disorders and inflammatory conditions.[1] This plant is selected because of its common use as food and medicinal remedies in Kani tribes. The decoction of the root of this plant is used by the tribes as an anti-arthritic and nerve tonic.[2] Preliminary phytochemical screening and antioxidant activity of *H. candolleanum* revealed the presence of phytochemical constituents like flavonoids, alkaloids, furanocoumarins, phenols, volatile oils, etc. and its free radical scavenging activity.[3] A number of furanocoumarins and two monoterpenoids were reported from the fruits and roots of *H. candolleanum*.[4] Furanocoumarins from its seeds exhibit antioxidant activity. There are reports on the isolation of monoterpenoids 2-exo, 3-endo-camphanediol, and 2-pinene-4, 10-diol from the seeds of *H. candolleanum*.[5]

Platelets play a prominent role in maintain homeostasis and thrombosis by regulated interactions between components of vessel wall and plasma proteins.[6] Platelets can adhere to the walls of the blood vessels, release bioreactive compounds, and aggregate to each other. These properties increase to a well established level in conditions of arterial thrombosis and atherogenesis.[7] Modern medical system generally prescribes blood thinning agents to mange several arterial disorders such as atherosclerosis, stokes, and myocardial infarction. The inappropriate blood clot formation leads to fatal cardiovascular diseases.[8] It is therefore important to prevent platelet dysfunctions that could lead to cardiovascular events. Mechanism of action and pharmacological efficacy of the current anti-platelet agents are still dicey and they are associated with the risk of severe or fatal bleeding.[9,10] The plant phytochemicals like flavonoids, alkaloids, tannins, and saponins are known to have anti-platelet and antioxidant activities.[11] Zulu medicinal plants *Protorhus longifolia*, *Bulbine natalensis*, and *Rapanea melanophloeos* can be used in the management of blood-clotting related diseases.[12] Literatures report that plants such as *Ocimum basilicum*[13] and *Nepeta juncea*[14] have anti-platelet aggregation activity. White and pink flowers of *Nelumbo nucifera* exert different levels of inhibitory action on platelets *in vitro*.[15] The clinical limitations and adverse side effects of blood diluting drugs fueled the search for new, safer, and effective anti-clotting agents of natural origin. Therefore, the present contribution was designed to evaluate the anti-platelet activity of methanol extract of *H. candolleanum* root.

8.2 MATERIALS AND METHODS

8.2.1 PREPARATION OF PLANT MATERIAL

The plant was collected from rocky grooves of Vagamon Hills, Kerala, India. A voucher specimen was kept in the herbarium of Navajyothi Sree Karunakara Guru Research Centre for Ayurveda and Siddha, Uzhavoor for further reference. The fresh roots of *H. candolleanum* were collected and washed thoroughly with water. The cleaned roots are chopped and then allowed for the complete shade drying and then ground to fine powder. About 50 g of dried powder was taken along with methanol and was extracted using soxhlet apparatus. The filtrate is dried by using rotary evaporator at 45 °C and the extract is used for further analysis.

8.2.2 DETERMINATION OF PLATELET AGGREGATION ACTIVITY

Platelet-rich plasma (PRP) and Tyrode buffer were used for the anti-platelet activity according to[16] Imran et al. PRP was prepared by centrifugation of citrated blood at 22 °C for 6 min, at 400 × *g*. Platelets were adjusted to 3.0 × 108 cell/ml with sterile saline. Tyrode buffer was prepared using sodium chloride 149 mM, potassium chloride 2.6 mM, sodium bicarbonate 9.5 mM, glucose 5.5 mM, sodium dihydrogen phosphate 0.5 mM, magnesium chloride 0.6 mM, and gelatin 0.25%. The PRP 0.13×10^{-7} for each assay was resuspended in Tyrode buffer (pH adjusted to 7.4 with 0.25 M HCl). Aggregation of the platelets was induced by $CaCl_2$ at a final concentration of 2 µM. Platelet aggregation was recorded by increasing transmittance value of spectrophotometric measurements. To determine the *in vitro* anti-platelet aggregation property, different concentrations (100, 200, 300, 400, and 500 µg/ml) of plant extract were added to the platelet suspension for 1 min exposure at 37 °C before treatment with platelet aggregating agents. The change in turbidity is observed and plotted on a recorder. Aspirin at 500 µg/ml was used as a standard.

8.3 RESULTS AND DISCUSSION

The functional abnormality of platelets leads to the generation of cardiovascular diseases such as arterial hypertension, atherosclerosis, and thrombosis. Increased platelet reactivity was reported in patients with hypertension or coronary heart disease. As part of finding suitable therapies to reduce abnormal hyperactivity of platelets in cardiovascular disorder, scientific world highly depends on medicinal plants.[17] The anti-platelet aggregation activity of root, leaf, and seed extracts was presented in Figures 8.1, 8.2, and 8.3. The extracts showed a concentration dependent inhibitory activity with a maximum activity at 500 µg/ml concentrations. Furthermore, the anti-platelet activity of root was relatively high (89.54%) compared to leaf and seed. Prevention of platelet aggregation was higher in root extract, compared to that of standard aspirin (IC50 47.77 µg/ml).

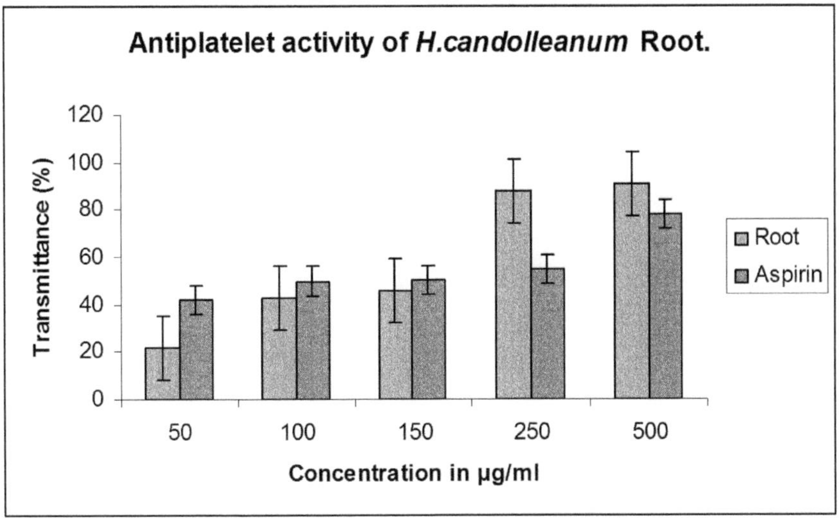

FIGURE 8.1 Anti-platelet aggregation activity of methanol extract of *H. candolleanum* root.

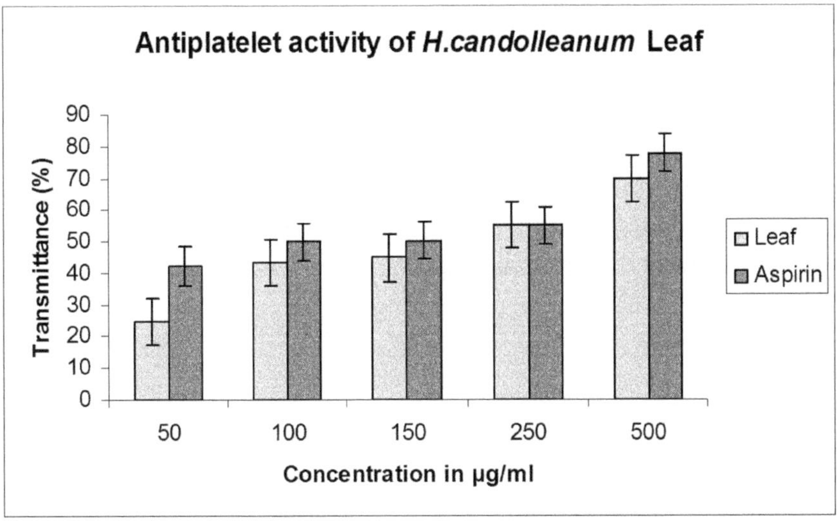

FIGURE 8.2 Anti-platelet aggregation activity of methanol extract of *H. candolleanum* leaf.

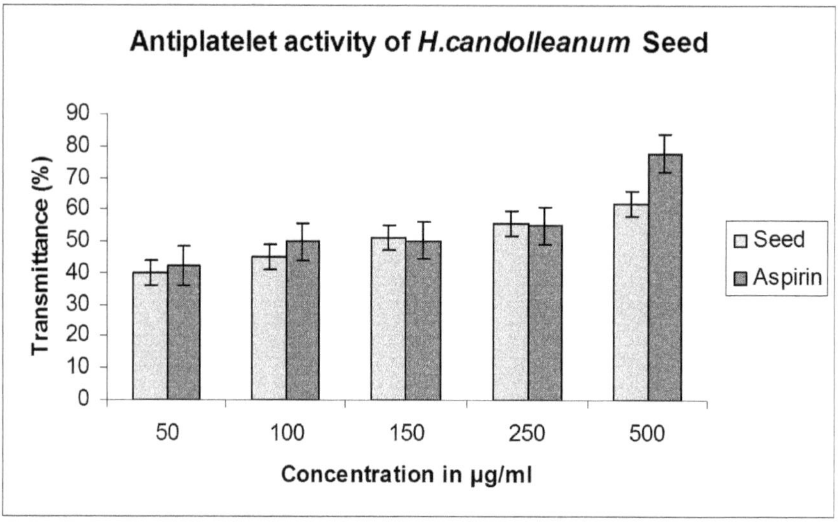

FIGURE 8.3 Anti-platelet aggregation activity of methanol extract of *H. candolleanum* seed.

8.4 CONCLUSION

The obtained data indicated that the methanol extracts of root, leaf, and seed of *H. candolleanum* possess potent anti-platelet activity limited to primary homeostasis in human blood. In addition, the anti-platelet activity of root is relatively high compared to that of leaf and seed. However, further studies are needed to confirm the mode of action and efficacy of all the three extracts in platelet aggregation.

KEYWORDS

- **homeostasis**
- **furanocoumarins**
- **phytochemicals**
- **monoterpenoids**
- **siddha**

REFERENCES

1. Mukherjee, P. K.; Constance, L. *Umbelliferae (Apiaceae) of India;* Oxford and IBH Publishing Company Pvt. Ltd: New Delhi, 1993; Vol. 243.
2. Saradamma, L.; Nair, C. P. R.; Bhatt, A. V.; Rajasekaran, S.; Lakshmi, N.; Nair, V. V. *All India Co-Ordinated Research Project on Ethno Botany. Technical Report (AICRP) Phase II;* Ministry of Environment and Forests (MOEF): Govt. of India, New Delhi. 1990; Vol. 243, pp 1987–90.
3. Aravind, H.; Rajesh, M. G. Evaluation of In Vitro Antioxidant and Antimicrobial Activity of *H. Candolleanum* (Wight et Arn.) Gamble. *Scientia.* **2012,** *8,* 65–71.
4. Susan, C.; Singh, O. V.; Sethuraman, M. G.; George, V. Coumarins from *Heracleum Candolleanum. Indian Drugs.* **2001,** *38,* 594–596.
5. Susan, C.; Sethuraman, M. G.; George, V. Monoterpenoids from the Seeds of *Heracleum Candolleanum. Fitoterapia.* **2000,** *71,* 616–617.
6. Saengkhae, C.; Arunnopparat, W.; Sungkhajorn, P.; Antioxidant Activity of *Nelumbo Nucifera Gaertn.* On Oxidative Stress-Induced Erythrocyte Hemolysis in Hypertensive and Normotensive Rats. *J. Physiol. Sci.* **2008,** *20,* 70–78.
7. Guyton, A. C.; Hall, J. E. *Textbook Of Medical Physiology,* 10th ed; Harcourt Asia Pvt. Limited: Singapore, 2000; pp 184– 222.
8. Heather, B.; Rebecca, J. F. Medline Plus Health Information. *Blood Clot;* 2001.
9. Hsieh, P. W.; Huang, T. L.; Wu, C. C.; Chiang, S. Z.; Wu, C. I.; Wu, Y. C. The Evaluation and Structure-Activity Relationships of 2-Benzoylaminobenzoic Esters and Their Analogues as Anti-Inflammatory and Antiplatelet Aggregation Agents. *Bioorg. Med. Chem. Lett.* **2007,** *17,* 1812–1817.
10. Fabre, J.; Gurney, M. E. Limitations of Current Therapies to Prevent Thrombosis: A Need for Novel Strategies. *Mol. Biosyst.* **2010,** *6,* 305–315.
11. Gilani, A. H.; Mehmood, M. H.; Janbaz, K. H.; Khan, A.; Saeed, S. A. Ethnopharmacological Studies on Antispasmodic and Antiplatelet Activities of *Ficus Carica. J. Ethnopharmacol.* **2008,** *119,* 1–5.
12. Mosa, R. A.; Lazarus, G. G.;Gwala, P. E.; Oyedeji, A. O. ; Opoku, A. R. *In Vitro* Anti-Platelet Aggregation, Antioxidant and Cytotoxic Activity of Extracts of Some Zulu Medicinal Plants. *J. Nat. Prod.* **2011,** *4,* 136–146.
13. Amrani, S.; Harnafi, H.; Gadi, D.; Mekhfi, H.; Legssyer, A.; Aziz, M.; Martin-Nizard F. ; Bosca, L. Vasorelaxant and Anti-Platelet Aggregation Effects of Aqueous *Ocimum Basilicum* Extract. *J. Ethnopharmacol.* **2009,** *125,* 157–162.
14. Hussain, J.; Khan, A. L.; Rehman, N.; Hamayun, M.; Shah, T.; Nisar, M.; Bano, T.; Shinwari, Z. K.; Lee, I. J. Proximate and Nutrient Analysis of Selected Vegetable Species: A Case Study of Karak Region Pakistan. *Afr. J. Biotechnol.* **2009,** *8,* 2725–2729.
15. Brindha Durairaj, B.; Dorai, A. Antiplatelet Activity of White and Pink *Nelumbo Nucifera Gaertn* Flowers. *Braz. J. Pharm. Sci.* **2010,** *46,* 579–583.
16. Imran, R. A.; Priya, B. L.; Chithra, R.; Shalini, K.; Vasanthi, J. *Invitro* Antiplatelet Activity Guided Fractionation of Aerial Parts of *Melothria Maderaspatana. Indian J. Pharm. Sci.* **2006,** *68,* 668–670.

17. Massberg, S.; Schurzinger, K.; Lorenz, M.; Konrad, I.; Schulz, C.; Plesnila, N. Platelet Adhesion via Glycoprotein II Integrin is Critical for Atheroprogression and Focal Cerebral Ischemia: An in Vivo Study in Mice Lacking Glycoprotein Iib. *Circulation.* **2005,** *8,*1180–1188.

CHAPTER 9

ROLE OF MEDICINAL PLANTS IN TARGETING IMPORTANT SIGNALING PATHWAYS IN CERVICAL CANCER

SAVITA PANDITA, RASHMI DESHPANDE, SHAMA APHALE, and RUCHIKA KAUL-GHANEKAR*

Interactive Research School for Health Affairs (IRSHA), Bharati Vidyapeeth University, Katraj-Dhankawadi, Pune-Satara Road, Pune 411043, Maharashtra, India

**Corresponding author. E-mail: ruchika.kaulghanekar@gmail.com, kaul_r@yahoo.com*

CONTENTS

ABSTRACT

Cervical cancer is one of the major health problems in women, representing the fourth most common cancer worldwide.[1] The main etiological factor for cervical cancer is persistent infection with the human papilloma virus (HPV), out of which HPV 16 and 18 account for 50–70% of cervical cancer cases. HPV infection leads to dysregulation of important signaling pathways that alter the expression of transcription factors which play vital role in normal cell function. These impaired signaling pathways thus, may serve as targets for cancer drug development. Despite advanced anticancer therapies, the issues of low survival rates, drug associated side effects and recurrence still persist.[3] In recent years, plants and herbs have been accepted as one of the main sources of chemopreventive drugs.[4] Thus, herbal medicines are being investigated for their use as adjunct to conventional therapies to manage the debilitating side effects associated with the latter. This review focuses on important signaling pathways that are reported to be targeted by medicinal plants in the management of cervical cancer. The pathways that have been described include p53 and Rb related pathways affected by HPV cell cycle regulation, angiogenesis, inflammation, PI3K/AKT/mTOR, and ras/raf/mitogen-activated protein kinase.

9.1 INTRODUCTION

Cervical cancer is the fourth most common cancer and leading cause of death in women globally.[1] It occurs usually in mid-life, mostly in the age group of 20–65 years and has a serious impact on woman's life. In India, it ranks as the second major cause of female cancer and leading cause of mortality.[1,5] According to HPV and related disease report 2014, around 122,844 new cervical cancer cases were diagnosed annually and 67,477 were reported to die from the disease in India.[5] Cervical cancer accounts for 17% of all cancer deaths among women aged between 30 and 69 years. Though cervical cancer is preventable, the risk is high in under developed countries due to lack of efficient screening programs.[6,7]

The major risk factor for the development of cervical cancer is persistent HPV infection.[8] The high-risk subtypes HPV 16 and 18 contribute to 70% of cervical cancers and are associated with cervical dysplasia or cervical intraepithelial neoplasia (CIN), known as squamous intraepithelial lesions (SIL), graded as low (LSIL) or high (HSIL),[9] The oncogenic activity of high risk HPV depends on the expression of the two oncoproteins E6 and E7,[8] These oncoproteins deregulate the host cell growth cycle by binding and inactivating tumor suppressor proteins, cell cyclins, and cyclin dependent kinases.[10] The complex interactions of E6 and E7 oncoproteins with many growth factor signaling pathways, angiogenesis and inflammation related markers as well as cell cycle checkpoints leads to genomic instability resulting into tumorigenesis.[8,9] Targeting of these pathways by novel drug candidates may lead to development of new strategies for cervical cancer management.

9.2 MEDICINAL PLANTS AS ANTICANCER DRUG CANDIDATES

The current treatment strategies for cervical cancer include various combinations of surgery, radiation therapy, and platinum based chemotherapy.[11] Despite these therapeutic options, it is associated with high mortality.[12] The major drawback of conventional treatment is its inability to distinguish between the cancer cells and the normal cells, therefore, leading to severe side-effects and dose limitations. Moreover, failure of chemotherapy to eliminate all tumor cells due to intrinsic or acquired drug resistance leads to tumor recurrence and metastasis.[13] In addition, due to high cost associated with the available cancer treatments, there is an increased demand for novel drug discovery from natural sources to manage the above side-effects.[14] Globally, medicinal plants are being used as complementary and alternative medicines (CAM) by cancer patients together with conventional treatments.[15,16] The advances in the medicinal plant studies have resulted in discovery of various plant extracts, fractions and pure compounds as potential anticancer drug candidates.[17] More than 60% of the drugs that are in the market are derived from natural sources including plants, marine organisms, and microorganisms.[18] The natural products from plants contain secondary metabolites (PSMs) such as alkaloids, flavonoids, phenolics, tannins, anthraquinones, and so on, which exhibit various biological properties including anticancer activity.[19,20] Many plant based anticancer agents including taxol, vincristine, vinblastine and topotecan have been in clinical use for a long time all over the world.[18] To identify lead anticancer compounds for prevention and treatment of cervical cancer efforts should be made to understand the signaling pathways that get altered during the cancer development.

9.3 SIGNALING PATHWAYS TARGETED BY MEDICINAL PLANTS IN CERVICAL CANCER

Cervical cancer occurs due to changes in multiple genes and signaling pathways.[21] Among several molecular pathways reported, the major pathways involved in cervical cancer have been described (Fig. 9.1). During the last decade, various studies have been carried out to investigate several molecular targets in cervical cancer.[22] Targeted therapies in conventional treatment act by inhibiting a specific molecule involved in a pathway thereby interfering either with proliferation or survival and in effect hindering the malignant transformation by inducing cell death or regulating cell cycle.[23] The drug resistance is a major hurdle in targeted approaches which can be overcome by combination treatments with natural products.[24,25] In this context, medicinal plants exhibit significant potential because of their ability to interact with different molecular pathways.[26,27] The general mechanism of action of any drug includes either affecting cell viability or inducing cell cycle arrest or modulating pro-apoptotic and anti-apoptotic proteins or by regulating signaling pathways involved in progression, metastasis and angiogenesis.[28,29] Various medicinal plants that have been reported to target these major signaling pathways (Fig.9.2) have been reviewed upon in following sections.

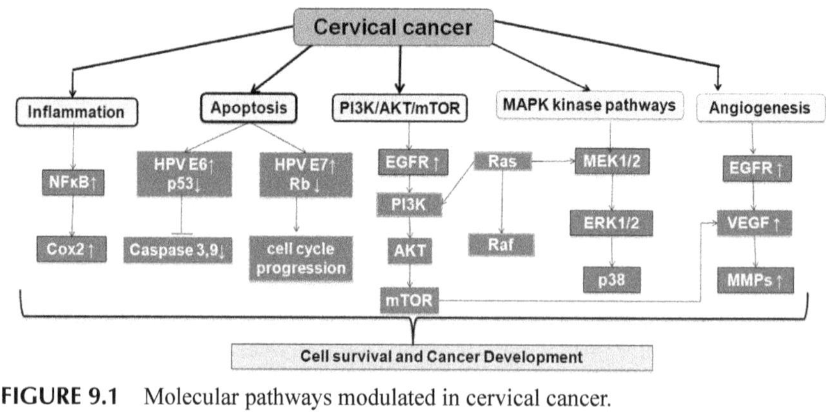

FIGURE 9.1 Molecular pathways modulated in cervical cancer.

Cervical cancer progression involves critical steps that affect various pathways that include inflammation, apoptosis, PI3K/AKT/mTOR, MAPK kinase and angiogenesis. NFκb and Cox-2 are the important inflammatory markers that are over expressed in cervical cancer. HPV E6 and E7 are the important viral oncoproteins that are essential for cancer cell transformation. E6 degrades p53 through ubiquitin-dependent proteasome pathway resulting into disruption of growth-inhibitory and apoptosis-inducing effects of p53 involving caspases 3 and 9. E7 inactivates Rb which causes loss of Rb/E2F complexes, thereby promoting cell cycle progression. PI3K activation may occur via Ras mutation or by increased expression of EGFR. Activation of PI3K/AKT/mTOR can increase VEGF leading to angiogenesis. VEGF activation may also increase expression of MMPs resulting into migration of cells. MAPK activation leads to downstream activation of ERK and p38 pathway, thereby leading to cell survival and cancer development.

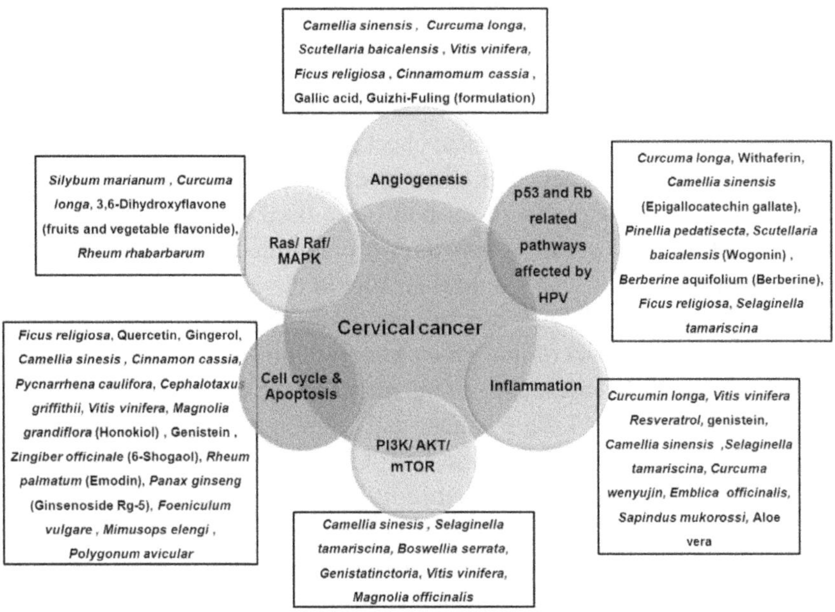

FIGURE 9.2 Various medicinal plants targeting important pathways in cervical cancer.

The figure shows various medicinal plants along with their molecular targets used in the management of cervical cancer.

9.3.1 P53 AND RB RELATED PATHWAYS AFFECTED BY HPV

Dysregulation of tumor suppressor p53 is mediated by HPV E6 oncoprotein via two mechanisms.[30] In one, E6 targets the degradation of p53 through ubiquitin dependent pathway wherein E6 binds to E6-associated protein (E6-AP), a cellular protein with known E3 ligase activity, leading to ubiquitination of p53 and its degradation by 26S proteasome.[31] In another mechanism, HPV E7 gene product binds to the hypophosphorylated form of retinoblastoma (Rb) family of proteins.[32] This binding disrupts the complex between phospho Rb (pRb) and cellular transcription factor E2F-1, resulting in its liberation that allows the transcription of cell cycle proliferating genes.[33] Various medicinal plants such as *Curcuma longa* (Withaferin A),[34,35] *Camellia sinensis* (Epigallocatechin gallate),[36] *Pinellia pedatisecta,*[37] *Scutellaria baicalensis* (Wogonin),[38] *Berberisaquifolium* (Berberine),[39] *Ficus religiosa,*[40] and *Selaginella tamariscina*[41] have been reported to target HPV oncogenes.

9.3.2 CELL CYCLE REGULATION AND APOPTOSIS

Cell cycle and apoptosis are critical checkpoints in cancer cells. Cell cycle involves a series of events that take place in a cell leading to its division and duplication. Cell cycle check points are used by the cell to monitor and regulate the cell cycle. Apoptosis or programmed cell death is a tightly regulated process that plays important role in development, homeostasis, as well as in antiviral defense mechanism.[42] Any defects in this process may lead to the development of malignant tumors.[43] It is now well documented that induction of cell cycle arrest and apoptosis by anticancer agents is an important strategy for killing cancer cells. A number of medicinal plants such as *Ficus religiosa,*[40] Quercetin,[44] [6]-Gingerol,[45] *Camellia sinensis,*[46,47] *Cinnamomum cassia,*[48] *Pycnarrhena cauliflora,*[49] *Cephalotaxus griffithii,*[50] *Vitis vinifera,*[9,51] *Magnolia grandiflora* (Honokiol),[52] Genistein,[53] *Zingiber officinale* (6-Shogaol),[54] *Rheum palmatum* (Emodin),[55] *Panax ginseng* (Ginsenoside Rg-5),[56] *Foeniculum vulgare,*[57] *Mimusops elengi,*[58] and *Polygonum aviculare*[59] have been reported to be effective in regulating cell cycle and apoptosis.

9.3.3 PHOSPHATIDYLINOSITOL 3 PHOSPHOINOSITIDE 3′ KINASE (PI3K)/SERINE-THREONINE KINASE (AKT)/ MAMMALIAN TARGET OF RAPAMYCIN (PI3K/AKT/MTOR) PATHWAY

The PI3K/AKT/mTOR pathway is an important intracellular signaling pathway that regulates cell proliferation and survival by controlling the cell cycle. It plays a central role in mediating diverse cellular functions like cell growth, proliferation, metabolism, survival, and angiogenesis.[60] An imbalance in AKT/mTOR pathway contributes to malignant transformation and is frequently observed in cervical cancer patients.[21,61,62] Thus, targeting this signal pathway offers a promising approach for cervical cancer therapy. Recently, it has been shown that chemoradiation response rate can be improved by using AKT inhibitors in patients with cervical cancer.[63] In clinical trials, various drugs have been shown to target PI3K (PI103andBGT226), AKT (PerifosineandGSK690693) and mTOR pathways (temsirolimus, everolimus, and ridaforolimus) pathways.[64,65] The use of phytochemicals to overcome chemoresistance and target this pathway is currently being evaluated for development of potential drugs against cervical cancer.[66] The medicinal plants that have been reported to target PI3K/AKT/mTOR in cervical cancer include *Camellia sinesis,*[67] *Selaginella tamariscina,*[68] *Boswellia serrata,*[69] *Genista tinctoria,*[70] *Vitis vinifera,*[71] and *Magnolia officinalis.*[72]

9.3.4 RAT SARCOMA (RAS)/RAPIDLY ACCELERATED FIBROSARCOMA (RAF)/MITOGEN-ACTIVATED PROTEIN KINASE (MAPK) PATHWAY

Mitogen-activated protein kinase (MAPK) cascade plays a key role in the regulation of normal cell proliferation, transformation, apoptosis and migration through activation of various transcription factors.[73] This pathway is often deregulated in cancers as a result of abnormalities in the RAS or RAF genes, thereby rendering it as a potential therapeutic target for cancer treatment. Targeting Ras-MAPK pathway in cancer has shown to improve therapeutic response.[74] Recently, several small-molecule inhibitors have been reported to target Ras (tipifarnib and lonafarnib), Raf (Sorafenib and PLX4032) and MAPK (AZD6244 and XL518).[64,65] Recurrence and metastasis due to resistance of cancer cells to chemotherapeutic agents represents a major problem for treatment of cervical cancer.[75] The use of herbal medicines as anti-cancer agents has been shown to produce beneficial effects in many cancer patients.[76] Different medicinal plants that have been reported to regulate Ras/Raf/MAPK pathway in cervical cancer include, *Silybum marianum,*[77] *Curcuma longa,*[78] and *Rheum rhabarbarum.*[79] Flavonoids such as 3,6-dihydroxyflavone, extracted from fruits and vegetables, have shown to down-regulate the MAPK, JNK, and ERK.[80]

9.3.5 ANGIOGENESIS PATHWAY

Angiogenesis (development of new blood vessels) is an essential process required for tissue development, reproduction and wound healing.[81] In cancer, it plays an important role in growth, progression, and metastasis of tumors. VEGF, EGFR, and MMPs are essential angiogenic markers.

9.3.5.1 VASCULAR ENDOTHELIAL GROWTH FACTOR (VEGF)

VEGF is a crucial factor involved in regulating angiogenesis that leads to progression of HPV induced cervical cancer.[4,9] Many studies have demonstrated that its expression correlates with more aggressive tumors.[82] VEGF inhibitors are agents that block the growth of malignant cells by inhibiting blood vessel formation through interference with signaling pathways involved in proliferation and metastasis of tumors. Currently bevacizumab, sunitinib, sorafenib, pazopanib, cediranib, brivanib, carboplatin, and paclitaxel with or without cediranib maleate are used as antiangiogenic drugs targeting VEGF pathway.[22,65,83] The use of anti-VEGF drugs is limited due to their serious side effects, hence, the use of herbs could have significant potential.[84] Various medicinal plants that have been shown to target VEGF pathway in cervical cancer include *Camellia sinensis,*[22,85] *Curcuma longa,*[22,78] *Scutellaria baicalensis,*[86] and *Vitis vinifera.*[51,87]

9.3.5.2 EPIDERMAL GROWTH FACTOR RECEPTOR (EGFR)

The Epidermal Growth Factor (EGF) family of Receptor Tyrosine Kinases is important in regulation of cell growth and survival. It comprises of four receptors: EGFR (HER1), ErbB-2/neu (HER2), ErbB3 (HER3) and ErbB4

(HER4).65 EGFR is a cell surface protein that binds to EGF leading to activation of a cascade of signal transduction pathways such as PI3K/Akt/mTOR, Ras/Raf/MAPK resulting in proliferation, invasion and angiogenesis. It is present in normal tissues but is also found to be over-expressed in many solid tumors, including cervical cancer.[83] Increased EGFR expression has been reported to be positively correlated with poor prognosis and tumor aggressiveness.[22] Oncogenic proteins, E6 and E7 encoded by HPV 16 have been shown to alter growth and differentiation of epithelial cells via EGFR pathway.[88] Inhibitors of EGFR, such as gefitinib,[65] lapatinib,[65] erlotinib,[65,89] nimotuzumab,[22] trastuzumab,[65] cetuximab,[22,65] and panitumumab[65] have proven to be efficacious and are being evaluated in cervical cancer patients. Various medicinal plants such as *Curcuma longa,*[82] *Camellia sinensis,*[22,67] *Ficus religiosa,*[40] *Cinnamomum cassia,*[48] and Gallic acid[90] have been shown to targetEGFR pathway.

9.3.5.3 MATRIX METALLOPROTEINASES (MMPS)

MMPs belong to a family of zinc proteases and have been found to be responsible for degradation of extracellular matrix that is required for cell migration, metastasis, and angiogenesis. Recent studies have indicated an association between the presence of MMPs and HPV in cervical cancer.[91,92] Elevated expression of MMP 2, 9, 13 and 15 have been reported in invasive cervical carcinomas.[93–95] Various medicinal plants have been reported to regulate MMP expression. A herbal formulation, Guizhi–Fuling decoction composed of *Cinnamomum cassia Blume, Paeonia lactiflora Pall, Paeonia suffruticosa Andrews, Prunus persica Batsch* and *Poria cocos Wolf*[96] has been shown to down regulate MMPs in cervical cancer. Other medicinal plants such as *Curcuma longa,*[97] *Ficus religiosa,*[40] and *Cinnamomum cassia*[48] have been shown to reduce the expression of MMP2.

9.3.6 INFLAMMATORY MARKERS ASSOCIATED WITH CERVICAL CANCER

9.3.6.1 COX-2

Numerous studies focus on relationship between inflammation and cancer.[98] Cyclooxygenase-2 (COX-2) is involved in inflammation, pathogenesis and progression of cancer by affecting cell proliferation, mitosis, cell adhesion, apoptosis, immune surveillance, and/or angiogenesis,[99,100] Moreover, *in vitro* and *in vivo* studies have shown that expression of COX-2 promotes expression of angiogenic factors VEGF and bFGF in cancer cells.[101,102] COX-2 is over-expressed in cervical cancer and is a biomarker for early detection.[103] Earlier studies have reported that COX-2 plays an important role in inflammation and its increased expression was found in precancerous intraepithelial lesions in cervical cancer.[98] Recent studies correlate Cox-2 expression with severity of cervical cancer precursor (CIN) lesions, invasive disease and lymph node metastasis. Medicinal plants such as *Curcumin longa,*[97] *Vitis vinifera* (resveratrol),[104] genistein,[105] *Camellia sinensis* (Epigallocatechin gallate),[106] and *Selaginella tamariscina* (amentoflavone)[107] have been shown to down regulate the expression of COX-2 resulting into decreased inflammation, angiogenesis and growth inhibition in cervical cancer.

9.3.6.2 NF-κB

The nuclear factor kB (NF-κB) is a transcription factor found to mediate several pathways and number of processes such as inflammation, cell survival, cell proliferation, invasion, angiogenesis, metastasis and chemoresistance.[108] HPV E6 and E7 have been reported to increase the activity of NF-kB.[22] Cervical cancer progression is positively associated with the activation of NF-κB and different target genes (VEGF and MMPs), which promote the proliferation and metastasis of cancer cells.[109] NF-κB has also been shown to regulate COX-2 expression in cancer cells. Increased oxidative stress in the cell due to exposure to environmental carcinogens may activate expression of NF-kB.[110] Consequently, NF-kB has emerged as a promising anti-cancer target. Epigallocatechin gallate (EGCG),[106] *Vitis vinifera* (Resveratrol),[104] *Curcuma wenyujin*[111] and some of the herbal formulations such as Basant [composed of different components such as diferuloylmethane (curcumin), purified extracts of *Emblica officinalis* (amla), purified saponins from *Sapindus mukorossi*, aloe vera and rose water][112,113] have been reported to reduce NF-κB activity. Reduction of this activity in turn hampered the growth of cancer cells though induction of apoptosis.[111]

9.4 CONCLUSION

Medicinal plants are composed of a plethora of bioactive phytochemicals having anticancer activity. It is evident from many clinical trials that phytochemicals exhibit excellent promise in the management of cervical cancer. Up till now there has been great advancement in elucidating the pathways involved in cervical cancer. Targeting multiple pathways to develop novel drugs to achieve better cure rates with limited or no toxicity to the patients could be possible with the use of medicinal plants and should be explored further.

KEYWORDS

- **cervical cancer**
- **signaling pathways**
- **medicinal plants**
- **cell cycle**
- **apoptosis**
- **angiogenesis**

REFERENCES

1. Bruni, L. ICO Information Centre on HPV and Cancer (HPV Information Centre). *Human Papilloma virus and Related Diseases in the World;* Summary Report 2014–02–20. (accessed Nov 27, 2014).
2. Ali, F.; Kuelker, R.; Wassie, B. Understanding Cervical Cancer in the Context of Developing Countries. *Ann. Trop. Med. Public. Health.* **2012,** *5,* 3–15.
3. Molassiotis, A.; Fernadez-Ortega, P.; Pud, D. et al. Use of Complementary and Alternative Medicine in Cancer Patients: a European Survey. *Ann. Oncol. ESMO.* **2005,** *16*(4), 655–63. Doi:10.1093/Annonc/Mdi110.
4. Kaefer, C. M.; Milner, J. A. The Role of Herbs and Spices in Cancer Prevention. **2009,** *19*(6), 347–361. Doi:10.1016/J.Jnutbio.2007.11.003.
5. Bruni, L. ICO Information Centre on HPV and Cancer (HPV Information Centre). *Human Papillomavirus and Related Diseases in India;* Summary Report 2014–02–20. (accessed Nov 27, 2014).

6. Singh, S.; Badaya, S. A Strategy to Increase the Uptake of Cervical Cancer Screening In India: A Lesson from the Ongoing Programs. *South Asian J. Cancer.* **2013,** *2*(4), 201.
7. Richter, K. L. Alternative Sampling Methods for Cervical Cancer Screening: Practical Perspectives from the Laboratory. *South Afr. J. Gynaecol. Oncol.* **2013,** *5*(2), S5–S9.
8. Moody, C. A.; Laimins, L. A. Human Papillomavirus Oncoproteins : Pathways to Transformation. *Nat. Rev. Cancer.* 2010; *10*(8), 550–560. Doi:10.1038/Nrc2886
9. Domenico, F.; Di, Foppoli, C.; Coccia, R.; Perluigi, M. Biochimica Et Biophysica Acta Antioxidants In Cervical Cancer : Chemopreventive And Chemotherapeutic Effects Of Polyphenols. *BBA - Molecular Basis Of Disease.* **2012,** *1822*(5), 737–747. Doi:10.1016/J.Bbadis.2011.10.005.
10. Guo, C.; Liu, K.; Luo, H.; Chen, H. et al. Potent Anti-Tumor Effect Generated by a Novel Human Papillomavirus (HPV) Antagonist Peptide Reactivating the Prb/E2F Pathway. *PLoS One*. **2011,** *6*(3). Doi:10.1371/Journal.Pone.0017734.
11. Tan, W. et al. Anti-Cancer Natural Products Isolated from Chinese Medicinal Herbs. *Chin. Med.* **2011,** *6*(1), 27.
12. Chaudhuri, R. S; Mandal, S. Current Status of Knowledge, Attitude and Practice (KAP) and Screening for Cervical Cancer in Countries at Different Levels of Development. *Asian Pac. J. Cancer Prev.* **2012,** *13*(9), 4221–4227.
13. Liang, X. J. et al. Circumventing Tumor Resistance to Chemotherapy by Nanotechnology. *Methods Mol. Biol.(Clifton, N.J.)* **2010,** *596,* 467–488.
14. Mohan, A. et al. Combinations of Plant Polyphenols & Anti-Cancer Molecules: A Novel Treatment Strategy for Cancer Chemotherapy. *Anticancer Agents Med. Chem.* **2013,** *13*(2), 281–95.
15. Liao, G. S. et al. Herbal Medicine and Acupuncture for Breast Cancer Palliative Care and Adjuvant Therapy. *Evid. Based Complement. Alternat. Med.* 2013, *2013,* 437948. DOI:10.1155/2013/437948.
16. Wheat, J; Currie, G. Herbal Medicine for Cancer Patients: An Evidence Based Review. *Internet J. Alternat. Med.* **2007,** *5*(2).
17. Dias, D. A.; Urban, S.; Roessner, U. A Historical Overview of Natural Products in Drug Discovery. *Metabolites*. **2012,** *2*(2), 303–336.
18. Kaur, R. et al. Plants as a Source of Anticancer Agents. *J. Nat. Prod. Plant Resour.* **2011,** *1*(1), 119–124.
19. Baikar, S.; Malpathak, N. Secondary Metabolites as DNA Topoisomerase Inhibitors: A New Era towards Designing of Anticancer Drugs. *Pharmacogn. Rev.* **2010,** *4*(7), 12–26.
20. Sakarkar, D.; Deshmukh, V. Ethnopharmacological Review of Traditional Medicinal Plants for Anticancer Activity. *Int. J. Pharm. Tech. Res.* **2011,** *3*(1), 298–308.
21. Wu, J. Phosphatidylinositol 3-Kinase Signaling as a Therapeutic Target for Cervical Cancer. *Curr. Cancer Drug Targets*. **2013,** *13*(2), 143–56.
22. Dwarampudi, L. P. et al. The Potential Therapeutic Targets for Cervical Cancer. *Int. J. Health Allied Sci.* **2013,** *2,* 69–74.
23. Topcul, M.; Cetin, I. Endpoint of Cancer Treatment: Targeted Therapies. *Asian Pac. J. Cancer Prev.* **2014,** *15*(11), 4395–4403.

24. Wang, S. et al. Evodiamine Synergizes with Doxorubicin in the Treatment of Chemoresistant Human Breast Cancer without Inhibiting P-Glycoprotein. *PLoS One.* **2014,** *9*(5), E97512.
25. Heer, H.; Mehan, S. Cellular Signals like MAPK/NF-Kb/M-TOR Mediated Drug Resistance: A Promising Concept in Cancer Research. *Pharmacologia.* **2013,** *4,* 414–427.
26. Yadav, V. R. et al. Targeting Inflammatory Pathways by Triterpenoids for Prevention and Treatment of Cancer. *Toxins.* **2010,** *2*(10), 2428–2466.
27. Chen, X. W. et al. Interaction of Herbal Compounds with Biological Targets: A Case Study with Berberine. *Scientific World J.* **2012,** 31. DOI:10.1100/2012/708292.
28. Poyil, P. K. et al. Cancer Prevention with Promising Natural Products: Mechanisms of Action and Molecular Targets. *Anti-Cancer Agents Med. Chem.* **2012,** *12,* 1159–1184.
29. Kma, L. Roles of Plant Extracts and Constituents in Cervical Cancer Therapy. *Asian Pac. J. Cancer Prev.* **2013,** *14*(6), 3429–3436.
30. Stewart, D.; Ghosh, A.; Matlashewski, G. Involvement of Nuclear Export in Human Papillomavirus Type 18 E6-Mediated Ubiquitination and Degradation of P53. *J. Virol.* **2005,** *79*(14), 8773–83. Doi:10.1128/JVI.79.14.8773–8783.2005.
31. Beaudenon, S.; Huibregtse, J. M. HPV E6, E6AP and Cervical Cancer. *BMC Biochem.* **2008,** *9* (Suppl 1), S4. Doi:10.1186/1471–2091—9–S1–S4.
32. Wang, J.; Sampath, A; Raychaudhuri, P.; Bagchi, S. Both Rb and E7 are Regulated by the Ubiquitin Proteasome Pathway in HPV-Containing Cervical Tumor Cells. *Oncogene.* **2001,** *20*(34), 4740–9. Doi:10.1038/Sj.Onc.1204655.
33. Singh, S.; Johnson, J.; Chellappan, S. Small Molecule Regulators of Rb-E2F Pathway as Modulators of Transcription. *Biochim.. Biophys. Acta.* **2010,** *1799*(10–12), 788–94. Doi:10.1016/J.Bbagrm.2010.07.004.
34. Diane, M. et al. Curcumin Suppresses Human Papillomavirus Oncoproteins, Restores p53, Rb, and PTPN13 Proteins and Inhibits Benzo[A]Pyrene-Induced Upregulation of HPV E7. *Mol. Carcinog.* **2011,** *50*(1), 47–57.
35. Munagala, R.; Kausar, H.; Munjal, C.; Gupta, R. C. Withaferin A Induces P53-Dependent Apoptosis by Repression of HPV Oncogenes and Upregulation of Tumor Suppressor Proteins in Human Cervical Cancer Cells. *Carcinogenesis.* **2011,** *32*(11), 1697–705. Doi: 10.1093/Carcin/Bgr192.
36. Zou, C. P. et al. Green Tea Compound in Chemoprevention of Cervical Cancer. *Int. J. Gynecol. Cancer.* **2010,** *20*(4), 617–624.
37. Li, G. L. et al. HPV E6 Down-regulation and Apoptosis Induction of Human Cervical Cancer Cells by a Novel Lipid-Soluble Extract (PE) from *Pinellia Pedatisecta* Schott *In Vitro. J. Ethnopharmacol.* **2010,** *132*(1), 56–64. Doi: 10.1016/J.Jep.2010.07.035.
38. Kim, M. S. et al. Wogonin Induces Apoptosis by Suppressing E6 and E7 Expressions and Activating Intrinsic Signaling Pathways in HPV-16 Cervical Cancer Cells. *Cell Biol. Toxicol.* **2013,** *29*(4), 259–72. Doi: 10.1007/S10565–013–9251–4.
39. Mahata, et al. Berberine Modulates AP-1 Activity to Suppress HPV Transcription and Downstream Signaling to Induce Growth Arrest and Apoptosis in Cervical Cancer Cells. *Mol. Cancer.* **2011,** *10,* 39.
40. Choudhari, A. S.; Suryavanshi, S. A.; Kaul-Ghanekar, R. The Aqueous Extract of Ficus Religiosa Induces Cell Cycle Arrest in Human Cervical Cancer Cell Lines SiHa

(HPV-16 Positive) and Apoptosis in HeLa (HPV-18 Positive). *PLoS One.* **2013,** *8*(7), E70127.

41. Lee, S. et al. The Bioflavonoid Amentoflavone Induces Apoptosis via Suppressing E7 Expression, Cell Cycle Arrest at Sub-G_1 Phase, and Mitochondria-Emanated Intrinsic Pathways in Human Cervical Cancer Cells. *J. Med. Food.* **2011,** *14*(7–8), 808–16. Doi: 10.1089/Jmf.2010.1428.
42. Lowe, S. W.; Lin, A. W. Apoptosis In Cancer. *Carcinogenesis.* **2000,** *21*(3), 485–495.
43. Bredesen, D. E.; Mehlen, P.; Rabizadeh, S. Apoptosis and Dependence Receptors: A Molecular Basis for Cellular Addiction. *Physiol. Rev.* **2004,** *84*(2), 411–430.
44. Bishayee, K. et al. Quercetin Induces Cytochrome-C Release and ROS Accumulation to Promote Apoptosis and Arrest the Cell Cycle in G2/M, In Cervical Carcinoma: Signal Cascade and Drug-DNA Interaction. *Cell Prolif.* **2013,** *46*(2), 153–163.
45. Chakraborty, D. et al. [6]-Gingerol Induces Caspase 3 Dependent Apoptosis and Autophagy in Cancer Cells: Drug–DNA Interaction and Expression of Certain Signal Genes in Hela Cells. *Eur. J. Pharmacol.* **2012,** *694*(1), 20–29.
46. Singh, M. et al. Tea Polyphenols Induce Apoptosis through Mitochondrial pathway and by Inhibiting Nuclear Factor-kappaB and Akt Activation in Human Cervical Cancer Cells. *Oncol. Res.* **2011,** *19*(6), 245–257.
47. Ahmad, N. et al. Green Tea Constituentepigallocatechin-3-Gallate and Induction of Apoptosis and Cell Cycle Arrest in Human Carcinoma Cells. *J. Natl. Cancer Inst.* **1997,** *89*(24), 1881–1886.
48. Koppikar, S. et al. Aqueous Cinnamon Extract (ACE-c) From Bark of *Cinnamomum Cassia* causes apoptosis through Loss of Mitochondrial Membrane Potential. *BMC Cancer.* **2010,** *10,* 210.
49. Masrianif, et al. Pycnarrhena Cauliflora Ethanolic Extract Induces Apoptosis and Cell Cycle Arrest in Hela Human Cervical Cancer Cells. *Int. J. Res. Pharm. Biomed. Sci.* **2013,** *4*(4), 1060–1068.
50. Moirangthem, et al. Antioxidant, Antibacterial, Cytotoxic, and Apoptotic Activity of Stem Bark Extracts of Cephalotaxus Griffithii Hook. F. *BMC Complement. Altern. Med.* **2012,** *12,* 30.
51. Kraft, T. E. et al. Fighting Cancer with Red Wine? Molecular Mechanisms of Resveratrol. *Crit. Rev. Food Sci. Nutr.* **2009,** *49,* 782–799.
52. Yang, G. L. et al. Effects of Honokiol on Proliferation and Apoptosis of Human Cervical Carcinoma Cell Line Hela In Vitro. *Sichuan. Da. Xue Xue Bao Yi Xue Ban.* **2008,** *39*(4), 558–62.
53. Wang, S. Y. et al. The Differential Inhibitory Effects of Genistein on the Growth of Cervical Cancer Cells In Vitro. *Neoplasma.* **2001,** *48*(3), 227–33.
54. Qun, L. et al. The Cytotoxicity Mechanism of 6-Shogaol-Treated HeLa Human Cervical Cancer Cells Revealed by Label-Free Shotgun Proteomics and Bioinformatics Analysis. *Evid. Based Complement. Alternat. Med.* **2012,** 278652, Doi:10.1155/2012/278652.
55. Yaoxian, W. et al. Emodin Induces Apoptosis of Human Cervical Cancer Hela Cells Via Intrinsic Mitochondrial and Extrinsic Death Receptor Pathway. *Cancer Cell Int.* **2013,** *13,* 71.
56. Liang, L. D. et al. Ginsenoside-Rg5 Induces Apoptosis and DNA Damage in Human Cervical Cancer Cells. *Mol. Med. Rep.* **2015,** *11,* 940–946.

57. Devika, V; Mohandass, S. Apoptotic Induction of Crude Extract of *Foeniculum Vulgare* Extracts on Cervical Cancer Cell Lines. *Int. J. Curr. Microbiol. Appl. Sci.* **2014,** *3*(3), 657–661.
58. Ganesh, G. et al. Cytotoxic and Apoptosis Induction Potential of *Mimusops Elengil.* In Human Cervical Cancer (SiHa) Cell Line. *J. King Saud Univ. Sci.* **2014,** *26,* 333–337.
59. Mohammad, R. et al. The Apoptotic and Cytotoxic Effects of *Polygonum avicular* Extract on Hela-S Cervical Cancer Cell Line. *Afr. J. Biochem. Res.* **2011,** *5*(14), 373–378.
60. Duenas-Gonzalez, A. et al. New Molecular Targets against Cervical Cancer. *Int. J. Womens Health.* **2014,** *6,* 1023–1031.
61. Soonthornthum, T. et al. Epidermal Growth Factor Receptor as a Biomarker for Cervical Cancer. *Ann. Oncol.* **2011,** *22,* 2166–2178.
62. Pal, I.; Mandal, M. PI3K and Akt as Molecular Targets for Cancer Therapy: Current Clinical Outcomes. *Acta Pharmacol. Sin.* **2012,** *33,* 1441–1458.
63. Chen, Y. J. et al. Total Synthetic Protoapigenone WYC02 Inhibits Cervical Cancer Cell Proliferation and Tumour Growth through PIK3 Signalling Pathway. *Basic Clin. Pharmacol. Toxicol.* **2013,** *113,* 8–18.
64. Liu, Y. et al. Liquiritigenin Inhibits Tumor Growth and Vascularization in a Mouse Model of HeLa Cells. *Molecules.* **2012,** *17,* 7206–7216.
65. Vici, P. et al. Emerging Biological Treatments For Uterine Cervical Carcinoma. *J. Cancer.* **2014,** *5*(2), 86–97.
66. Ji, J.; Zheng, P. S. Activation of mTOR Signaling Pathway Contributes to Survival of Cervical Cancer Cells. *Gynecol. Oncol.* **2010,** *117,* 103–8.
67. Sah J.; Balasubramanian, S. et al. Epigallocatechin-3-Gallate Inhibits Epidermal Growth Factor Receptor Signaling Pathway. Evidence for Direct Inhibit if ERK ½ and AKT Kinases. *J. Biol. Chem.* **2004,** *79*(13), 12755–12762.
68. Lee, S; Kim, H. et al. The Bioflavonoid Amentoflavone Induces Apoptosis Via Suppressing E7 Expression, Cell Cycle Arrest at Sub-G_1 Phase, And Mitochondria-Emanated Intrinsic Pathways in Human Cervical Cancer Cells. *J. Med. Food.* **2011,** *14*(7–8), 808–16. Doi: 10.1089/Jmf.2010.1428.
69. Bhushan S. et al. Activation of P53/P21/PUMA Alliance and Disruption of PI-3/Akt in Multimodal Targeting of Apoptotic Signaling Cascades in Cervical Cancer Cells by a Pentacyclic Triterpenediol from Boswellia Serrata. *Mol. Carcinog.* **2009,** *48*(12), 1093–108. Doi: 10.1002/Mc.20559.
70. Kim, S. H.; Kim, Y. B. et al. Genistein Inhibits Cell Growth by Modulating Various Mitogen Activated Protein Kinases and Akt in Cervical Cancer Cells. *Ann. N Y Acad. Sci.* **2009,** *1171,* 495–500.
71. Sexton, E.; Themsche, C. et al. Resveratrol Interferes with AKT Activity and Triggers Apoptosis in Human Uterine Cancer Cells *Mol. Cancer.* **2006,** *5,* 45. Doi: 10.1186/1476–4598–5–45.
72. Hyun, S.; Kim, M. et al. The Peroxisome Proliferator-Activated Receptor-Gamma Agonist 4-Omethylhonokiolinduces Apoptosis by Triggering the Intrinsic Apoptosis Pathway and Inhibiting the PI3K/Akt Survival Pathway in SiHa Human Cervical Cancer Cells. *J. Microbiol. Biotechnol.* MB Papers in Press, Jan 7, 2015DOI: 10.4014/Jmb.1411.11073

73. Ramachandran, R. et al. AKT Inhibitors Promote Cell Death in Cervical Cancer through Disruption of mTOR Signaling and Glucose Uptake. *PLoS One.* **2014,** *9*(4), 1–12.
74. Farrand, L. et al. Phytochemicals: A Multitargeted Approach to Gynecologic Cancer Therapy. *Biomed Res. Int.* **2014,** Article ID 890141, 10 Pages: DOI:10.1155/2014/890141.
75. Munshi, A.; Ramesh, R. Mitogen-Activated Protein Kinases And Their Role In Radiation Response. *Genes. Cancer.* **2013,** *4*(9–10), 401–408.
76. Santarpia, L.; Lippman, S. L.; El-Naggar, A. K. Targeting the MA P K- RAS-RAF Signaling Pathway in Cancer Therapy. *Expert Opin. Ther. Targets.* **2012,** *16*(1), 103–119.
77. Huang, Q. et al. Silymarin Augments Human Cervical Cancer Hela Cell Apoptosis Via P38/JNK MAPK Pathways In Serum-Free Medium. *J. Asian Nat. Prod. Res.* **2005,** *7*(5), 701–709.
78. Binion, D. G.; Otterson, M. F.; Rafiee, P. Curcumin Inhibits VEGF-Mediated Angiogenesis in Human Intestinal Microvascular Endothelial Cells through COX-2 And MAPK Inhibition. *Gut.* **2008,** *57,* 1509–1517.
79. Zhen, Y. Z. et al. Rheinlysinate Inhibits Cell Growth by Modulating Various Mitogen-Activated Protein Kinases in Cervical Cancer Cells. *Oncol. Lett.* **2011,** *2,* 129–133,
80. Eunjung, L. et al. Cytotoxic Activity of 3,6-Dihydroxyflavone in Human Cervical Cancer Cells and its Therapeutic Effect on C-Jun N-Terminalkinase Inhibition. *Molecules.* **2014,** *19,* 13200–13211; Doi:10.3390molecules190913200.
81. Wu, M. P.; Chou, C. Y. Angiogenesis, Thrombospondin-1 and Cervical Carcinogenesis. *Taiwane. J. Obstet. Gynecol.* **2005,** *44*(2), 128–138. Doi:10.1016/S1028–4559 (09) 60124–8.
82. Pornphrom, Y. C. et al. Antitumor and Antiangiogenic Activities of Curcumin in Cervical Cancer Xenografts in Nude Mice. *Biomed Res. Int.* **2014,** ***2014,*** 12. DOI:10.1155/2014/817972.
83. Ramalho, A. S. et al. Molecular Targets for Therapeutic Interventions in Human Papillomavirus-Related Cancers (Review). *Oncol. Rep.* **2010,** *24,* 1419–1426.
84. Jeong, S. J. et al. Antiangiogenic Phytochemicals and Medicinal Herbs. *Phytother. Res.* 2010; DOI: 10.1002/Ptr.3224.
85. Zhang, Q.; Tang, X.; Lu, Q.; Zhang, Z.; Rao, J.; Le, A. D., Green Tea Extract and (-)-Epigallocatechin-3-Gallate Inhibit Hypoxia- and Serum-Induced HIF-1 alpha Protein Accumulation and VEGF Expression in Human Cervical Carcinoma and Hepatoma Cells. *Mol. Cancer Ther.* **2006,** *5*(5), 1227–1238.
86. Yang, L. et al. Wogonin Induces G1 Phase Arrest through Inhibiting Cdk4 and cyclin D1 Concomitant with an Elevation in p21Cip1 in Human Cervical Carcinoma HeLa Cells. *Biochem. Cell Biol.* **2009,** *87,* 933–942.
87. Tang, X. et al. Overexpression of Human Papillomavirus Type 16 Oncoproteins Enhances Hypoxia-Inducible Factor 1 Alphaprotein Accumulation and Vascular Endothelial Growth Factor Expression in Human Cervical Carcinoma Cells. *Clin. Cancer Res.* **2007,** *13,* 2568–2576.
88. Ward, M. D.; Leahy, D. J. Kinase Receiver-Activator Preference in ErbB Heterodimers Determined by Intracellular Regions and Not Coupled to Extracellular Asymmetry. *J. Biol. Chem.* **2014,** DOI: 10.1074/Jbc.M114.612085.

89. Woodworth, C. D. et al. Inhibition of the Epidermal Growth Factor Receptor by Erlotinib Prevents Immortalization of Human Cervical Cells by Human Papillomavirus Type 16. *Virol.* **2011,** *421*(1), 19–27.
90. Zhao, B.; Hu, M. Gallic Acid Reduces Cell Viability, Proliferation, Invasion and Angiogenesis in Human Cervical Cancer Cells. *Oncol. Lett.* **2013,** *6*(6), 1749–1755.
91. Rajkumar, T.; Sabitha, K.; Vijayalakshmi, N.; Shirley, S.; Bose, M. V.; Gopal, G.; Selvaluxmy, G. Identification and Validation of Genes Involved in Cervical Tumourigenesis. *BMC Cancer.* **2011,** *11,* 80. Doi:10.1186/1471–2407–11–80.
92. Hagemann, T. et al. Molecular Profiling of Cervical Cancer Progression. *Br. J. Cancer.* **2007,** *96*(2), 321–8. Doi:10.1038/Sj.Bjc.6603543.
93. Ung, Y. H.; Eki, M. U. Correlation Between Vascular Endothelial Growth Factor-C Expression and Invasion Phenotype in Cervical Carcinomas. *Int. J. Cancer.* **2002,** *343,* 335–343. Doi:10.1002/Ijc.10193.
94. Deryugina, E. I.; Quigley, J. P. Matrix Metalloproteinases and Tumor Metastasis, *Cancer Metastasis. Rev.* **2006,** 9–34. Doi:10.1007/S10555–006–7886–9.
95. Boccardo, E.; Lepique, A. P.; Villa, L. L. The Role of Inflammation in HPV. *Carcinogenesis.* 2010; *31*(11), 1905–1912. Doi:10.1093/Carcin/Bgq176.
96. Yao, Z.; Shulan, Z. Inhibition Effect of Guizhi-Fuling-Decoction on the Invasion of Human Cervical Cancer. *J. Ethnopharmacol.* **2008,** *120,* 25–35.
97. Maher, D. M. et al. Curcumin Suppresses Human Papillomavirus Oncoproteins, Restores P53, Rb, And Ptpn13 Proteins and Inhibits Benzo[A]Pyrene-Induced Upregulation of HPV E7. *Mol. Carcinog.* **2011,** *50*(1), 47–57.
98. Young, J. L. et al. Cyclooxygenase-2 in Cervical Neoplasia: A Review. *Gynecol. Oncol.* **2008,** *109*(1), 140–5. Doi:10.1016/J.Ygyno.2008.01.008.
99. Trappen, P. O. et al. A Model for Co-Expression Pattern Analysis of Genes Implicated in Angiogenesis and Tumour Cell Invasion in Cervical Cancer. *Br. J. Cancer.* **2002,** 537–544. Doi:10.1038/Sj.Bjc.6600471.
100. Harris, R. E. Cyclooxygenase-2 (Cox-2) and the Inflammogenesis of Cancer. *Subcell Biochem.* **2007,** *42,* 93–126.
101. Kim, M. H. et al. Expression of Cyclooxygenase-1 and -2 Associated with Expression of VEGF in Primary Cervical Cancer and at Metastatic Lymph Nodes. *Gynecol. Oncol.* **2003,** *90*(1), 83–90. Doi:10.1016/S0090–8258(03)00224–5.
102. Sreekanth, C. N. et al. Molecular Evidences for the Chemosensitizing Efficacy of Liposomal Curcumin in Paclitaxel Chemotherapy in Mouse Models of Cervical Cancer. *Oncogene.* **2011,** *30*(28), 3139–3152. Doi:10.1038/Onc.2011.23.
103. Saldivar, J. S.; Lopez, D.; Feldman, R. A.; Tharappel-Jacob, R.; de la Rosa, A.; Terreros, D.; Baldwin, W. S. COX-2 Overexpression as a Biomarker of Early Cervical Carcinogenesis: a Pilot Study. *Gynecol. Oncol.* **2007,** *107(*1 Suppl 1), S155–62. Doi:10.1016/J.Ygyno.2007.07.023.
104. Aggarwal, B. B. et al. Role of Resveratrol in Prevention and Therapy of Cancer: Preclinical and Clinical Studies. *Anticancer Res.* **2004,** *24*(5A), 2783–840.
105. Wang, J. et al. Both Rb and E7 are Regulated by the Ubiquitin Proteasome Pathway in HPV-Containing Cervical Tumor Cells. *Oncogene.* **2001,** *20*(34), 4740–4749. Doi:10.1038/Sj.Onc.1204655.
106. Zou, C. P. et al. Green Tea Compound in Chemoprevention of Cervical Cancer. *Int. J. Gynecol. Cancer.* **2010,** *20*(4), 617–624.

107. Lee, S. et al. The Bioflavonoid Amentoflavone Induces Apoptosis Via Suppressing E7 Expression, Cell Cycle Arrest at Sub-G_1 Phase, And Mitochondria-Emanated Intrinsic Pathways in Human Cervical Cancer Cells. *J. Med. Food.* **2011,** *14*(7–8), 808–16. Doi: 10.1089/Jmf.2010.1428.
108. Hoesel, B.; Schmid, J. A. The Complexity of NF- KB Signaling in Inflammation and Cancer. *Mol. Cancer.* **2013,** *12*(1), 1. Doi:10.1186/1476–4598–12–86.
109. Huang, A. et al. Involvement of Matrix Metalloproteinases in the Inhibition of Cell Invasion and Migration through the Inhibition of NF- KB by the New Synthesized Ethyl 2- [N - P -Chlorobenzyl- (2 ' - (JOTO1007) in Human Cervical Cancer Caski Cells, *Vivo.* **2009,** *23,* 23, 613–619.
110. Kim, S.; Oh, J. Involvement of NF- KB and AP-1 in COX-2 Upregulation by Human Papillomavirus 16 E5 Oncoprotein. *Carcinogenesis.* **2009,** *30,* 753–757.
111. Lim, C. et al. Curcuma Wenyujin Extract Induces Apoptosis and Inhibits Proliferation of Human Cervical Cancer Cells In Vitro and In Vivo. *Integr. Cancer Ther.* **2010,** *9*(1), 36–49. Doi: 10.1177/1534735409359773.
112. Talwar, G. P. et al. A Novel Polyherbal Microbicide with Inhibitory Effect on Bacterial, Fungal and Viral Genital Pathogens. *Int. J. Antimicrob. Agents.* **2008,** *32*(2), 180–185.
113. Basu, P. et al. Clearance of Cervical Human Papilloma Virus Infection by Topical Application of Curcumin and Curcumin Containing 120 Polyherbal Cream: A Phase II Randomized Controlled Study. *Asian Pac. J. Cancer Preven.* **2013,** *14*(10), 5753–5759.

CHAPTER 10

AUDIO VISUAL ENTRAINMENT AND ACUPRESSURE THERAPY FOR INSOMNIA

G. HEMA, MARIYA YELDHOS, SOWMYA NARAYANAN, and L. DHIVYALAKSHMI*

Department of Biomedical Engineering, Sri Ramakrishna Engineering College, Anna University, Coimbatore, Tamil Nadu, India

**E-mail: dhiviyalakshmi.lakshmipathy@srec.ac.in*

CONTENTS

ABSTRACT

Insomnia is one of the most prevalent psychological disorders worldwide. Some of the deficiencies of the current treatments of insomnia are: side effects in the case of sleeping pills and high costs in the case of psychotherapeutic treatment. In this paper, we propose a device which provides a combination of audiovisual entrainment (AVE) and acupressure therapy for insomnia. This device provides drug-free treatment of insomnia through a user friendly and portable device that enables relaxation of brain and muscles, with certain advantages such as low cost, and wide accessibility to a large number of people. Tools adapted toward the treatment of insomnia are audio, visual, and acupressure points unit. Audio unit consists of continuous exposure to binaural beats of a particular frequency of audible range, visual unit comprises of flash of LED light, and the acupressure points were found to be as GB-20, GV-16, and B-10.

10.1 INTRODUCTION

In today's competitive world, stress is inevitable. This leads to conditions like insomnia (lack of sleep) of which many are unaware. Such conditions cause a lot of physiological as well as psychological harm. Insomnia is one of the most common sleep disorders, with a prevalence of 40% in adults. As of now, insomnia is primarily treated using sleeping pills. These are harmful in the long run as they suppress one stage of the sleep cycle and essentially cause long-term damage in the name of temporary relief and high costs in the case of psychotherapeutic treatment.

10.2 OBJECTIVE

The main objective of developing this project is to provide drug-free treatment for insomnia through audiovisual entrainment (AVE) and acupressure techniques by means of a user friendly and portable device that enables relaxation of brain and muscles.

10.3 BRAINWAVES

The brain is made up of billions of brain cells called neurons, which communicate by means of electrical signals. The combination of millions of neurons sending signals at once produces an enormous amount of electrical activity in the brain, which can be detected using sensitive electrodes that measure electricity levels over areas of the scalp. The combination of electrical activity of the brain is commonly called a brainwave pattern, because of its cyclic, wave-like nature. Brainwaves are divided into bandwidths to describe their function but are best thought of as a continuous spectrum of consciousness. The brainwaves change according to actions and emotions. When slower brainwaves are dominant one may feel tired, slow, or dreamy. The higher frequencies are dominant when one feels active or alert. The brainwaves are classified based on frequency as alpha, beta, theta, and delta. They are depicted in Figure 10.1.

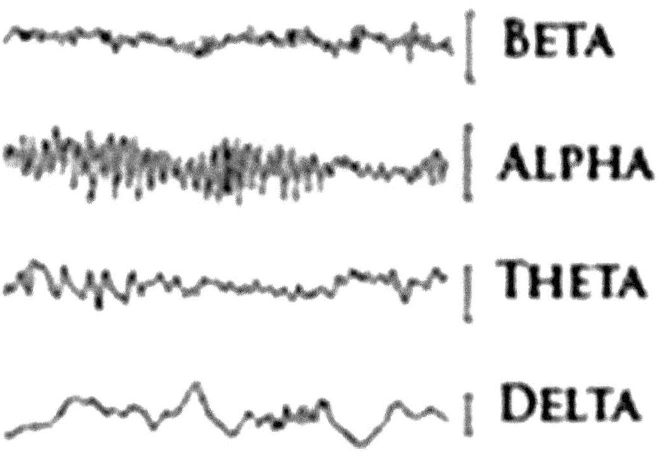

FIGURE 10.1 Brainwaves observed in the human brain.

Alpha waves (8–12 Hz) - Alpha brainwaves are present during quietly flowing thoughts, but not quite meditation. Alpha is the resting state for the brain. Alpha waves aid overall mental coordination, calmness, alertness, mind/body integration, and learning.

Beta waves (12–38 Hz) - Beta brainwaves dominate the normal waking state of consciousness when attention is directed toward cognitive tasks and the outside world. Beta is a "fast" activity, present when we are alert, attentive, engaged in problem solving, judgment, decision making, and engaged in focused mental activity.

Theta waves (3–8 Hz) - Theta brainwaves occur most often in sleep but are also dominant in the deep meditation. It acts as the gateway to learning and memory. In theta, the senses are withdrawn from the external world and focused on signals originating from within. It is that twilight state which is normally experienced while drifting off to sleep.

Delta waves (0.5–3 Hz) - Delta brainwaves are the slowest but loudest brainwaves. They are generated in deepest meditation and dreamless sleep. Healing and regeneration are stimulated in this state, and that is why deep restorative sleep is so essential to the healing process.

10.4 SLEEP

It is a widely perceived notion that sleep is a passive, dormant part of our daily lives. However, the human brain is actually very active during sleep. Moreover, sleep affects our physical and mental health in various ways. Nerve signaling chemicals called neurotransmitters determine whether we are asleep or awake by acting on neurons in the brain. The neurons in the brainstem produce neurotransmitters such as serotonin and norepinephrine that keep some parts of the brain active while we are awake. There is a chemical called adenosine that builds up in blood while we are awake and causes drowsiness. This chemical gradually breaks down while we are asleep.

10.4.1 THE SLEEP CYCLE

The brain passes through various stages during sleep which is collectively known as the sleep cycle. There are five stages of sleep, namely: 1, 2, 3, 4, and REM which progress in a repetitive, cyclic manner. This is illustrated in Figure 10.2.

During stage 1, which is light sleep, one drifts in and out of sleep and can be awakened easily. The eyes move very slowly and muscle activity slows. People awakened from stage 1 sleep often remember fragmented visual images. Many also experience sudden muscle contractions called hypnic myoclonia, often preceded by a sensation of starting to fall. When entering stage 2 sleep, the eye movements stop and brain waves become slower, with occasional bursts of rapid waves called sleep spindles. In stage 3, extremely slow brain waves called **delta waves** begin to appear, interspersed with smaller, faster waves. By stage 4, the brain produces delta waves almost exclusively. It is very difficult to wake someone during stages 3 and 4, which together are called deep sleep. There is no eye movement or muscle activity. When the brain switches into REM sleep, the breathing becomes more rapid, irregular, and shallow, the eyes jerk rapidly in various directions, and the limb muscles become temporarily paralyzed. Heart rate and blood pressure are shown to increase. This is the stage of the sleep cycle in which dreams occur.

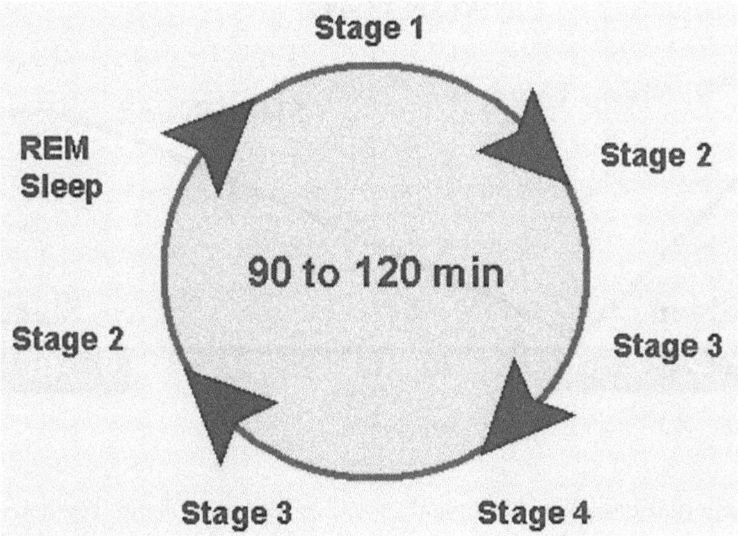

FIGURE 10.2 Stages of the sleep cycle.

The first REM sleep period usually occurs about 70–90 min after falling asleep. A complete sleep cycle takes 90–110 min on average. The first sleep cycles each night contain relatively short REM periods and long periods of deep sleep. As the night progresses, REM sleep periods increase in length while deep sleep decreases. By morning, people spend nearly all their sleep time in stages 1, 2, and REM.

10.4.2 SLEEP AND CIRCADIAN RHYTHM

Sleep is regulated by two body systems: sleep/wake homeostasis and the circadian biological clock. When awake for a long period of time, sleep/wake homeostasis signals that a need for sleep is accumulating and that it is time to sleep. It also helps to maintain enough sleep throughout the night to make up for the hours of being awake. If this restorative process existed alone, it would mean that one would be most alert as our day was starting out, and that the longer one was awake, the more one would feel like sleeping. In this way, sleep/wake homeostasis creates a drive that balances sleep and wakefulness. This phenomenon is portrayed in the diagram Figure 10.3.

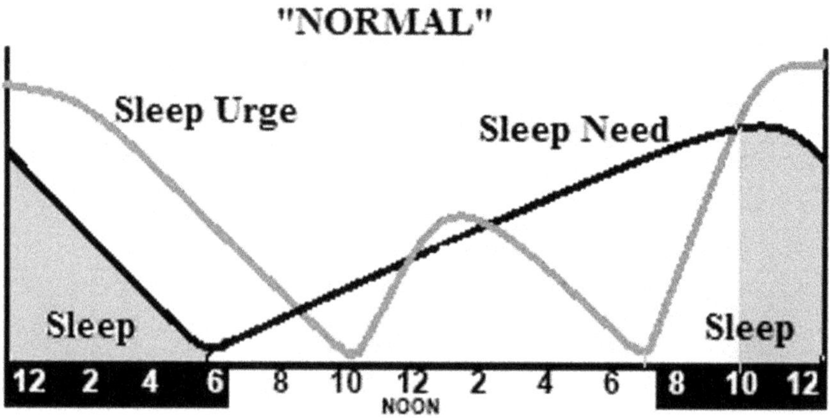

FIGURE 10.3 Normal circadian sleep rhythm.

The internal circadian biological clock, on the other hand, regulates the timing of periods of sleepiness and wakefulness throughout the day. The circadian rhythm dips and rises at different times of the day, so adults' strongest sleep drive generally occurs between 2:00–4:00 am and in the afternoon between 1:00–3:00 pm, although there is some variation from individual to individual. The sleepiness experienced during these circadian dips would be less intense if one has had sufficient sleep, and more intense when sleep deprived. The circadian rhythm also causes more alertness at certain points of the day, despite long periods of wakefulness where sleep/

wake restorative process would otherwise cause sleepiness. The diagrammatic representation of this clock is portrayed in Figure 10.4.

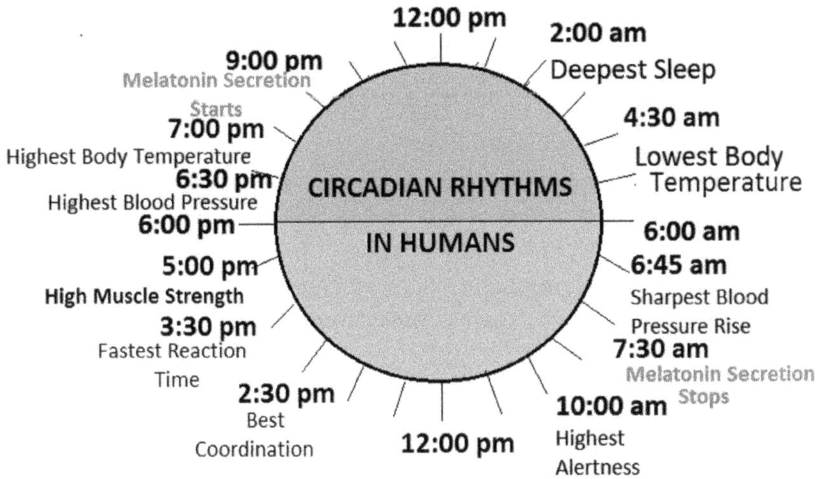

FIGURE 10.4 The biological clock in human beings.

The circadian biological clock is controlled by a part of the brain called the suprachiasmatic nucleus (SCN), a group of cells in the hypothalamus that respond to light and dark signals. From the optic nerve of the eye, light travels to the SCN, signaling the internal clock that it is time to be awake. The SCN signals to other parts of the brain that control hormones, body temperature and other functions that play a role in making us feel sleepy or awake.

In the mornings, with exposure to light, the SCN sends signals to raise body temperature and produce hormones like cortisol. The SCN also responds to light by delaying the release of other hormones like melatonin, which is associated with sleep onset and is produced when the eyes signal to the SCN that it is dark. Melatonin levels rise in the evening and stay elevated throughout the night, promoting sleep.

Onset of conditions like insomnia can occur when the circadian rhythm is disrupted by keeping long and irregular hours. Because of this, it is important to keep a regular sleep schedule and allow plenty of time for quality sleep, allowing these two vital biological components, namely, the sleep/wake restorative process and the circadian rhythm to regulate sleep.

10.5 CAUSES OF INSOMNIA

Insomnia is a general term that refers to difficulty in falling asleep. This condition may be caused by a wide variety of factors including medical factors, psychiatric issues, and brain conditions. There are many medical conditions that can lead to insomnia. In some cases, a medical condition itself causes insomnia, while in other cases, symptoms of the condition cause discomfort that can make it difficult for a person to sleep.

Examples of medical conditions that can cause insomnia are:

- Nasal/sinus allergies
- Gastrointestinal problems such as reflux
- Endocrine problems such as hyperthyroidism
- Arthritis
- Asthma
- Neurological conditions such as Parkinson's disease
- Chronic pain
- Low back pain

Medications such as those taken for the common cold and nasal allergies, high blood pressure, heart disease, thyroid disease, birth control, asthma, and depression can also cause insomnia. In addition, insomnia may be a symptom of underlying sleep disorders. For example, restless legs syndrome, a neurological condition in which a person has an uncomfortable sensation of needing to move his or her legs can lead to insomnia. Sleep apnea is another sleep disorder linked to insomnia. With sleep apnea, a person's airway becomes partially or completely obstructed during sleep, leading to pauses in breathing and a drop in oxygen levels. This causes a person to wake up briefly but repeatedly throughout the night. People with sleep apnea sometimes report experiencing insomnia.

Insomnia can be caused by psychiatric conditions such as depression. Psychological struggles can make it hard to sleep, insomnia itself can bring on changes in mood, and shifts in hormones and physiology can lead to both psychiatric issues and insomnia at the same time. Sleep problems may represent a symptom of depression, and the risk of severe insomnia is much higher in patients with major depressive disorders. Studies show that insomnia can also trigger or worsen depression. It is important to know that symptoms of depression and insomnia can be linked, and one can make the other worse. Fortunately both are treatable, regardless of which came first.

Most adults have had some trouble sleeping because they feel worried or nervous, but for some it's a pattern that interferes with sleep on a regular basis. Anxiety symptoms that can lead to insomnia include:

- Tension
- Getting caught up in thoughts about past events
- Excessive worrying about future events
- Feeling overwhelmed by responsibilities
- A general feeling of being over stimulated

These symptoms of general anxiety can make it difficult to sleep. Anxiety may be associated with onset insomnia (trouble falling asleep), or maintenance insomnia (waking up during the night and not being able to return to sleep). In either case, the quiet and inactivity of night often brings on stressful thoughts or even fears that keep a person awake. When this happens for many nights, one might start to feel anxiousness, dread, or panic at just the prospect of not sleeping. This is how anxiety and insomnia can feed each other and become a cycle that should be interrupted through treatment. There are cognitive and mind-body techniques that help people with anxiety settle into sleep, and overall healthy sleep practices that can improve sleep for many people with anxiety and insomnia.

10.6 TREATMENT OF INSOMNIA

Insomnia is a curable disorder and is treated in various ways ranging from medication to counseling. There are many different types of sleep aids for insomnia, including over-the-counter (non-prescription) and prescription medications. Major classes of prescription insomnia medications include benzodiazepine hypnotics, non-benzodiazepine hypnotics, and melatonin receptor agonists. These drugs are useful for temporary relief but in the long run, they affect the REM stage of the sleep cycle and cause imbalance. This causes dependency on the pills as one is unable to fall asleep naturally. Continuous use of such medications causes irreversible damage to the kidneys and liver.

There are psychological and behavioral techniques that can be helpful for treating insomnia. Relaxation training, stimulus control, sleep restriction, and cognitive behavioral therapy (CBT) are some examples. Relaxation training, or progressive muscle relaxation, teaches the person to systematically tense and relax muscles in different areas of the body. This helps to calm the body and induce sleep. Other relaxation techniques that help many people sleep involve breathing exercises, mindfulness, meditation techniques, and guided imagery. Stimulus control helps to build an association between the bedroom and sleep by limiting the type of activities allowed in the bedroom. An example of stimulus control is going to bed only when you are sleepy, and getting out of bed if you have been awake for 20 min or more. This helps to break an unhealthy association between the bedroom and wakefulness. Sleep restriction involves a strict schedule of bedtimes and wake times and limits time in bed to only when a person is sleeping. CBT includes behavioral changes, but it adds a cognitive or "thinking" component. CBT works to challenge unhealthy beliefs and fears around sleep and teach rational, positive thinking. There is a good amount of research supporting the use of CBT for insomnia. For example, in one study, patients with insomnia attended one CBT session via the internet per week, for six weeks. After the treatment, these people had improved sleep quality. However, such treatment comes at an expensive price and requires continuous sessions with a specialist.

10.6.1 PROPOSED DEVICE AND METHODOLOGY

This project aims in designing a device which provides a combination of AVE and acupressure based compression therapy for insomnia. This device provides drug-free treatment of insomnia through a user friendly and portable device that provides relaxation to the brain and muscles, with certain advantages such as low cost, and wide accessibility to a large number of people.

Tools adapted toward the treatment of insomnia:

- **Audio unit**
    - How: Continuous exposure to binaural beats of a particular frequency of audible range.
    - Why: Binaural beats are preferred over various other auditory stimuli as they are proved to have a therapeutic effect and are a vital component of AVE.

- **Visual unit**
  - How: Flash of red colored LED light.
  - WHY: Red colored light is used as a form of light therapy to stimulate melatonin generation which in turn aids sleep.

- **Acupressure points**
  - How: Acupressure points are stimulated using massage vibrators.
  - Why: The points selected are associated with sleep and relaxation. These points are Governing Vessel (GV) 16, Gall Bladder (GB) 20, and Bladder (B) 10.

Bright light therapy or phototherapy is more widely used to treat seasonal affective disorder, but is also an effective method of adjusting sleep-wake timing [1]. Light therapy is often used to synchronize sleep patterns with the external day and night. In people with a delayed circadian rhythm, the internal biological clock can be shifted to an earlier position and aligned with the external environment through exposure to appropriately timed light in the morning. Similarly, for people whose internal clocks are set too early, the internal clock can be shifted to a later time with evening light exposure. The timing of light treatment with respect to the position of the internal clock is critical. **From this it is inferred that light therapy can be used to reset the body's internal clock.**

When light is pulsed into the eyes or tones pulsed into the ears, the nerve pathways from the eyes and ears carry the evoked potentials into the thalamus. When a repetitive stimulus of the proper frequency and sufficient strength to excite the thalamus is present, their frequency signature is shown in the EEG. AVE dissociates those experiencing PTSD away from destructive distressing rumination, increases blood flow, normalizes brain wave and neurotransmitter production, calms the limbic system, restores the adrenals, and produces somatic relaxation. The subjective benefits of AVE are reduced anxiety, improved sleep, improved mood, increased energy, improved relationships with family and civilians, reduced physical problems, improved productivity and reduced dependence for medications or self-medicating on alcohol and recreational drugs. **From this, it is inferred that AVE can be used to produce relaxation of the brain waves and induce sleep. It is observed that entrainment occurs best near the natural alpha frequency from 9 to 11 Hz.**

Melatonin is well recognized for its role as a potent antioxidant and is directly implicated in the free radical theory of aging[2]. Moreover, melatonin has been shown to retard age-related increases in lipid peroxidation and oxidative damage. Melatonin protects hepatic mitochondrial respiratory chain activity in senescence-accelerated mice and to act directly upon the immune system. The red light treatment has also been successfully implemented in the clinical setting for its effectiveness in reducing various conditions like ADHD, post-traumatic stress disorder and insomnia. From this, it is inferred that red light is associated with melatonin generation which in turn induces sleep.

Acupuncture therapy, commonly used in clinical practice in oriental cultures, has the potential to produce a positive effect with patients experiencing insomnia[3]. Acupuncture treatment methods for insomnia used various meridian points on the whole body. The use of complementary therapies for insomnia may enable individuals to experience improved health and increase their quality of life. Here the research was done by randomizing the clinical trials to determine the effectiveness of acupuncture. **From this, it is inferred that acupuncture therapy has the potential to produce a positive effect on people experiencing insomnia.**

Insomnia is one of the most common sleep disorder with a prevalence of 40% in adults[4]. It is generally believed that 10–15% of the adult population suffers from chronic insomnia, and an additional 25–35% has transient or occasional insomnia. Nondrug therapy including acupuncture is commonly used by patients with insomnia. The mechanism of acupuncture treatment may be regulating yin and yang to reinforce health and eliminate the pathogenic, thus improving sleep. **From this, it is inferred that acupuncture appears to be effective in treatment of insomnia.**

Inferences

1. Light therapy can be used in order to control the biological clock and thereby cause drowsiness.
2. AVE can be used to manipulate the brainwaves into a state of sleep. The delta waves that are observed during sleep can be mimicked using this technique.
3. Red light can be used to stimulate melatonin generation which in turn induces sleep.
4. Acupuncture therapy has a positive effect on insomnia patients. As acupressure follows the same principles, it can be used to the same effect.

5. Acupuncture is found to be effective in insomnia therapy.

10.6.2 AUDIO VISUAL AND ACUPRESSURE UNIT

In this device, two fundamental concepts, namely AVE and acupressure have been used. AVE is achieved using separate audio unit, which consists of a binaural beat generator and visual unit, by means of which light therapy is provided. Acupressure therapy is provided using a separate massage unit, in which the acupressure points are stimulated by vibrators. The overall block diagram combining these three units is given below as Figure 10.5.

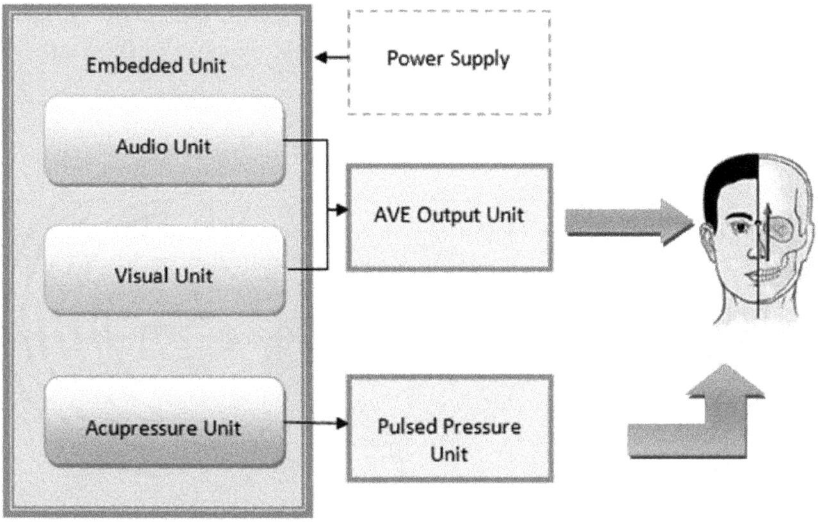

FIGURE 10.5 Overall block diagram of the therapy unit.

10.6.2.1 AUDIO UNIT

10.6.2.1.1 Binaural Beats

Binaural beats are used for the audio unit. They are one of the key components of AVE. Binaural beats are auditory processing artifacts caused by specific physical stimuli. This effect was discovered in 1839 by Heinrich Wilhelm Dove and earned greater public awareness in the late 20th century based on claims coming from the alternative medicine community that binaural beats could help induce relaxation, meditation, and other desirable mental states.

The effect on the brainwaves depends on the difference in frequencies of each tone: For example, if 100 Hz was played in one ear and 110 in the other, then the binaural beat would have a frequency of 10 Hz. The brain produces a phenomenon resulting in low-frequency pulses in the amplitude and sound localization of a perceived sound when two tones at slightly different frequencies are presented separately, one to each of a subject's ears, using stereo headphones. A beating tone will be perceived, as if the two tones mixed naturally, out of the brain. The frequencies of the tones must be below 1000 Hz for the beating to be noticeable. The difference between the two frequencies must be small (less than or equal to 30 Hz) for the effect to occur; otherwise, the two tones will be heard separately, and no beat will be perceived. This concept is illustrated in Figure 10.6.

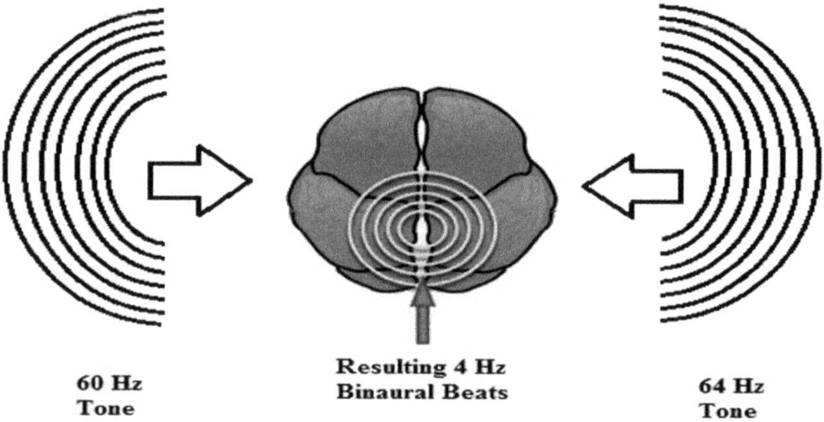

FIGURE 10.6 Generation of 4 Hz binaural beats.

Binaural beats may influence functions of the brain in ways besides those related to hearing. This phenomenon is called "frequency following response." The concept is that if one receives a stimulus with a frequency in the range of brain waves, the predominant brainwave frequency is said to be likely to move toward the frequency of the stimulus and this process is called entrainment. This is the principle behind the audio unit of the device.

10.6.2.1.2 Description of Audio Unit

The audio unit consists of two frequency generators, each of which produces a different frequency in order to create binaural beats. The sound is repeated at regular intervals and is controlled by a microcontroller. The output of the frequency generators is given to the brain using padded headphones in order to ensure patient comfort. The volume can be controlled by the user as per their convenience. As two different frequencies are generated, one is given to each ear. The frequencies used are 60 and 64 Hz. The difference between these two frequencies is 4 Hz which lies within the delta wave range (0–4 Hz). As delta waves are associated with sleep, this causes the brain waves to be lulled into a state of relaxation.

10.6.2.2 VISUAL UNIT

10.6.2.2.1 Audio Visual Entrainment

The visual unit is used to complete the phenomenon of AVE. This utilizes the binaural beats discussed in the audio unit as well as visual stimuli produced in the visual unit. AVE, a subset of brainwave entrainment, uses flashes of lights and pulses of tones to guide the brain into various states of brainwave activity. AVE devices are often termed light and sound machines or mind machines. Altering brainwave activity is believed to aid in the treatment of psychological and physiological disorders.

All of our senses (except smell) access the brain's cerebral cortex via the thalamus, and because the thalamus is highly innervated with the cortex, sensory stimulation can easily influence cortical activity. Touch, photic, and auditory stimulation are capable of affecting brain wave activity. A large area of skin must be stimulated to affect brainwaves, which leaves both auditory and photic stimulation as the most effective and easiest means of affecting brain activity. Therefore, mind machines are typically in the form of light and sound devices.

Auditory or visual stimulation can take a variety of forms, generating different subjective and clinical effects. AVE involves organized, repetitive stimulation at a particular frequency for a specific period of time, and the frequency of stimulation is reflected within the EEG. This is called "open loop" stimulation, or free-running entrainment, and it does not require continuous monitoring. "Close loop" AVE would involve visual and auditory stimulation in response to one's EEG similar to biofeedback.

10.6.3 LIGHT THERAPY AND MELATONIN STIMULATION

The pattern of waking during the day when it is light and sleeping at night when it is dark is a natural part of human life. A key factor in how human sleep is regulated is exposure to light or to darkness. Exposure to light stimulates a nerve pathway from the retina in the eye to an area in the brain called the hypothalamus. There, a special centre called the suprachiasmatic nucleus (SCN) initiates signals to other parts of the brain that control hormones, body temperature and other functions that play a role in making us feel sleepy or wide awake.

Melatonin is a natural hormone made by the pineal gland, a small gland located above the middle of the brain. During the day the pineal is inactive. When the sun goes down and darkness occurs, the pineal is activated by the SCN and begins to produce melatonin, which is released into the blood. Usually, this occurs around 9 pm. As a result, melatonin levels in the blood rise sharply and drowsiness sets in. The melatonin level in the blood stays elevated for about 12 h after which it falls back to low daytime levels by about 9 am. Daytime levels of melatonin are barely detectable. This process is illustrated in Figure 10.7.

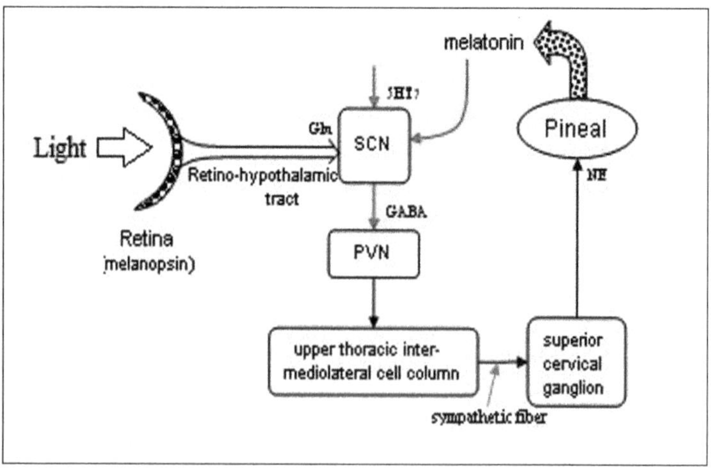

FIGURE 10.7 Light therapy and melatonin stimulation.

Bright light therapy can be used to treat insomnia, by promoting melatonin generation which in turn induces sleep[5]. The light stimulation is given in the evening in order to maintain the circadian rhythm. The color used here is red which activates the pineal gland and causes production of melatonin.

10.6.4 DESCRIPTION OF VISUAL UNIT

The visual unit consists of an eyepiece fitted with red LEDs that glow in a periodic manner, emitting light at regular intervals in a pulsed sequence. This flashing of light is controlled by a microcontroller. This is used to enhance the effect of the binaural beats and bring about AVE. The eyepiece is padded with two layers of sponge material. This is done in order to shield the eye from excessive light and heat produced by the LED. It also adds to patient comfort. Red colored light is chosen particularly because it enhances melatonin generation, which in turn is associated with inducing sleep.

10.6.4.1 SELECTION OF SHIELDING MATERIAL

In the visual unit, it was found that direct contact between the human eyelid and the LED would lead to adverse effects such as heating and overexposure. In order to avoid these harmful outcomes, the eyepiece was padded with shielding material. So as to decide which material would best shield the human eye from heat, a simple study was carried out. Here, five red LEDs were taken of which four were covered with various shielding materials and one was taken as the control device. The LEDs were turned on at the same time and the heat dissipation was measured at 15 min intervals using a thermistor. The materials studied were sponge, cotton, polyester, and sponge lined with cotton. Ultimately sponge lined with cotton was found to be the most effective shielding material. The comparison is depicted graphically in Figure 10.8.

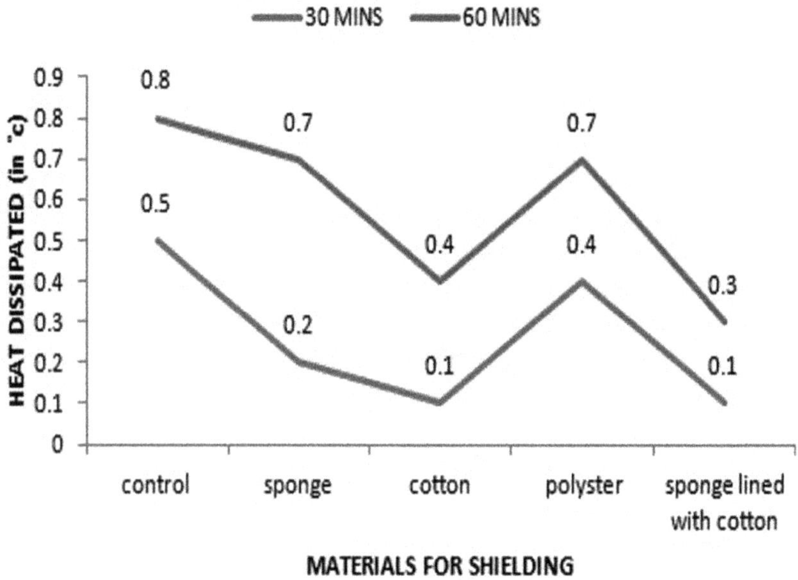

FIGURE 10.8 Graphical analysis of shielding material selection.

10.6.5 ACUPRESSURE UNIT

10.6.5.1 ACUPRESSURE CONCEPTS

Acupressure is an ancient Chinese technique used as alternative medicine[6]. Although numerous acupressure points exist in the body that can induce sleep, the following points have been selected after consultation with experts and bearing in mind other considerations such as device design, patient comfort, and a smaller target area.

The chosen acupressure points are GV 16, GB 20, and B 10. GV 16 stands for "Governing Vessel 16" and is known as the Wind Mansion. It is located directly below the occipital protuberance on the posterior midline of the head. This point has been chosen as it if considered to promote communication between the head and body and eliminate fear and negative thoughts, thereby inducing a relaxed state of mind.

GB 20 stands for "Gall Bladder 20" and is also known as the Wind Pool. The location of this point is in a depression between the upper portion of the sternocleidomastoid muscle and the trapezius, level with GV 16. It is associated with relief of head and neck pain, muscle relaxation in these areas and all issues associated with the brain.

B 10 stands for "Bladder 10" and is known as the Heavenly Pillar. It is located about a half-inch from the base of the skull on the muscles bordering the spine; this point can relieve the fatigue and emotional distress of insomnia. Thorough research has proved that the selected points, aside from being proven to induce sleep, have other advantages such as balancing out of the sympathetic and parasympathetic nervous system, reducing stress and inducing relaxation throughout the body.

The 5 points that have been selected for the acupressure unit are anatomically depicted in Figure 10.9.

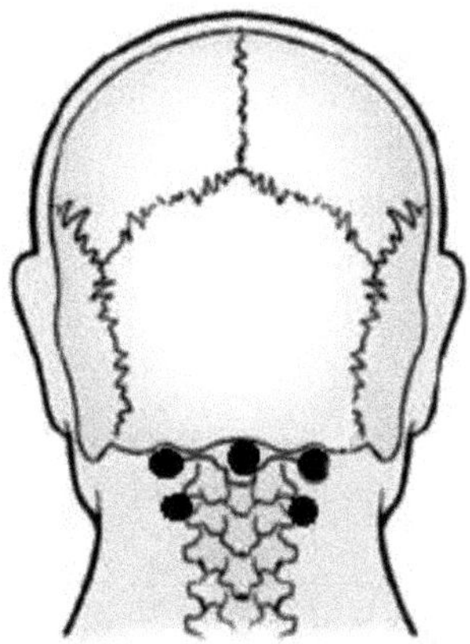

FIGURE 10.9 Acupressure points for insomnia.

10.6.5.2 DESCRIPTION OF ACUPRESSURE UNIT

In this device, acupressure concepts are used to treat insomnia in a non-invasive user-friendly method. The acupressure points associated with sleep are massaged in a continuous manner using a specially designed vibrator that is used to stimulate the particular points. The vibrator consists of five miniature mobile motors capable of continuous motion about an axis. The motors are attached to a woolen neckpiece and are stitched in place. The arrangement of the motors is based on the location of the acupressure points. The speed of the motor can be controlled by means of a potentiometer.

10.6.5.3 HARDWARE DESIGN

In this device, the hardware implementation is carried out using five major components. They are:

- Power supply
- PIC microcontroller
- 555 timer
- Light emitting diode
- Massage vibrator

10.6.5.4 POWER SUPPLY UNIT

The power supply units are mainly designed to convert high voltage AC mains electricity into a suitable low voltage supply for electronic circuits and other devices. The power supply unit can be divided into a series of blocks with each block performing specific function. The blocks include transformer, rectifier, filter, and regulator units (Fig. 10.10).

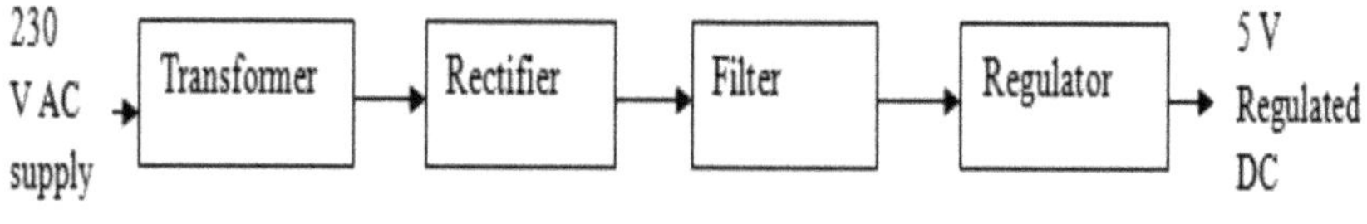

FIGURE 10.10 Block diagram of power supply unit.

The 230 V mains AC supply is converted into low voltage by the step down transformer. The secondary of the transformer is connected to rectifier which delivers a rectified DC output. The DC output is filtered using a simple resistor, capacitor network which provides a DC output. The output of the filter is connected to a regulator to provide a regulated DC voltage of about 5 V. The regulator consists of three pins namely input pin for connecting input, ground pin, and an output pin. The step down transformer used in this work provides a 12–0–12 V at output.

10.6.5.4.1 Microcontroller (PIC16F887A)

PIC 16F887A is an enhanced CMOS flash based eight bit microcontroller with 256 bytes of EEPROM memory provided with two comparators, 14 channels of analog to digital (A/D) convertor, a synchronous serial port and an Enhanced Universal Asynchronous Receiver Transmitter (EUSART). This controller features 14 KB of program memory which facilitates control of multiple operations by a single controller. The A/D convertor caters the sensing operation and the EEPROM memory facilitates reprogramming up to 1000 times. These features make PIC 16F887 ideal for controlling the flashing of the LED lights and to synchronize with the binaural beats.

Specification of microcontroller (PIC16F887A)

- Operating speed 20 MHZ oscillator/clock input
- Direct, indirect, and relative addressing modes
- Software selectable frequency range 8 MHZ to 31 KHZ
- Operating voltage range 2.2–5.5 V
- Industrial and extended temperature range
- Operating current 11 μA @ 32 KHZ
- Watch dog timer current 1 μA @ 2.0 V

10.6.6 PIN DESCRIPTION FOR INSOMNIA THERAPY

The 40 PINS in PIC 16F887 are grouped into five ports namely A, B, C, D, and E containing eight PINS in each port. The role of PORT is to receive information from external source such as sensor or to send information to external elements. The corresponding data registers for these ports are TRIS A, TRIS B, TRIS C, TRIS D, and TRIS E, respectively. In this work, the PIN 2 in port A is connected to the potentiometer, which controls the speed of the massage vibrator. The port D containing PIN 19 is connected to the red color LED which gives flashes of light in certain time interval (Fig. 10.11). The PIN 15 belonging to port C is used to control the vibrator unit. The port B containing the PINS 33 and 34 is connected to frequency generator circuit, which produces binaural beats of 60 and 64 Hz. Figure 10.12 shows the pin description of PIC 16F887.

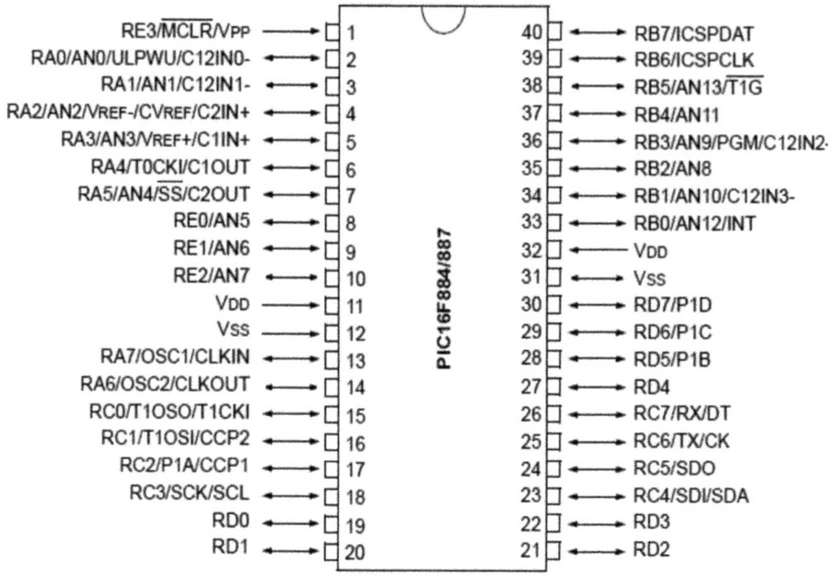

FIGURE 10.11 PIN diagram of PIC 16F887A.

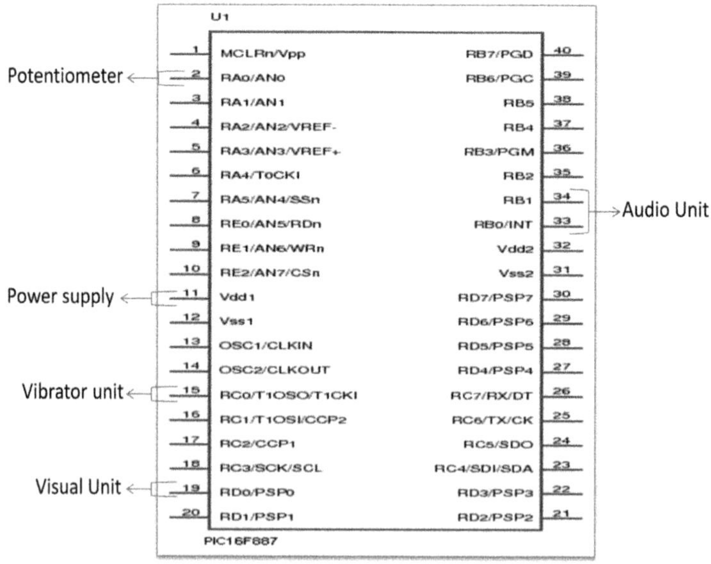

FIGURE 10.12 PIN description of PIC 16F887.

10.6.6.1 555 TIMER

The 555 timer is an integrated circuit (a circuit built on a piece of semi conductor material that performs a defined function) which can be used in many applications which require oscillator, pulse generation, or timer controlled devices. The 555 timer has three operating modes; monostable, astable, and bistable. This utilizes the 555 in astable mode, thus we will focus on the basics of astable operation. In astable mode, the 555 outputs a constant stream of rectangular pulses. The rectangular pulses will be outputted at a specific frequency that is defined by the components that are placed in between the pins of the 555 timer. Figure 10.13 shows the pin description of 555 timer.

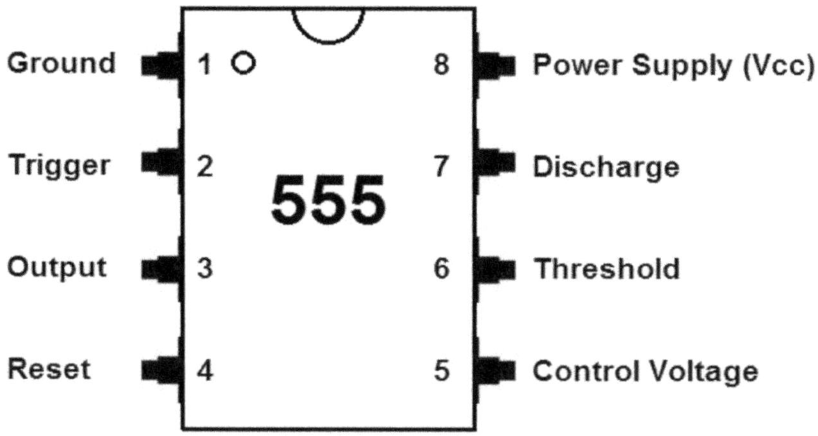

FIGURE 10.13 Pin description of 555 timer.

The frequency 60 and 64 Hz are generated using 555 timer. Trigger pin is connected to 33rd and 34th pin of microcontroller. The output is taken from 3rd pin of 555 timer and connected to headphones to listen binaural beats.

10.6.6.2 MASSAGE VIBRATOR

Precision Microdrives Model 304-015 are small in size, they can still be powerful enough to be used in massaging and stimulation applications.

PicoVibe™ motors are popular for use in hand held products because their variety of shapes and sizes makes them easy for design and mounting. They primarily contain smaller eccentric rotating mass motors, aimed at lighter or handheld applications. Figure 10.14 shows the precision micro drives vibrator model 304-015 used for acupressure therapy.

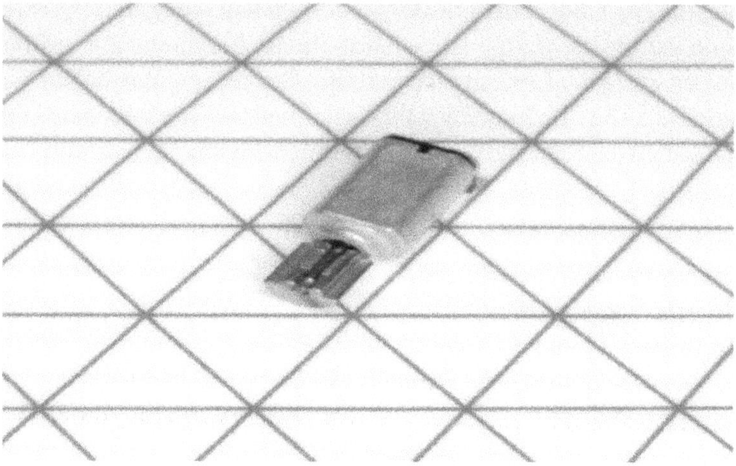

FIGURE 10.14 Precision microdrives vibrator model 304-015.

The specifications of the vibrator used in this work are:

- Body diameter: 4.1 mm [+/−0.2]
- Body length: 6.8 mm [+/−0.2]
- Counter weight radius: 1.4 mm [+0.08/−0.1]
- Counter weight length: 3 mm [+/−0.1]
- Shaft orientation: inline
- Rated operating voltage: 2.5 V
- Rated vibration speed: 11,000 rpm [+/−2500]
- Typical rated operating current: 25 mA
- Typical normalized amplitude: 0.25 G

10.6.6.3 LIGHT EMITTING DIODE

A light emitting diode (LED) is a two-lead semiconductor light source. It is a basic p-n junction diode, which emits light when activated. When a fitting voltage is applied to the leads, electrons are able to recombine with electron holes within the device, releasing energy in the form of photons. This effect is called electroluminescence, and the color of the light (corresponding to the energy of the photon) is determined by the energy band gap of the semiconductor. Figure 10.15 shows the LED used in visual unit.

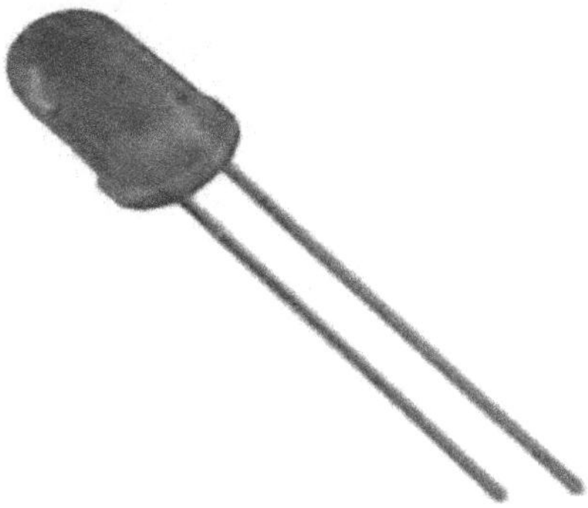

FIGURE 10.15 LED used in visual unit.

An LED is often small in area (less than 1 mm^2) and integrated optical components may be used to shape its radiation pattern. In this device the LED is used in order to indicate proper functioning of components as well as a part of the visual therapy unit.

10.7 RESULTS AND DISCUSSION

The result or outcome of the project is analyzed by testing it on patients of insomnia and analyzing the electroencephalogram of the patient to check whether the delta wave (pertaining to sleep) appears. This was done and the results were analyzed.

10.8 RESULT ANALYSIS

In order to analyze the efficiency of the device used in the treatment of insomnia it was tested on various test subjects. The outcome was mostly positive. Thus, the device AVE and acupressure therapy for insomnia is effective.

The efficiency of the device used in treating insomnia was examined by conducting case study at Sri Ramakrishna Hospital, Coimbatore under the guidance of Dr. S Ananth, Consultant Psychiatrist, Counselor and Therapist, Sri Ramakrishna Hospital, Coimbatore with patients suffering from insomnia. The patient selection was based on the type and cause of insomnia. Mostly, patients suffering from mild ailments and simple insomnia were preferred. The patients who had insomnia due to underlying clinical conditions were not considered for the study.

The study was conducted in a simple yet efficient manner. The subjects were initially given a questionnaire to diagnose the disease. Then, they were given a trial of the instrument and the EEG was taken in both awake and in sleeping states. The subject was then questioned on the quality of sleep and as to whether the device assisted in falling asleep.

Questionnaire

The patients were initially subjected to this questionnaire in order to diagnose insomnia and get a basic idea of the patient history and lifestyle.

INSOMNIA ASSESMENT

S. NO.	QUESTIONS	YES	NO	MAYBE
1.	Do you have trouble falling asleep?			
2.	Do you wake up un-refreshed?			
3.	Do you take medications to help you sleep?			
4.	Do you use alcohol to help you sleep?			
5.	Do you have any medical conditions that disrupts your sleep?			
6.	Do you tend to feel nervous or worried?			
7.	Are you shift worker or is your sleep schedule irregular?			
8.	Do you have any unusual behavior or movements during sleep (E.g.: sleep walking, kicking etc)			
9.	Do you snore, gasp, snort or choke in your sleep?			
10.	Do you have difficulty staying awake during the day?			

Feedback form

After the trial of the device, patients were asked for their feedback in order to assess the quality of relaxation provided.

FEEDBACK FORM
AUDIO VISUAL ENTRAINMENT AND ACUPRESSURE THERAPHY FOR INS OMNIA

NAME: AGE:

1. Did you feel relaxed while using the device?
   ☐ Soothing ☐ No effect ☐ Disturbing
2. How did the light in the visual unit affect your sleep?
   ☐ Soothing ☐ No effect ☐ Disturbing
3. How did the sound in the audio unit affect your sleep?
   ☐ Soothing ☐ No effect ☐ Disturbing
4. How did the acupressure affect your sleep your sleep?
   ☐ Soothing ☐ No effect ☐ Disturbing
5. How long did it take you to fall a sleep>
6. What was the duration of your sleep?

PATIENT 1 (Fig. 10.16)

- Name : Marappa Gounder. N
- Age : 76 years
- Therapy duration : 10 min
- Sleep duration : 20 min

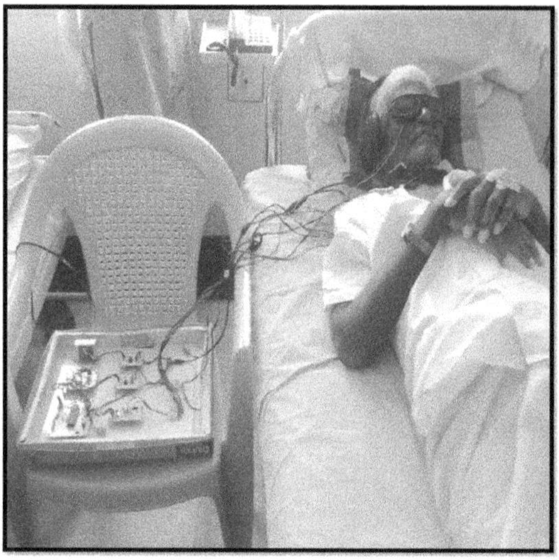

FIGURE 10.16 Testing of device in patient 1.

PATIENT 2 (Fig. 10.17)

- Name : Shanmuga Sundaram. S
- Age : 47 years
- Therapy duration : 15 min
- Sleep duration : 30 min

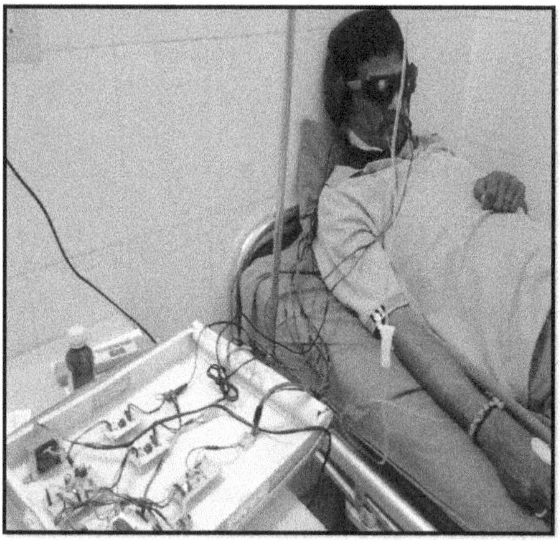

FIGURE 10.17 Testing of device in patient 2.

10.9 CONCLUSION AND FUTURE SCOPE

10.9.1 CONCLUSION

The therapy for insomnia using AVE and acupressure techniques has been successfully implemented and tested in patients. The device successfully induced relaxation in the patient followed by sleep. The advantage of this device is that therapeutic effect can be achieved without the aid of drugs and its portability ensures ease of use by patients.

10.9.2 FUTURE SCOPE

This device has been successfully implemented in patients.

10.10 DEVELOPMENTS FOR COMMERCIALIZATION

This device can be modified from the prototype used in the clinical trial room to a commercial product that can be distributed in medical markets all over the world.

- Rather than a separate PCB board, the circuit can be miniaturized and mounted within the acupressure unit. This improves portability.
- The use of wires can be minimized and a smaller, wireless model of the device can be designed.
- Different modes in the device can be made available to the user such that they are in control of the duration of each form of therapy. In this way, each patient can custom design their own course of therapy. Pre-set modes will also be available for easy operation.
- The device can be controlled using a mobile phone. This is one of the latest trends in technology and would make the device significant in the current market scenario.
- By miniaturization, the budget can be brought down further and the device will become more economically accessible to a greater number of people.

KEYWORDS

- **acupressure**
- **insomnia**
- **entrainment**
- **binaural beats**

REFERENCES

1. Siever, D.; Evans, J. Audio-Visual Entrainment: History, Physiology, and Clinical Studies. In *Handbook of Neurofeedback: Dynamics and Clinical Applications;* **2007** pp. 155–183.
2. Yeager, R. L.; Oleske, D. A.; Sanders, R. A.; Watkins, J. B. 3rd.; Eells, J. T.; Henshel, D. S. Melatonin as a Principal Component of Red Light Therapy. *Med. Hypothesis.* **2007,** *69*(2), 372–376.
3. Sok, S. R.; Erlen, J. A.; Kim, K. B. Effects of Acupuncture Therapy on Insomnia. *J. Adv. Nurs.* **2003,** *44*(4), 375–384.
4 Cao, H.; Pan, X.; Li, H.; Liu, J. Acupuncture for Treatment of Insomnia: A Systematic Review of Randomized Controlled Trials. *J. Altern. Complement. Med.* **2009,** *15*(11), 1171–1186.
5. Shirani, A.; St Louis, E. K. Illuminating Rationale and Uses for Light Therapy. *J. Clin. Sleep Med.* **2009,** *5*(2), 155–163.
6. Clark, M. T.; Clark, R. J.; Toohey, S.; Bradbury-Jones, C. Rationales and Treatment Approaches Underpinning the Use of Acupuncture and Related Techniques for Plantar Heel Pain: A Critical Interpretive Synthesis. *Acupunct. Med.* **2016,** acupmed-2015.

CHAPTER 11

A REVIEW ON MEDICINAL PLANTS USED IN CARDIOPROTECTIVE REMEDIES IN TRADITIONAL MEDICINE

S. SARANYA and V. VIJAYA PADMA*

Translational Research Laboratory, Department of Biotechnology, Bharathiar University, Coimbatore 641046, Tamil Nadu, India

**Corresponding author. E-mail: vvijayapadma@rediffmail.com*

CONTENTS

ABSTRACT

Cardiovascular diseases (CVD) are the number one cause of mortality worldwide; it can be developed due to use of some chemotherapeutic drugs, change of life style and some disease conditions. The drugs which induce cardiotoxicity include anthracyclines, isoproterenol, trastuzumab, 5-fluorouracil, cyclophosphamide (CP) and heavy metals like arsenic (As), cadmium, and lead. These drugs induce oxidative stress resulting in free radical generation which in turn causes cardiac injury. About 80% of the world population relies on the use of traditional medicine to combat different types of CVD. Recent studies have focused on various plant extracts, herbs, and polyherbal formulations to treat CVD. Medicinal plants possess antioxidant, anti-inflammatory and cardioprotective activity that prove useful in ameliorating the cardiotoxicity. The current review discusses the cardioprotective efficacy of various phytochemicals from medicinal plants.

11.1 INTRODUCTION

Cardiovascular diseases (CVD) are the leading cause of death in developing countries. CVD causes over 1.5 million deaths in the European Union (EU) and is the main cause of years of life lost from early death. CVD include coronary heart disease, myocardial infarction (MI), peripheral artery disease, rheumatic heart disease, and congenital heart disease.[1] Coronary heart disease is the most common type of heart disease, killing more than 385,000 people annually.[2] More than half of the deaths due to heart disease were reported in men.[2] The risk factors for the growing burden of CVD includes hypertension, dyslipidemia, diabetes, obesity, change of life style, physical inactivity, use of tobacco and some chemotherapeutics.[3] The drugs which induce cardiotoxicity include anthracyclines, isoproterenol, trastuzumab, 5-fluorouracil, CP and heavy metals like arsenic, cadmium, and lead. These drugs enhance the formation of free radicals leading to oxidative stress, which results in cardiac damage.[4]

Natural compounds and food products derived from medicinal plants have been widely used in ayurveda and siddha as a source of medicine for treating various CVD. Some 7000 natural compounds are currently used in modern medicine; most of these had been used for centuries by traditional healers.[5] Recently, attention has been focused on phytochemicals, such as flavonoids, phenolic diterpenes, alkaloids, and xanthone derived from different plant species as potential therapeutic agents in the prevention and management of CVD due to their antioxidant nature.[6] Efforts are being focused on promising phytochemicals from medicinal plants that have been tested in cardiotoxicity models.

11.2 CARDIOPROTECTIVE EFFECT OF MEDICINAL PLANTS

In Indian traditional medicine system, plant and plant formulations have been used to treat CVD for a long time. Many plants have been used in the traditional medicinal system for the treatment and management of cardiotoxicity. Some of them are *Allium sativum*, *Amaranthus viridis*, *Calotropis procera*, *Hybanthus enneaspermus*, *Inula racemosa*, *Nelumbo nucifera*, *Radix paeoniae rubrae*, *Rhodobryum roseum*, *Sida cordifolia*, *Spondias mombin*, and *Terminalia chebula*.

Natural compounds with cardioprotective activity include saffron (*Crocus sativus*), embelin (*Embelia ribes*), rutin (*Coriandrum sativum*), berberine (*Coptis chinensis*), piperine (*Rhodobryum roseum*), naringenin (*Citrus paradisi*), baicalein (*Scutellaria baicalensis*), silibinin (*Silybum marianum*), mangiferin (*Mangifera indica*), and puerarin (*Pueraria lobata*) (Table 11.1). Table 11.2 shows the various phytoconstituents derived from plant source.

TABLE 11.1 Chemical Constituents of Cardioprotective Medicinal Plants.

Plant name	Family	Chemical constituents
Aegle marmelos Ref.[7]	Rutaceae	Aegelin, alloimperatorin, marmelide, marmeline, marmelosin, marmesin, psoralen, skimming, tannic acid, xanthotoxol, and β-sitosterol.
Amaranthus viridis Ref.[8]	Amaranthaceae	Flavonoids, quercetin, saponins, glycosides, terpenoids, amino acids, alkaloids, carbohydrates, phenolic compounds, and proteins.
Andrographis paniculata Ref.[9]	Acanthaceae	Alkaloids, saponins, tannins, glycosides, fixed oils, phlobatannins, and simple sugars.
Artemisia afra Ref.[10]	Asteraceae	Flavone (acacetin), sesquiterpene (12α, 4α-dihydroxybishopsolicepolide), diterpene (phytol), and triterpenes.

TABLE 11.1 *(Continued)*

Plant name	Family	Chemical constituents
Azadirachta indica Ref.[11]	Meliaceae	Alkaloids, flavonoids, tannins, saponins, glycosides, anthraquinones, terpenes, and carbohydrate.
Calotropis procera Ref.[12]	Asclepiadaceae	Anthocyanins, Sterols, Glycosides, and Alkaloids.
Carica papaya Ref.[13]	Caricaceae	α-tocopherol, lycopene, benzyl isothiocyanate, papain, chymopapain, cystatin, ascorbic acid, cyanogenic glycosides, glucosinolates, alkaloids (carpain and carpasemine), triterpenes, organic acids and flavonoids, sulfurous compounds (benzyl isothiocyanate), total ascorbic acid, total dietary fiber, and pectin.
Cassia auriculata Ref.[14]	Caesalpiniaceae	Fatty acid esters, fatty acid amide, triterpene, diterpene alcohols, phytol terpenoids, tannin, flavonoids, saponin, cardiac glycosides, steroids, grape seed oil, n-hexadecanoic acid, 9-octadecenoic acid (E)-,E,Z-1,3,12-nonadecatriene, and stearic acid.
Cissampelos pareira Ref.[15]	Menispermaceae	Alkaloids, flavonoids, glycosides, steroids, sterols, tannins, and essential oils.
Cladosiphon okamuranus	Chordariaceae	Fucoidan, fucose, uronic acid, monosaccharides, and sulfate.
Colebrookea oppositifolia Ref.[16]	Lamiaceae	Alkaloid, carbohydrate, glycoside, saponins, proteins, amino acids, phytosterols, fixed oils, fats, phenolic compounds, flavonoids, and terpenoids.
Commiphora mukul Ref.[17]	Burseraceae	Guggulsterones (4, 17 (20) - pregndiene-3, 16-dione), diterpenes, sterols, steroids, esters, and higher alcohols.
Coriandrum sativum Ref.[18]	Apiaceae	Rutin, ferulic acid, gallic acid, chlorogenic acid, caffeic acid, quercetin, isoquercetin, β-carotenoids, α and β-pinene, camphor, citronellol, coriandrol, p-cymene, geraniol, geranyl acetate, limonene, linalool, myrcene, α and β-phellandrene, and terpinene.
Crataegus oxyacantha Ref.[19]	Rosaceae	Amines (β-phenylethylamine, tyramine, and acetylcholine) triterpene saponins (Oleanolic acid, ursolic acid, and crataegolic acid), flavonoids, glycosides (quercetin, hyperoside, rutin, and vitexin), monomeric catechins, and Oligomeric proanthocyanidins.

TABLE 11.1 *(Continued)*

Plant name	Family	Chemical constituents
Crocus sativus Ref.[20]	Iridaceae	Crocetin, crocetin di-glucose ester, crocetin gentiobiose glucose ester, and crocin.
Daucus carota Ref.[21]	Umbelliferae	Flavonoids (Apigenin-4-o-β-glucoside) and glycosides (apigenin-7-o-β galactopyranosyl β-D mannopyranoside).
Ficus hispida Ref.[22]	Moraceae	Phenanthroindolizidine alkaloids, n-alkanes, coumarins, triterpenoids, hispidin, oleanolic acid, bergapten, β-amyrin, β-sitosterol, and lupeol acetate.
Flacourtia indica Ref.[23]	Salicaceae	Flavonoids, tannins, polysaccharides, β-sitosterol, β-sitosterol-β-D-glucopyranoside, ramontoside, butyrolactone lignin disaccharide, flacourside, methyl 6-O-(E)-p-coumaroyl glucopyranoside, 6-O-(E)-p-coumaroyl glucopyranose, coumarins (scoparone and aesculetin) and flacourtin.
Ginkgo biloba Ref.[24]	Ginkgoaceae	Flavonoid glycosides (kaempferol, quercitin, and isorhamnetin), diterpene lactones (Ginkgolides A, B, C, M, J, and bilobalide), and biflavones (ginkgetin, isoginkgetin, and bilobetin).
Hybanthus enneaspermus Ref.[25]	Violaceae	Aurantiamide acetate, isoarborinol, β-sitosterol, and triterpene.
Inula racemosa Ref.[26]	Asteraceae	Tannins, terpenes, flavonoids, pinene, alantolactones, cymene, ionone, isoledene, and elemene.
Ixora coccinea Ref.[27]	Rubiaceae	Steroids, tannins, flavonoids, glycosides, and alkaloids.
Nelumbo nucifera Gaertn Ref.[28]	Nelumbonaceae	Alkaloids (dauricine, lotusine, nuciferine, pronuciferine, liensinine, isoliensinine, roemerine, nelumbine, and neferine).
Phyllanthus urinaria Ref.[29]	Euphorbiaceae	Polyphenols, lignans, flavonoids, gallic acid, and ellagic acid.
Premna mucronata Ref.[30]	Verbenaceae	Flavonoids (luteolin, apigenin, and hispidulin).
Premna serratifolia Ref.[31]	Verbenaceae	Alkaloids, steroids, flavonoids, phenolic compounds, and glycosides specifically iridoid glycosides.
Rhodobryum roseum Ref.[32]	Bryaceae	Uridine, methyl piperate, piperine, caffeic acid, and methyl ester.

TABLE 11.1 *(Continued)*

Plant name	Family	Chemical constituents
Salvia miltiorrhiza Ref.[33]	Lamiaceae	Single phenolic acids (protocatechuic aldehyde, protocatechuic acid, caffeic acid, and danshensu) and polyphenolic acids (rosmarinic acid, lithospermic acid, salvianolic acid A, and salvianolic acid B).
Saussurea lappa Ref.[34]	Compositae	Flavonoids, terpenoids, alkaloids, and phytosterols.
Semecarpus anacardium Ref.[35]	Anacardiaceae	Alkaloids, carbohydrates, flavonoids (Biflavonoids, biflavone A, C, A1, A2, tetrahydrorobustaflavone, jeediflavone, semecarpuflavone, gulluflavone, bhilawanol, and amentoflavone), cardiac glycosides, proteins, saponins, tannins, and terpenoids.
Sida cordifolia Ref.[36]	Malvaceae	Alkaloids, oils, resin acid, mucin, potassium nitrate, sympathomimetic amines, ephedrine, pseudoephedrine (vasoconstrictor), vasicinone, vasicinol, vasicine (bronchodilator), steroids, flavonoids, and saponins.
Stachys schimperi Ref.[37]	Lamiaceae	Rutin, kaempferol, isorhamnetin, luteolin, hypersoid, and isoflavonoid daidzein; phenolic acids: (E)-hydroxylcinnamic acid, hydroxy-4-phenylbutanoic acid, syringic acid, vanillic acid, ferulic acid, p-coumaric acid, isoscutellarein, 7-O-[2″-O-(6‴-acetyl)-β-D-allopyranosyl-β-D-glucopyranoside, flavonoid, and glycoside.
Trichosanthes cucumerina Ref.[38]	Cucurbitaceae	Isoflavone glucoside, 5, 6, 6'-trimethoxy-3', 4'-methylene– dioxyisoflavone, 7- O -beta- D-(2"-O-pcoumaroyl glucopyranoside), cucurbitacin B, cucurbitacin E, isocucurbitacin B, 23, 24-dihydroisocucurbitacin B, 23, 24-dihydrocucurbitacin E, sterols 2 β-sitosterol, stigmasterol, α-carotene, and β-carotene.
Tylophora indica Ref.[39]	Asclepiadaceae	Alkaloids, phytosterols, saponins, amino acids, and flavonoids.
Viscum album Ref.[40]	Viscaceae	Flavonoids (quercetin), terpenoids (beta-amyrin, resin acids, beta-sitosterol, stigmasterol, and sterol A), amines, and phenolic compounds.

11.2.1 MECHANISM INVOLVED

Cardioprotective effects of plant-derived phytoconstituents were analyzed by various biochemical parameters and molecular mechanism. Phytoconstituents restored the altered antioxidants such as SOD, CAT, GPx, GST, and GSH levels to near normal status. Cardiac markers (LDH, CK-MB, SGOT, SGPT, and ALP) were significantly decreased in plant extracts treated groups.[41] When compared to isoproterenol treated group, plant extracts showed a relevant decrease in serum total cholesterol, TG, PL, LDL-C, VLDL-C, and a significant rise in HDL-C.[7] Jayalakshmi et al.[19] reported that the phytoconstituents offered cardioprotection by improving mitochondrial antioxidant status and mitochondrial function in rat heart.

Phytochemicals from medicinal plants have been tested in various cardiotoxicity models such as Aflatoxin, Arsenic, CP, adriamycin/DOX induced cardiotoxicity and isoproterenol induced MI in rat model, and so forth.[42–44]

11.3 AFLATOXIN INDUCED CARDIOTOXICITY

Aflatoxins are produced by *Aspergillus flavus* and *A. parasiticus* as toxic fungal metabolites. There are four types of naturally occurring aflatoxins such as aflatoxin B1 (AFB1), aflatoxin B2 (AFB2), aflatoxin G1 (AFG1), and aflatoxin G2 (AFG2). Among these, aflatoxin B1 is more toxic which contaminate foodstuffs. Aflatoxins possess mutagenic, teratogenic, carcinogenic, and immunosuppressive properties which result in liver, kidney, and heart damage. Hepatic cytochrome P450 enzyme system activates the AFB1 leading to the generation of toxic metabolite such as AFB1-8, 9-epoxide. This epoxide, subsequently binds to nucleophilic sites in DNA, resulting in the formation of major adduct 8, 9-dihydro8-(N7guanyl)-9-hydroxy-AFB1 (AFB1 N7-Gua), which is involved in the toxic mechanism of AFs.[45] Generation of reactive oxygen species such as hydroxyl radical, superoxide anion, and hydrogen peroxide as result of this metabolism in the liver is also responsible for AF induced toxicity.[13]

TABLE 11.2 Protective Effect of Medicinal Plants.

Plant/family name	Dose administered mg/kg	Treatment period	Extract	Parameters studied
Carica papaya Caricaceae Ref[1]3	250 mg/kg	14 d	Aqueous and Ethanolic (Fruit)	Decreased myocardial and kidney damage with decrease in serum marker levels and intracellular calcium and improved antioxidant status.
Camellia sinensis (Theaceae)	200 mg/kg	21 d	Aqueous (Leaf)	
Carum carvi (Umbelliferae)	2 mg/kg		(Seed)	
Alpinia galangal (Zingiberaceae)	1 mg/kg		(Rhizomes)	
Cinchona officinalis (Rubiaceae)	1 g/kg		(Bark)	
Boswellia serrata (Frankincense) Ref[4]5	1.25 g/kg		(Resin)	

11.4 ANTHRACYCLINES INDUCED CARDIOTOXICITY

Cardiovascular toxicity can be induced by various antineoplastic drugs. Anthracyclines are the best recognized agents, which cause cardiac damage (Table 11.3). Doxorubicin (DOX)/Adriamycin (trade name for DOX) and other anthracyclines are widely used in cancer treatment. DOX is a potent antitumor drug, but its clinical use is limited due to cardiotoxicity. DOX treatment induces morphological changes in heart mitochondria. It inhibits cytochrome oxidase as binding to cardiolipin.[46] The mechanism underlying DOX induced cardiotoxicity include: free radical generation, impaired adrenergic regulation, the release of vasoactive amines, and the suppression of muscle specific genes.[47] Other possible mechanisms are the induction of apoptosis, changes in lipid profile, mitochondrial DNA damage, changes in ATP production, downregulation of mRNA, expression for sarcoplasmic reticulum calcium ATPase, and histological changes in the myocardium.[48]

TABLE 11.3 Anthracyclines Induced Cardiotoxicity.[49]

Antineoplastic agent	Major cardiac side effect
Daunorubicin/doxorubicin	Acute/chronic CHF (congestive heart failure)
Cyclophosphamide/ifosfamide	Myocarditis, CHF
Paclitaxel/docetaxel	Hypotension, hypertension, bradycardia, atrial and ventricular arrhythmia.
Fluorouracil	MI, angina, hypotension, and coronary vasospasm
Rituximab	Hypotension, hypertension, and arrhythmia
Arsenic trioxide	QT prolongation and tachycardia
Trastuzumab	CHF
Thalidomide	Pulmonary hypertension
Etoposide	MI and hypotension
Vinca alkaloids	MI and autonomic cardioneuropathy
Pentostatin	MI, CHF, and acute arrhythmia
Cytarabine	Arrhythmia, pericarditis, and CHF
Interferon (at high doses)	Arrhythmia, dilated cardiomyopathy, and ischemic heart disease
Busulfan	Endocardial fibrosis
Cisplatin	Acute MI

The *in vitro* and *in vivo* studies have suggested that DOX induce cardiac toxicity through apoptosis, necrosis and other form of cell death called autophagy. DOX treatment induces apoptosis via an intrinsic and extrinsic pathway. In the extrinsic pathway; caspase 8 was activated by binding of death ligands (FasL, TNF-α, and TRAIL) with their receptors leads to subsequent activation of caspase 3, which results in cell death. The intrinsic pathway is mediated by mitochondrial cytochrome c release (Table 11.4). The cytochrome c forms a complex called apoptosome with the adaptor protein apoptosis protease activator protein-1 (Apaf-1), dATP, and caspase 9 in cytosol. This apoptosome activates caspase 9 results in DNA fragmentation.[50] Recent studies have shown that DOX treatment significantly increased the cardiac expression of pro-inflammatory cytokine, inflammatory cell infiltration, and necrosis in rat hearts. The increased generation of ROS leads to mitochondrial calcium accumulation, promotes MPT pore opening, causes mitochondrial swelling and ATP depletion, and hence triggers necrotic cell death.[51,52]

TABLE 11.4 Protective Effect of Medicinal Plants.

Plant/family name	Dose administered mg/kg	Treatment period	Extract	Parameters studied
Allium sativum Amaryllidaceae Ref[44]	250 mg/kg	28 d	Hydro-alcoholic (garlic)	Decreased kidney, liver and cardiac marker levels in serum and lipid peroxidation with concomitant increased in antioxidant status and improved lipid profile.
Bombax ceiba Malvaceae Ref.[43]	150, 300, and 450 mg/kg	6 d/week for 4 weeks	Aqueous (flower)	
Citrus hystrix Rutaceae Ref.[53]	500 and 1000 mg/kg	11 d	70% Ethanolic (fruit)	
Citrus paradisi Rutaceae Ref.[54]	25 mg/kg	7 d	Naringenin	
Colebrookea oppositifolia Lamiaceae Ref[16]	250 and 500 mg/kg	28 d	Methanolic (leaf)	
Curcuma longa Zingiberaceae Ref[55]	200 mg/kg	7 d	Aqueous and alcoholic (Rhizome)	
Flacourtia indica Salicaceae Ref[23]	250 and 500 mg/kg	14 d	90% Ethanolic (leaf)	
Gnetum bucholzianum Gnetaceae Ref[56]	2.5 mg/kg	28 d	Aqueous (leaf)	
Schisandra fructus Schisandraceae Ref.[57]	30 and 300 µg/ml	24 h	Ethanolic (fruit)	
Silybum marianum Asteraceae Ref.[58]	50 mg/kg	7 d	Silymarin	

TABLE 11.4 *(Continued)*

Plant/family name	Dose administered mg/kg	Treatment period	Extract	Parameters studied
Stachys schimperi Lamiaceae Ref.[37]	100 mg/kg	10 d	Methanolic (aerial part)	
Vaccinium macrocarpon Ericaceae Ref.[59]	100 mg/kg	10 d	Methanolic (fruit)	
Nardostachys jatamansi Valerianaceae Ref[60]	500 mg/kg	7 d	Ethanolic (root)	
Trichosanthes cucumerina Cucurbitaceae Ref.[38]	500 and 1000 mg/kg	49 d	Methanolic (fruit)	
Scutellaria baicalensis Lamiaceae Ref[61]	25 μM	24 h	Baicalein	
Eremosparton songoricum Vass. Fabaceae Ref[62]	20 μg/ml	24 h	Methanolic (chrysoeriol)	Improved cardiac tissue morphology, mitochondrial function, cell-membrane, and lysosomal membrane integrity.
Phyllanthus urinaria Euphorbiaceae Ref.[29]	1 and 10 μg/ml	48 h	Ethanolic (aerial part)	Improved heart function as evaluated b the heart rate, systolic, diastolic and mean arterial blood pressure and serum cardiac marker enzyme activities.
Ixora coccinea Rubiaceae Ref.[27]	200 and 400 mg/kg	7 d	Methanolic (leaf)	The dissipated mitochondrial potential and increased DNA fragmentation were ameliorated.

TABLE 11.4 *(Continued)*

Plant/family name	Dose administered mg/kg	Treatment period	Extract	Parameters studied
Lycium barbarum Solanaceae Ref.[63]	200 mg/kg	10 d	Aqueous (fruit)	
Coptis chinensis Ranunculaceae Ref.[64]	60 mg/kg	14 d	Berberine	Decreased oxidative stress and improved antioxidant activity in H9C2 cells. Inhibition of ROS mediated mitochondrial apoptosis induced by DOX.
Salvia miltiorrhiza Lamiaceae Ref.[33]	40 mg/kg	3 d	70% Methanolic (root)	Decreased myocardial tissue damage as evident from histopathology, ECG and mean arterial blood pressure measurement and increased activities of antioxidants.

11.5 ARSENIC INDUCED CARDIOTOXICITY

Arsenic (As) is one of the most widely studied elements in the field of metal intoxication after lead (Pb). It has been used in the treatment of a number of cancers, syphilis, and tuberculosis for many years.[65] Arsenic is a naturally occuring element distributed in water, soil, air, and food and exist in two forms such as inorganic [trivalent meta-arsenite (As^{3+}) and pentavalent arsenate (As^{5+})] and organic. Trivalent form of arsenic is more toxic than the pentavalent form. In Asian countries, India and Bangladesh are more susceptible to arsenic toxicity. Continuous exposure to arsenic leads to hyper generation of reactive oxygen species which results in cardiovascular complications and peripheral vascular disorders. Arsenic induced cardiotoxicity is associated with free radical generation, changes in cardiac ion channels and apoptosis.[66–69]

Recent reports suggest that different types of CVD result from oxidative stress.[70,71] The reactive oxygen species formation is more common in arsenic induced cardiotoxicity.[72]

Vascular endothelial dysfunction (VED) is known as loss of balance between the endothelium mediated vasodilation and vasoconstriction. The main factors that cause VED include: reduced synthesis and release of NO, hyper generation of ROS, inactivation of eNOS, and reduction in the free radical scavengers. VED is a hallmark of atherosclerotic risk and also associated with various chronic disorders such as atherosclerosis, hypertension, heart failure, and diabetic nephropathy. Arsenite activates NADPH oxidase and increases peroxynitrite formation which results in excessive ROS generation. The possible mechanism underlying arsenic induced apoptosis is through the activation of epidermal growth factor (EGF), p38 mitogen activated protein kinase (p38 MAPK, JNK, and p53 followed by $p21^{Cip1/Waf1}$activation. Thus excessive generation of ROS triggers a vascular injury, resulting in VED (Table 11.5).[73]

11.6 CYCLOPHOSPHAMIDE INDUCED CARDIOTOXICITY

Cyclophosphamide (CP) is widely used as an antineoplastic and immunosuppressant agent. It is used for the treatment of chronic and acute leukemias, multiple myeloma, lymphomas, rheumatic arthritis and as immunosuppressive agent for bone marrow transplantation. High dose

TABLE 11.5 Protective Effect of Medicinal Plants.

Plant/family name	Dose administered mg/kg	Treatment period	Extract	Parameters studied
Corchorus olitorius Tiliaceae Ref.[74]	50 and 100 mg/kg	15 d	Aqueous (leaf)	Improved cardiac function through decreased myocardial damage with decreased serum marker levels, increased membrane ATPase activities, improved antioxidant and mito-chondrial enzyme activities and lipid profile.
Salvia miltiorrhiza Lamiaceae Ref[75]	2 mg/kg	14 d	Salvianolic acid B	
Silybum marianum Asteraceae Ref[76]	75 mg/kg	28 d	Silibinin	
Terminalia arjuna Combretaceae Ref[77]	20 mg/kg	4 d	Chloroform-Methanolic (bark)	

CP associated cardiotoxicity occurs within 10 d of its administration.[78] The two active metabolite of CP are phosphoramide mustard and acrolein. CP is activated by hepatic P450 enzyme. The major active circulating metabolite called 4-hydroxycyclophosphamide is generated by hydroxylation, which is converted intracellularly to aldophosphamide. Aldophosphamide is metabolized to phosphoramide mustard and acrolein. Of these, phosphoramide mustard is associated with therapeutic effect of CP, while, acrolein is believed to be responsible for its cytotoxic effects. The mechanism underlying CP induced cardiotoxicity is associated with generation of free radicals by these metabolites.[22] CP induced oxidative stress disrupts the inner mitochondrial membrane of heart leading to the permeability of calcium ions (Table 11.6).[79]

11.7 ISOPROTERENOL INDUCED CARDIOTOXICITY

Isoproterenol ((L-b-(3,4-dihydroxyphenyl)-a-isopropyl amino ethanol hydrochloride), a synthetic ß -adrenoceptor agonist induces cardiotoxicity in the form of MI in rats as a result of disturbance in physiological balance between production of free radicals and antioxidative defense system.[82] High levels of circulating ISO leads to cardiac toxicity along with alterations in Ca^{2+}homeostasis, resulting in extensive myocardial necrosis, lipid peroxidation, and a decrease in ATP and creatine phosphate stores.[83–86]

Isoproterenol is also well known to generate free radicals and to stimulate lipid peroxidation, which may be a causative factor for irreversible damage to the myocardial membrane (Table 11.7).[87]

11.8 CONCLUSION AND FUTURE PROSPECTUS TO ENHANCE THE USE OF MEDICINAL PLANTS

The cardioprotective effect of medicinal plants is due to the presence of various phytochemicals called flavonoids, phenolic diterpenes, and alkaloids. The therapeutic significance of different plants and their extracts were tested in animal models with different cardiotoxicity models. The results indicate that plant extracts and some plant formulations have the ability to prevent/treat cardiac damages. The present_review on the cardioprotective efficacy of the medicinal plants suggests that they do play an important role in the treatment of CVD. However, most of the

TABLE 11.6 Protective Effect of Medicinal Plants.

Plant/family name	**Dose administered mg/kg**	**Treatment period**	**Extract**	**Parameters studied**
Crataeva nurvala Capparidaceae Ref[8]0	50 mg/kg	10 d	Methanolic (stem bark)	
Ficus hispida Moraceae Ref[2]2	400 mg/kg	10 d	Methanolic (leaf)	Restoration of myocardial and endothelial cell morphology, maintenance of lysosomal membrane integrity and thiol status in heart tissue.
Saraca indica Caesalpiniaceae Ref[8]1	200 and 400 mg/kg	10 d	Ethanolic (bark)	Decreased serum marker levels and inhibition of lipid peroxidation and augmentation of endogenous antioxidants in cardiac tissue.
Viscum album Viscaceae Ref[4]0	250 mg/kg	10 d	80% Methanolic (leaf)	Decreased genotoxicity and improved antioxidant status.

TABLE 11.7 Protective Effect of Medicinal Plants.

Plant/family name	Dose administered mg/kg	Treatment period	Extract	Parameters studied
Acorus calamus Araceae Ref.[42]	100 and 200 mg/kg	30 d	70% Ethanolic (rhizome)	Restoration of cardiomyocyte morphology and contractile function, increase in the enzymic and non-enzymic antioxidant levels in heart tissue. Decreased serum cardiac marker enzyme level.
Amaranthus viridis Amaranthaceae Ref.[8]	300 mg/kg	45 d	Methanolic (leaf)	
Calotropis procera Asclepiadaceae Ref.[12]	100, 200, 300, and 400 mg/kg	30 d	70% Ethanolic (latex)	
Cissampelos pareira Menispermaceae Ref.[15]	100 and 200 mg/kg	30 d	70% Ethanolic (root)	
Coleus forskohlii Lamiaceae Ref.[88]	50 mg/kg	30 d	80% Ethanolic (root)	
Cyperus rotundus Cyperaceae Ref.[89]	150 and 300 mg/kg	28 d	80% Ethanolic (rhizome)	
Erythrina stricta Papilionaceae Ref.[90]	200 mg/kg	28 d	Ethanolic (leaf)	
Evolvulus alsinoides Convolvulaceae Ref.[91]	100 and 200 mg/kg	30 d	Methanolic (aerial part)	
Indigofera tinctoria Fabaceae Ref.[92]	100 and 200 mg/kg	28 d	Hydro-alcoholic (leaf)	
Lagenaria siceraria Cucurbitaceae Ref.[93]	125, 250, and 500 mg/kg	30 d	90% Ethanolic (fruit)	

TABLE 11.7 *(Continued)*

Plant/family name	Dose administered mg/kg	Treatment period	Extract	Parameters studied
Nelumbo nucifera Gaertn Nelumbonaceae Ref.[28]	10 mg/kg	30 d	Methanolic (leaf)	
Orthosiphon stamineus Lamiaceae Ref.[94]	100 and 200 mg/kg	14 d	Methanolic (leaf)	
Oxalis corniculata Oxalidaceae Ref.[95]	250 mg/kg	30 d	Aqueous (leaf)	
Punica granatum Punicaceae Ref.[96]	100 and 300 mg/kg	21 d	Butanolic (fruit)	
Saussurea lappa Compositae Ref.[34]	100, 200, and 300 mg/kg	28 d	Aqueous (root)	
Semecarpus anacardium Anacardiaceae Ref.[35]	100 and 500 mg/kg	21 d	Ethanolic (nuts)	
Sida cordifolia Malvaceae Ref.[36]	100 and 500 mg/kg	30 d	Hydro-alcoholic (leaf)	
Spondias mombin Anacardiaceae Ref.[97]	100 and 250 mg/kg	30 d	Hydro-alcoholic (leaf)	
Trichopus zeylanicus Trichopodaceae Ref.[98]	500 mg/kg	28 d	70% Ethanolic (leaf)	
Tylophora indica Asclepiadaceae Ref.[39]	100 and 200 mg/kg	30 d	Hydro- alcoholic (leaf)	
Vitis vinifera Vitaceae Ref.[99]	500 mg/kg	28 d	70% Ethanolic (seed)	

TABLE 11.7 *(Continued)*

Plant/family name	Dose administered mg/kg	Treatment period	Extract	Parameters studied
Zingiber officinale Zingiberaceae Ref.[100]	200 mg/kg	20 d	Ethanolic (rhizome)	
Crocus sativus Iridaceae Ref.[20]	200, 400, and 800 mg/kg	30 d	Aqueous (saffron stigma)	
Inula racemosa Asteraceae Ref.[26]	400, 600, and 800 mg/kg	10 d	Ethanolic (root)	
Linum usitatissimum Linaceae Ref.[101]	500mg/kg	8 days	50% Ethanolic (seed)	
Ocimum basilicum Lamiaceae Ref.[102]	40 mg/kg	2 d	96% Ethanolic (leaf)	
Premna serratifolia Verbenaceae Ref.[31]	100 mg/100 g	28 d	90% Ethanolic (stem-bark and stem-wood)	Decreased myocardial damage and improved cardiac function as manifested in the form of increased heart rate, PRI and ECG values decreased arterial pressure and increased left ventricular end diastolic pressure. Decreased activities of serum cardiac marker levels, the serum iron binding capacity, maintained membrane ATPase activities, and glycoprotein levels in the heart tissue.
Aegle marmelos Rutaceae Ref.[7]	150 mg/kg	45 d	Aqueous (fruit)	
Artemisia afra Asteraceae Ref.[10]	100 and 200 mg/kg	30 d	Aqueous (leaf)	
Cassia auriculata Caesalpiniaceae Ref.[14]	250 mg/kg	12 d	Aqueous and ethanolic (flower)	
Coriandrum sativum Apiaceae Ref.[18]	100, 200, and 300 mg/kg	28 d	80% Methanolic (seed)	

TABLE 11.7 *(Continued)*

Plant/family name	Dose administered mg/kg	Treatment period	Extract	Parameters studied
Daucus carota Umbelliferae Ref.[21]	250 and 500 mg/kg	28 d	Aqueous (root)	Decreased the blood glucose level and improved lipid profile. Decreased serum cardiac marker enzyme level, restoration of antioxidant status and maintenance ECG pattern, hemodynamic values and decreased levels of glycoproteins and maintained membrane ATPase activities.
Myristica fragrans Myristicaceae Ref.[103]	100 mg/kg	30 d	Aqueous (seed)	
Picrorhiza kurroa Scrophulariaceae Ref.[104]	80 mg/kg	15 d	Ethanolic (rhizome and root)	
Terminalia pallida Combretaceae Ref.[105]	100, 300, and 500 mg/kg	30 d	Ethanolic (fruit)	
Gleditsia sinensis Fabaceae Ref.[106]	15 and 30 mg/kg	15 min	75% Ethanolic (fruit)	
Pueraria lobata Fabaceae Ref.[107]	600 and 1200 mg/kg	40 d	Puerarin	Decreased myocardial ischemia through protection from apoptosis. Prevention of myocardial cell damage and inflammation by decreasing the protein expression. A significant reduction in vascular reactivity to various agonists and lipid peroxidation (MDA). Maintenance of cardiac cell and lysosomal membrane integrity with decrease in decrease in Kreb's cycle enzymes, and inhibition of apoptosis.
Garcinia mangostana Clusiaceae Ref.[108]	200 mg/kg	6 d	Methanolic (fruit)	
Crataegus oxyacantha Rosaceae Ref.[19]	0.5 ml/100 g	30 d	Ethanolic (fruit)	

studies focused on biochemical parameters and mitochondrial enzymes. Few studies have attempted to identify the mechanism of cardioprotective effect of various medicinal plants in different cardio toxicity models. Much remains to be understood regarding the molecular mechanism of cardioprotection offered by phytoconstituents in different forms of cardiotoxicity. Determination of the role of medicinal plants against cardiotoxin induced inflammation, necrosis and tissue damage by analyzing the cell signaling, cell cycle, and so forth through gene profiling/expression studies is warranted for finding the complete cure for CVD.

KEYWORDS

- **cardiovascular diseases**
- **chemotherapeutics**
- **medicinal plants**
- **antioxidants**

REFERENCES

1. WHO, Fact Sheet on Cardiovascular Diseases. In *Cardiovascular Diseases*, **2007**; pp 317.
2. CDC, *Heart Disease Fact Sheet;* 2014.
3. Petersen, S.; Peto, V.; Rayner, M.; Leal, J.; Luengo, F. R.; Gray, A. *European Cardiovascular Disease Statistics;* British Heart Foundation: London, **2005**; pp 200.
4. Miolo, G. M.; Mura, N. L.; Nigri, P.; Murrone, A.; Ronch, L. D.; Viel, E.; Veronesi, A.; Lestuzzi, C. The Cardiotoxicity of Chemotherapy: New Prospects for an Old Problem. *Radiol. Oncol.* **2006,** *40,* 149–161.
5. Eddouks, M.; Chattopadhyay, D.; De Feo, V.; Cho, W. C. Medicinal Plants in the Prevention and Treatment of Chronic Diseases 2013. *Evid. Based Complement. Alternat. Med. Ecam.* **2014,** *2014*, 180981.
6. Pauletti, P. M.; Castro-Gamboa, I.; Siqueira, S. D. H.; Young, M. C. M.; Tomazela, D. M.; Eberlin, M. N.; De Silva Bolzani, V. New Antioxidant C-Glucosylxanthones from the Stems of *Arrabidaea samydoides. J. Nat. Prod.* **2003,** *66,* 1384–1387.
7. Krushna, G.; Kareem, M.; Devi, K. Antidyslipidaemic Effect of *Aegle marmelos* Linn. Fruit on Isoproterenol Induced Myocardial Injury in Rats. *Int. J. Pharmacol.* **2008,** *6,* 19.

8. Saravanan, G.; Ponmurugan, P. *Amaranthus Viridis* Linn Extract Ameliorates Isoproterenol-Induced Cardiac Toxicity in Rats by Stabilizing Circulatory Antioxidant System. *Oxid. Antioxid. Med. Sci.* **2012,** *1,* 69–73.
9. Ojha, S. K.; Nandave, M.; Kumari, S.; Arya, D. S. Antioxidant Activity of *Andrographis Paniculata* in Ischemic Myocardium of Rats. *Global. J. Pharm.* **2009,** *3,* 154–157.
10. Sunmonu, T. O.; Afolayan, A. J. Protective Effect of *Artemisia Afra Jacq.* on Isoproterenol-Induced Myocardial Injury in Wistar Rats. *Food. Chem. Toxicol.* **2010,** *48,* 1969–1972.
11. Peer, P. A.; Trivedi, P. C.; Nigade, P. B.; Ghaisas, M. M.; Deshpande, A. D. Cardioprotective Effect of *Azadirachta Indica* A. Juss. on Isoprenaline Induced Myocardial Infarction in Rats. *Int. J. Cardiol.* **2008,** *126,* 123–126.
12. Ahmed, K. K. M.; Rana, A. C.; Dixit, V. K. Effect of *Calotropis Procera* Latex on Isoproterenol Induced Myocardial Infarction in Albino Rats. *Phytomedicine.* **2004,** *11,* 327–330.
13. Mannaa, F. A.; Abdel-Wahhab, K. G.; Abdel-Wahhab, M. A. Prevention of Cardiotoxicity of Aflatoxin B1 via Dietary Supplementation of Papaya Fruit Extracts in Rats. *Cytotechnology.* **2014,** *66,* 327–334.
14. Manimegalai, S.; Venkatalakshmi, P. Cardioprotective Effect of *Cassia auriculata* Linn., Petal Extract on Isoproterenol Induced Myocardial Infarction in Male Albino Rats. *IJPSR.* **2012,** *3,* 848–852.
15. Singh, B. K.; Pillai, K. K.; Kohli, K.; Haque, S. E. Effect of *Cissampelos pareira* Root Extract on Isoproterenol-Induced Cardiac Dysfunction. *J. Nat. Med.* **2013,** *67,* 51–60.
16. Pallab, K. H.; Kush, B.; Kumar, B. A.; Kishor, T. B.; Singh, N. D.; Girraj, T.; Kumar, S. D.; Shivani, G. *In Vitro -In Vivo* Evaluation of Cardioprotective Effect of the Leaf Extract of *Colebrookea oppositifolia Sm. J. Global Trend. Pharm. Sci.* **2011,** *2,* 310–324.
17. Ojha, S. K.; Nandave, M.; Arora, S.; Mehra, R. D.; Joshi, S.; Narang, R.; Arya, D. S. Effect of *Commiphora mukul* Extract on Cardiac Dysfunction and Ventricular Function in Isoproterenol-Induced Myocardial Infarction. *Indian. J. Exp. Biol.* **2008,** *46,* 646–652.
18. Patel, D. K.; Desai, S. N.; Gandhi, H. P.; Devkar, R. V.; Ramachandran, A. V. Cardio Protective Effect of *Coriandrum sativum* L. On Isoproterenol Induced Myocardial Necrosis in Rats. *Food Chem. Toxicol.* **2012,** *50,* 3120–3125.
19. Jayalakshmi, R.; Thirupurasundari, C. J.; Devaraj, S. N. Pretreatment with Alcoholic Extract of *Crataegus oxycantha* (AEC) Activates Mitochondrial Protection During Isoproterenol - Induced Myocardial Infarction in Rats. *Mol. Cell. Biochem.* **2006,** *292,* 59–67.
20. Sachdeva, J.; Tanwar, V.; Golechha, M.; Siddiqui, K. M.; Nag, T. C.; Ray, R.; Kumari, S.; Arya, D. S. *Crocus sativus* L. (Saffron) Attenuates Isoproterenol-Induced Myocardial Injury Via Preserving Cardiac Functions and Strengthening Antioxidant Defense System. *Exp. Toxicol. Pathol.* **2012,** *64,* 557–564.
21. Muralidharan, P.; Balamurugan, G.; Pavan Kumar. Inotropic and Cardioprotective Effects of *Daucus carota* Linn. on Isoproterenol-Induced Myocardial Infarction. *Bangladesh. J. Pharmacol.* **2008,** *3,* 74–79.

22. Shanmugarajan, T. S.; Arunsundar, M.; Somasundaram, I.; Krishnakumar, E.; Sivaraman, D.; Ravichandiran, V. Cardioprotective Effect of *Ficus hispida* Linn. on Cyclophoaphamide Provoked Oxidative Myocardial Injury in a Rat Model. *Int. J. Pharm.* **2008,** *4,* 78–87.
23. Palani, S.; Jayakumar, M.; Karthi, S.; Raja, S. Protective Effects of *Flacourtia indica* on Doxorubicin-Induced Cardiotoxicity in Rats. *Toxicol. Environ. Chem.* **2012,** *94,* 1014–1025.
24. Panda, V. S.; Naik, S. R. Cardioprotective Activity of *Ginkgo biloba* Phytosomes in Isoproterenol-Induced Myocardial Necrosis in Rats: A Biochemical and Histoarchitectural Evaluation. *Exp. Toxicol. Pathol.* **2008,** *60,* 397–404.
25. Radhika, S.; Smila, K. H.; Muthezhilan, R. Cardioprotective Activity of *Hybanthus enneaspermus (Linn.)* on Isoproterenol Induced Rats. *Indian. J. Fund. Appl. Life. Sci.* **2011,** *1,* 90–97.
26. Shirole, T. S.; Jagtap, A. G.; Phadke, A. S.; Velhankar, R. D. Preventive Effect of Ethanolic Extract of *Inula racemosa* on Electrocardiographic, Biochemical & Histopathological Alteration in Isoproterenol Induced Myocardial Infarction in Rats. *Int. J. Res. Pharmacol. Phytochem.* **2013,** *3,* 13–22.
27. Momin, F. N.; Kalai, B. R.; Shikalgar, T. S.; Naikwade, N. S. Cardioprotective Effect of Methanolic Extract of *Ixora coccinea* Linn. Leaves on Doxorubicin Induced Cardiac Toxicity in Rats. *Indian. J. Pharmacol.* **2012,** *44,* 178–183.
28. Subashini, R.; Rajadurai, M. Evaluation of Cardioprotective Efficacy of *Nelumbo nucifera* Leaf Extract on Isoproterenol-Induced Myocardial Infarction in Wistar Rats. *Int. J. Pharm. Pharm. Sci.* **2011,** *2,* 285–294.
29. Chularojmontri, L.; Wattanapitayakul, S. K.; Herunsalee, A.; Charuchongkolwongse, S.; Niumsakul, S.; Srichairat, S. Antioxidative and Cardioprotective Effects of *Phyllanthus urinaria* L. on Doxorubicin-Induced Cardiotoxicity. *Biol. Pharm. Bull.* **2005,** *28,* 1165–1171.
30. Hardik, S.; Hital, S.; Kirti, P.; Tejal, G. Cardioprotective Effect of Flavonoids Rich Fraction of *Premna mucronata* on Isoproterenol–Induced Myocardial Infarction in Wistar Rats. *Int. J. Phyto. Pharm.* **2014,** *5,* 95–108.
31. Rajendran; Rekha; Basha, N. S. Cardioprotective Effect of Ethanol Extract of Stem-Bark and Stem-Wood of *Premna serratifolia* Lin. (Verbenaceae). *Res. J. Pharm. Technol.* **2008,** *1,* 487–491.
32. Hu, Y.; Guo, D. H.; Liu, P.; Rahman, K.; Wang, D. X.; Wang, B. Antioxidant Effects of a *Rhodobryum Roseum* Extract and its Active Components in Isoproterenol-Induced Myocardial Injury in Rats and Cardiac Myocytes against Oxidative Stress-Triggered Damage. *Pharmazie*. **2009,** *64,* 53–57.
33. Jiang, B.; Zhang, L.; Li, M.; Wu, W.; Yang, M.; Wang, J.; Guo, D. Salvianolic Acids Prevent Acute Doxorubicin Cardiotoxicity in Mice Through Suppression of Oxidative Stress. *Food. Chem. Toxicol.* **2008,** *46,* 1510–1515.
34. Saleem, T. S.; Lokanath, N.; Prasanthi, A.; Madhavi, M.; Mallika, G.; Vishnu M. N. Aqueous Extract of *Saussurea lappa* Root Ameliorate Oxidative Myocardial Injury Induced by Isoproterenol in Rats. *J. Adv. Pharm. Technol. Res.* **2013,** *4,* 94–100.
35. Asdaq, S. M. B.; Chakraborty, M. Myocardial Potency of *Semecarpus anacardium* Nut Extract against Isoproterenol Induced Myocardial Damage in Rats. *Int. J. Pharm. Sci. Rev. Res.* **2010,** *2,* 10–13.

36. Kubavat, J. B.; Asdaq, S. M. Role of *Sida Cordifolia* L. Leaves on Biochemical and Antioxidant Profile during Myocardial Injury. *J. Ethnopharmacol.* **2009,** *124,* 162–165.
37. Abdel-Sattar, E.; El-Gayed, S. H.; Shehata, I.; Ashour, O. M.; Nagy, A. A.; Mohamadin, A. M. Antioxidant and Cardioprotective Activity of *Stachys Schimperi Vatke* against Doxorubicin-Induced Cardiotoxicity. *Bull. Fac. Pharm. Cairo Univ.* **2012,** *50,* 41–47.
38. Shah, S. L.; Mali, V. R.; Zambare, G. N.; Bodhankar, S. L. Cardioprotective Activity of Methanol Extract of Fruit of *Trichosanthes cucumerina* on Doxorubicin-Induced Cardiotoxicity in Wistar Rats. *Toxicol. Int.* **2012,** *19,* 167–172.
39. Asdaq, S. B.; Sowmya, S. K. Effect of Hydroalcoholic Extracts of *Tylophora indica* Leaves in Isoprenaline- Induced Myocardial Damage in Rat Heart. *Iran. J. Pharmacol.* **2010,** *9,* 15–20.
40. Sekeroglu, V.; Aydin, B.; Sekeroglu, Z. A. *Viscum Album* L. Extract and Quercetin Reduce Cyclophosphamide-Induced Cardiotoxicity, Urotoxicity and Genotoxicity in Mice. *Asian Pac. J. Cancer. Prev.* **2011,** *12,* 2925–2931.
41. Rajaprabhu, D.; Rajesh, R.; Jeyakumar, R.; Buddhan, S.; Ganesan, B.; Anandan, R. Protective Effect of *Picrorhiza kurroa* on Antioxidant Defense Status in Adriamycin-Induced Cardiomyopathy in Rats. *J. Med. Plant. Res.* **2007,** *1,* 80–85.
42. Singh, B. K.; Pillai, K. K.; Kohli, K.; Haque, S. E. Isoproterenol-Induced Cardiomyopathy in Rats: Influence f *Acorus calamus* Linn.: A. Calamus Attenuates Cardiomyopathy. *Cardiovasc. Toxicol.* **2011,** *11,* 263–271.
43. Patel, S. S.; Verma, N. K.; Rathore, B.; Nayak, G.; Singhai, A. K.; Priya Singh. Cardioprotective Effect of *Bombax ceiba* Flowers against Acute Adriamycin-Induced Myocardial Infarction in Rats. *Braz. J. Pharmacog.* **2011,** *21,* 704–709.
44. Alkreathy, H.; Damanhouri, Z. A.; Ahmed, N.; Slevin, M.; Osman, A. B. M.; Ali, S. S. Aged Garlic Extract Protects Against Doxorubicin-Induced Cardio toxicity in Rats. *Food. Chem. Toxicol.* **2010,** *48,* 951–956.
45. Abdulmajeed, N. A. Therapeutic Ability of Some Plant Extracts on Aflatoxin B1 Induced Renal and Cardiac Damage. *Arabian. J. Chem.* **2011,** *4,* 1–10.
46. Gille, L.; Nohl, H. Analyses of the Molecular Mechanism of Adriamycin-Induced Cardiotoxicity. *Free. Radic. Biol. Med.* **1997,** *23,* 775–782.
47. Wakade, A. S.; Shah, A. S.; Kulkarni, M. P.; Juvekar, A. R. Protective Effect of *Piper Longum* L. on Oxidative Stress Induced Injury and Cellular Abnormality in Adriamycin Induced Cardiotoxicity in Rats. *Indian. J. Exp. Biol.* **2008,** *46,* 528–533.
48. Jones, R. L.; Swanton, C.; Ewer, M. S. Anthracycline Cardiotoxicity. *Expert. Opin. Drug. Saf.* **2006,** *5,* 791–809.
49. Chanan-Khan, A.; Srinivasan, S.; Czuczman, M. S. Prevention and Management of Cardiotoxicity from Antineoplastic Therapy. *J. Support. Oncol.* **2004,** *2,* 251–266.
50. Zhang, Y. W.; Shi, J.; Li, Y. J.; Wei, L. Cardiomyocyte Death In Doxorubicin-Induced Cardiotoxicity. *Arch. Immunol. Ther. Exp.* **2009,** *57,* 435–445.
51. Dorn, G. W. Apoptotic and Non-Apoptotic Programmed Cardiomyocyte Death in Ventricular Remodelling. *Cardiovasc. Res.* **2009,** *81,* 465–473.
52. Gustafsson, A. B.; Gottlieb, R. A. Heart Mitochondria: Gates of Life and Death. *Cardiovasc. Res.* **2008,** *77,* 334–343.

53. Putri, H.; Nagadi, S.; Larasati, Y. A.; Wulandari, N.; Adam H. Cardioprotective and Hepatoprotective Effects of *Citrus Hystrix* Peels Extract on Rats Model. *Asian Pac. J. Trop. Biomed.* **2013,** *3,* 371–375.
54. Arafa, H. M.; ABD-Ellah, M. F.; Hafez, H. F. Abatement by Naringenin of Doxorubicin Induced Cardiac Toxicity in Rats. *J. Egypt. Natl. Cancer Inst.* **2005,** *17,* 291–300.
55. El-Sayed, E. M.; Abd El-Azeem, A. S.; Afify, A. A.; Shabana, M. H.; Ahmed, H. H. Cardioprotective Effects of *Curcuma longa* L. Extracts against Doxorubicin-Induced Cardiotoxicity in Rats. *J. Med. Plant. Res.* **2011,** *5,* 4049–4058.
56. Johnkennedy, N.; Ifeoma, U. H. Cardioprotective Effect of *Gnetum bucholzianum* Leaf Extract against Doxorubicin Cardiomyopathy in Wistar Rats. *Int. J. Med. Sci.* **2012,** *1,* 61–64.
57. Choi, E. H.; Lee, N.; Kim, H. J.; Kim, M. K.; Chi, S. G.; Kwon, D. Y.; Chun, H. S. *Schisandra Fructus* Extract Ameliorates Doxorubicin-Induce Cytotoxicity in Cardiomyocytes: Altered Gene Expression for Detoxification Enzymes. *Genes Nutr.* **2008,** *2,* 337–345.
58. El-Shitany, N. A.; El-Haggar, S.; El-Desoky, K. Silymarin Prevents Adriamycin-Induced Cardiotoxicity and Nephrotoxicity in Rats. *Food. Chem. Toxicol.* **2008,** *46,* 2422–2428.
59. Elberry, A. A.; Abdel-Naim, A. B.; Abdel-Sattar, E. A.; Nagy, A. A.; Mosli, H. A.; Mohamadin, A. M.; Ashour, O. M. Cranberry (*Vaccinium macrocarpon*) Protects against Doxorubicin-Induced Cardiotoxicity in Rats. *Food. Chem. Toxicol.* **2010,** *48,* 1178–1184.
60. Subashini, R.; Gnanapragasam, A.; Senthilkumar, S.; Yogeeta, S. K.; Devaki, T. Protective Efficacy of *Nardostachys Jatamansi* (Rhizomes) on Mitochondrial Respiration and Lysosomal Hydrolases During Doxorubicin Induced Myocardial Injury in Rats. *J. Health. Sci.* **2007,** *53,* 67–76.
61. Chang, W. T.; Li, J.; Haung, H. H.; Liu, H.; Han, M.; Ramachandran, S.; Shao, Z. H. Baicalein Protects against Doxorubicin-Induced Cardio Toxicity by Attenuation of Mitochondrial Oxidant Injury and JNK Activation. *J. Cell Biochem.* **2011,** *112,* 2873–2881.
62. Zhe, L.; Xiao-Dong, S.; Ying, X.; Xiao-Jian, W.; Hui, Y.; Yong-Yi, B.; Jun-Hao, L.; Chan-Na, Z.; Ru-Tai, H. Protective Effect of Chrysoeriol against Doxorubicin-Induced Cardiotoxicity *in Vitro. Chin. Med. J.* **2009,** *122,* 2652–2656.
63. Xin, Y. F.; Wan, L. L.; Peng, J. L.; Guo, C. Alleviation of the Acute Doxorubicin-Induced Cardiotoxicity by *Lycium barbarum* Polysaccharides through the Suppression of Oxidative Stress. *Food. Chem. Toxicol.* **2011,** *49,* 259–264.
64. Zhao, X.; Zhang, J.; Tong, N.; Liao, X.; Wang, E.; Li, Z.; Luo, Y.; Zuo, H. Berberine Attenuates Doxorubicin Induced Cardio Toxicity in Mice. *J. Int. Med. Res.* **2011,** *39,* 1720–1727.
65. Zhu, J.; Chen, Z.; Lallemand-Breitenbach, V.; De The, H. "How Acute Promyclocytic Leukaemia Revived Arsenic." *Nat. Rev. Cancer.* **2002,** *2,* 705–713.
66. Chang, S. I.; Jin, B.; Youn, P.; Park, C.; Park, J. D.; Ryu, D. Y. Arsenic Induced Toxicity and the Protective Role of Ascorbic Acid in Mouse Testis. *Toxicol. Appl. Pharmacol.* **2007,** *218,* 196–203.

67. Hei, T. K.; Liu, S. X.; Waldren, C. Mutagenicity of Arsenic in Mammalian Cells: Role of Reactive Oxygen Species. *Proc. Natl. Acad. Sci.* **1998,** *95,* 8103–8104.
68. Zhao, X. Y.; Li, G. Y.; Liu, Y.; Chai, Chen, J. X.; Zhang, Y.; Du, Z. M.; Lu, Y. J.; Yan, B. F. Resveratrol Protects against Arsenic Trioxide Induced Cardiotoxicity *in Vitro* and *in Vivo*. *Br. J. Pharmacol.* **2008,** *154,* 105–113.
69. Shi, H.; Shi, X.; Liu, K. J. Oxidative Mechanism of Arsenic Toxicity and Carcinogenesis. *Mol. Cell. Biochem.* **2004,** *255,* 67–78.
70. Dhalla, N. S.; Temsah, R. M.; Netticadan, T. Role of Oxidative Stress in Cardiovascular Diseases. *J. Hypertens.* **2000,** *18,* 655–673.
71. Haidara, M. A.; Yassin, H. Z.; Rateb, M.; Ammar, H.; Zorkani, M. A. Role of Oxidative Stress in Development of Cardiovascular Complications in Diabetes Mellitus. *Curr. Vasc. Pharmacol.* **2006,** *4,* 215–227.
72. Bashir, S.; Sharma, Y.; Irshad, M.; Dutta-Gupta, S.; Dogra, T. D. Arsenic-Induced Cell Death in Liver and Brain of Experimental Rats. *Basic. Clin. Pharmacol. Toxicol.* **2006,** *98,* 38–43.
73. Balakumar, P.; Kaur, J.; Arsenic Exposure and Cardiovascular Disorders: An Overview. *Cardiovasc. Toxicol.* **2009,** *9,* 169–176.
74. Das, A. K.; Ranabir Sahu, Dua, T. K.; Bag, S; Gangopadhyay, M.; Sinha, M. K.; Dewanjee, S. Arsenic-Induced Myocardial Injury: Protective Role of *Corchorus olitorius* Leaves. *Food. Chem. Toxicol.* **2010,** *48,* 1210–1217.
75. Wang, M.; Sun, G.; Wu, P.; Chen, R.; Yao, F.; Qin, M.; Luo, Y.; Sun, H.; Zhang, Q.; Dong, X.; Sun, X. Salvianolic Acid B Prevents Arsenic Trioxide-Induced Cardiotoxicity *in Vivo* and Enhances Its Anticancer Activity *in Vitro*. *Evid. Based Complement. Alternat. Med.* **2013,** *2013,* 1–9.
76. Muthumani, M.; Milton Prabu, S. Silibinin Potentially Attenuates Arsenic-Induced Oxidative Stress Mediated Cardiotoxicity and Dyslipidemia in Rats. *Cardiovasc. Toxicol.* **2014,** *14,* 83–97.
77. Manna, P.; Sinha, M.; Sil, P. C. Arsenic-Induced Oxidative Myocardial Injury: Protective Role of Arjunolic Acid. *Arch. Toxicol.* **2008,** *82,* 137–149.
78. Goldberg, M. A.; Antin, J. H.; Guinan, E. C.; Rappeport, J. M. Cyclophosphamide Cardiotoxicity: An Analysis of Dosing as a Risk Factor. *Blood.* **1986,** *68,* 1114–1118.
79. Souid, A. K.; Tacka, K. A.; Galvan, K. A.; Penefsky, H. S. Immediate Effects of Anticancer Drugs on Mitochondrial Oxygen Consumption. *Biochem. Pharmacol.* **2003,** *66,* 977–987.
80. Sudharsan, P. T.; Mythili, Y.; Selvakumar, E.; Varalakshmi, P. Lupeol and its Ester Ameliorate the Cyclophosphamide Provoked Cardiac Lysosomal Damage Studied in Rat. *Mol. Cell. Biochem.* **2006,** *282,* 23–29.
81. Viswanatha Swamy, A. H. M.; Patel, U. M.; Koti, B. C.; Gadad, P. C.; Patel, N. L.; Thippeswamy, A. H. M. Cardioprotective Effect of *Saraca indica* against Cyclophosphamide Induced Cardiotoxicity in Rats: A Biochemical, Electrocardiographic and Histopathological Study. *Indian. J. Pharmacol.* **2013,** *45,* 44–48.
82. Zhou, R.; Xu, Q.; Zheng, P.; Yan, L.; Zheng, J.; Dai, G. Cardioprotective Effect of Fluvastatin on Isoproterenol-Induced Myocardial Infarction in Rat. *Eur. J. Pharmacol.* **2008,** *586,* 244–250.
83. Ramos, K.; Acosta, D. Cytotoxic Actions of Isoproterenol in Cardiac Cells: Protective Effects of Anti-Oxidants. In *CRC Handbook of Free Radicals and Antioxidants*

in Biomedicine; Miquel, J., Quintanilha, A. T. M., Weber, H., Eds.; CRC Press: Boca Raton, **1989**; Vol. 2, pp 177–185.

84. Dhalla, K. S.; Rupp, H.; Beamish, R. E.; Dhalla, N. S. Mechanisms of Alterations on Cardiac Membrane Ca^{2+} Transport Due to Excess Catecholamines. *Cardiovasc. Drug. Ther.* **1996,** *10,* 231–238.
85. Rupp, H.; Dhalla, K. S.; Dhalla, N. S. Mechanisms of Cardiac Cell Damage Due to Catecholamines: Significance of Drugs Regulating Central Sympathetic Outflow. *J. Cardiovasc. Pharmacol.* **1994,** *24,* S16–S24.
86. Dhalla, N. S.; Yates, J. C.; Naimark, B.; Dhalla, K. S.; Beamish, R. E.; Ostadal, B. Cardiotoxicity of Catecholamines and Related Agents. In *Cardiovascular Toxicology;* Daniel Acosta, J., Ed.; Raven Press: New York; **1992**; pp 239–281.
87. Chatelain, P.; Gremel, M.; Brotelle, R. Prevention by Amiodarone of Phospholipid Depletion in Isoproterenol-Induced Ischemia in Rats. *Eur. J. Pharmacol.* **1987,** *144,* 83–90.
88. Ahsan, F.; Siddiqui, H. H.; Mahmood, T.; Srivastav, R. K.; Nayeem, A. Evaluation of Cardio Protective Effect of *Coleus Forskohlii* against Isoprenaline Induced Myocardial Infarction in Rats. *Indian J. Pharm. Biol. Res.* **2014,** *2,* 17–25.
89. Raza, S. M.; Tomar, V.; Siddiqui, H. H. Cardio-Protective Effect of Alcoholic Extract of *Cyperus Rotundus* Rhizome on Isoproterenol Induced Myocardial Necrosis in Rats. *Int. J. Pham. Sci. Res.* **2012,** *3,* 2535–2538.
90. Kuppusamy, A.; Varadharajan, S.; Josey, C.; John, H.; Sherin, D.; Chirakkan, D.; Athiyappan, G. Cardioprotective Effect of *Erythrina stricta* Leaves on Isoproterenol-Induced Myocardial Infarction in Rat. *Bangladesh. J. Pharmacol.* **2010,** *5,* 1–4.
91. Sudhakumari Kumar, A. H. V.; Javed, A.; Jaiswal, M.; Talkad, M.S. Cardioprotective Effects in Methanolic Extract of *Evolvulus alsinoides* Linn on Isoproterenol - Induced Myocardial Infarction in Albino Rats. *Int. J. Basic Med. Sci. Pharm.* **2012,** *2,* 53–57.
92. Nagasaraswathi, M.; Rafi Khan, P.; Aleemuddin, M. A.; Gopi Chand, K.; Sravani, K. Effect of *Indigofera tinctoria* Linn against Isoproterenol Induced Myocardial Infarction on Albino Wistar Rats. *J. Curr. Chem. Pharm. Sci.* **2013,** *3,* 222–230.
93. Vijayakumar, M.; Selvi, V.; Krishnakumari, S. Cardioprotective Effect of *Lagenaria Siceraria* (Mol) on Antioxidant Tissue Defense System against Isoproterenol Induced Myocardial Infarction in Rats. *J. Ethnopharmacol.* **2010,** *1,* 207–210.
94. Maheswari, C.; Umadevi, M.; Anudeepa, J.; Ramya, R.; Narayanan, R. V. Cardioprotective Effect of *Orthosiphon Stamineus* on Isoproterenol Induced Myocardial Infarction in Rat. *Int. J. Pharm. Technol.* **2011,** *3,* 2896–2904.
95. Abhilash, P. A.; Nisha, P.; Prathapan, A.; Nampoothiri, S. V.; Cherian, L. O.; Sunitha, T. K.; Raghu, K. G. Cardioprotective Effects of Aqueous Extract of *Oxalis corniculata* in Experimental Myocardial Infarction. *Exp. Toxicol. Pathol.* **2011,** *63,* 535–540.
96. Mahalaxmi, M.; Pankaj, P.; Ghadi, P.; Kasture, S. Cardioprotective Potential of *Punica granatum* Extract in Isoproterenol-Induced Myocardial Infarction in Wistar Rats. *J. Pharmacol. Pharmacother.* **2010,** *1,* 32–37.
97. Akinmoladun, A. C.; Obuotor, E. M.; Barthwal, M. K.; Dikshit, M.; Farombi, E. O. Ramipril-Like Activity of *Spondias mombin* Linn against No-Flow Ischemia and Isoproterenol Induced Cardio Toxicity in Rat Heart. *Cardiovasc. Toxicol.* **2010,** *10,* 295–305.

98. Velavan, S.; Selvarani, S.; Adhithan, A. Cardioprotective Effect of *Trichopus zeylanicus* against Myocardial Ischemia Induced by Isoproterenol in Rats. *Bangladesh. J. Pharmacol.* **2009,** *4,* 88–91.
99. Velavan, M. T.; Aegil, I.; Gokulakrishnan, K. Protective Effect of *Vitis Vinifera* against Myocardial Ischemia Induced by Isoproterenol in Rats. *Pharmacol..* **2008,** *3,* 958–967.
100. Nazam, A. M.; Bhandari, U.; Pillai, K. K. Ethanolic *Zingiber officinale* R. Extract Pretreatment Alleviates Isoproterenol Induced Oxidative Myocardial Necrosis in Rats. *Indian J. Exp. Biol.* **2006,** *44,* 892–897.
101. Zanwar, A. A.; Hegde, M. V.; Bodhankar, S. L. Cardioprotective Activity of Flax Lignan Concentrate Extracted from Seeds of *Linum usitatissimum* in Isoprenalin Induced Myocardial Necrosis in Rats. *Interdisp. Toxicol.* **2011,** *4,* 90–97.
102. Fathiazad, F.; Matlobi, A.; Khorrami, A.; Hamedeyazdan, S.; Soraya, H.; Hammami, M.; Maleki-Dizaji, N.; Garjani, A. Phytochemical Screening and Evaluation of Cardioprotective Activity of Ethanolic Extract of *Ocimum basilicum* L.(Basil) against Isoproterenol Induced Myocardial Infarction in Rats. *Daru.* **2012,** *20,* 87.
103. Kareem, M. A.; Krushna, G. S.; Hussain, S. A.; Devi, K. L. Effect of Aqueous Extract of Nutmeg on Hyperglycaemia, Hyperlipidaemia and Cardiac Histology Associated with Isoproterenol-Induced Myocardial Infarction in Rats. *Trop. J. Pharm. Res.* **2009,** *8,* 337–344.
104. Senthil Kumar, S. H.; Anandan, R.; Devaki, T.; Santhosh Kumar, M. Cardioprotective Effects of *Picrorrhiza kurroa* against Isoproterenol Induced Myocardial Stress in Rats. *Fitoterapia.* **2001,** *72,* 402–405.
105. Shaik, A. H.; Rasool, S. N.; Reddy, V. K. A.; Kareem, A. M.; Krushna, S. G. Cardioprotective Effect of HPLC Standardized Ethanolic Extract of *Terminalia pallida* Fruits against Isoproterenol-Induced Myocardial Infarction in Albino Rats. *J. Ethnopharmacol.* **2012,** *141,* 33–40.
106. Wu, J.; Li, J.; Zhu, Z.; Li, J.; Huang, G.; Tang, Y.; Gao, X. Protective Effects of Echinocystic Acid Isolated from *Gleditsia sinensis* Lam. against Acute Myocardial Ischemia. *Fitoterapia.* **2010,** *81,* 8–10.
107. Chen, R.; Xue, J.; Xie, M. Puerarin Prevents Isoprenaline-Induced Myocardial Fibrosis in Mice by Reduction of Myocardial TGF-B 1 Expression. *J. Nutr. Biochem.* **2012,** *23,* 1080–1085.
108. Pandima Devi, S.; Kannan, V. Ameliorative Prospective of Alpha-Mangostin, A Xanthone Derivative from *Garcinia mangostana* against β-Adrenergic Catecholamine-Induced Myocardial Toxicity and Anomalous Cardiac TNF-α And COX-2 Expressions in Rats. *Exp. Toxicol. Pathol.* **2008,** *60,* 357–364.

CHAPTER 12

SCOPE OF NON-INVASIVE SURGERY OF SHUSHRUT IN THE PRESENT ERA WITH SPECIAL REFERENCE TO KELOIDS

J. N. MISHRA*

Faculty of Ayurveda, Lucknow University, Lucknow 226007, Uttar Pradesh, India

*E-mail: jn.mishra@yahoo.co.in, dr.jn.mishra.lko@gmail.com

CONTENTS

ABSTRACT

A successful keloid management is ready to peep through newly modified non-invasive, bloodless, painless, and non-infective technique developed by Prof. J. N. Mishra, Lucknow, India borrowing knowledge from Sushrut. It has bright future for alike conditions subject to developing newer techniques to approach deep tissues of cavities and vessels. In this preliminary study four cases of keloid of different parts of the body were treated successfully with the pressure gradient technique with maximum follow-up of 27 years.

12.1 INTRODUCTION

Elephinstono says, "Hindu surgery is as remarkable as their medicine." Ancient surgeons conducted amputations, practiced dichotomy, abdominal laparotomy, herniorrhaphy, fistulotomy, set fractures and dislocations, and foreign body extraction. There are certain surgical conditions which are incurable such as cancer and keloid etc. Keloid may not be inducted into malignancy but the behavior is reckoned to line up the cancer like, since the management is frustrating due to recurrence and psycho-social reasons. Keloid formation occurs as a result of pathological wound healing. Despite the high prevalence of keloid in general population, they remain on the more challenging dermatologic condition to manage. More than a cosmetic nuisance they are often symptomatic and can have a significance psycho-social burden on the patient. Although multiple treatment modalities exist; no single treatment has proven widely effective. In fact, recurrence following treatment is generally the rule. Combination therapy is likely the optimal strategy. Lee et al.[7] evaluated 20 patients with keloid and found that more than 80% of patients experience keloid associated with pruritus and pain. Many reports indicate a severe negative impact on quality of life from unknown reasons, keloid occurs more frequently among blacks, Hispanics and Asians, and less commonly Caucasians.[9,1]

Intense research is under way to better understand the pathophysiology of the abnormal processes leading to keloid formation. For now our greatest weapon lies in patient's education, combination therapy, and prevention. The latest approach to this is counseling against body piercing and should avoid elective cosmetic procedure with a risk for scaring and the use of silicon gel sheet following surgical excision to reduce recurrence.

The author has developed the pressure gradient technique out of modified Kharsutra of Prof. P. J. Deshpandey, BHU, Varanasi, India. The technique has been found quite successful which also explores its scope in other alike surgical conditions. The present technique is certainly going to shift the surgical domain from minimal invasive surgery to non-invasive surgery.

12.2 REVIEW

The title "father of Indian surgery" is bestowed upon great surgeon Sushrut. The surgery is dominated by skill which is recognized since the Indian history. There is reference available that Indians used quill of the feather attached to an animal bladder to suck out purulent material.[6] Tribes of India and South Africa used indigenous method of sealing minor injuries by applying termites or scarabs. In sixteenth century, French surgeon Ambroise Pare gave a better understanding of surgery elaborating its different objects such as elimination of superfluous tissue, restoration of dislocation, separation of pathological union, joining the pathological division and repairing the defect of nature. Sushrut is known for an early innovation of rhino-plastic surgery. The ligature was introduced as hemostat by Alexandrian surgeon (300 BC). Galen[16] used ligature and known to be the king of the catgut suture. There are three obstacles of surgery—bleeding, pain, and infection.

The advances in the surgery have transformed from risky "art" into scientific discipline. After the invention of laser, cryosurgery, endoscopic surgery, and microsurgery the operations have become easier and fruitful, but still there are some conditions which need innovative research and remedy and here ayurvedic parasurgical procedure may still contribute much in many surgical conditions such as fistula-in-ano, piles, polyps, keloid, and similar other conditions. The Sushrut concept has advantages like minimum post-operative pain, no bleeding, no hospitalization, no recurrence, and no stricture formation.

Keloid scar is a chronic inflammation but recurrence is the rule. This is followed by trauma to the skin, insect bites, acne, and chicken pox etc. Conventional management has many options namely surgical excision, skin grafting, interlesional steroid injection as a combined therapy. Though the combined therapy is most successful in present scenario.[12,15,2,14] However, there are adverse effects of steroid such as atrophy of skin, hypo-pigmentation, telangiectasis, necrosis, ulceration, and cushingoid disappointed the therapy.[14,13,12] Radiation therapy is used as monotherapy or as adjuvant after excision,[15] its carcinogenic nature and adverse effect of radiation therapy restrict to continue its wide spread use. Silicon sheet application was first used in 1983. The advantage of this technique is non-invasive but required prolonged application.[17] Laser and cryo therapies are widely used for the treatment of keloids and hypertrophic scars but the response rate is not up to the mark.[4,3] Cryosurgery alone has a response rate not to the satisfaction but in combination with steroid the response is remarkable.[5] Intralesional interferon injection modulates the growth factor composition.[11] Several other studies have failed to demonstrate long term efficacy in the management of keloid.[11]

The treatment of keloid remains challenging clinical problem despite of numerous proposed therapy reported in literature. Presently there is no consensus in the present scenario to treat the keloid. Surgical excision followed by interlesional steroid injection seems to be the most widely used and effective treatment modality. Conclusively, it may be said that the keloids are still difficult to treat due to high recurrence rate regardless of kind of conventional therapy. The author has developed the non-invasive pressure gradient technique to meet the challenge.

12.3 METHOD

This technique, since being in preliminary stage has been applied on only polypus keloid bearing body, fundus, and neck. For this purpose a cotton thread has been used having hard core but outer soft and cushioned so that it may not injure the tissues in contact. The thickness of the thread was 0.5 mm. The thread has been applied on the neck of the keloid with pressure gradient technique using slip loose knot method to the extent before feeling of the pain. Every third day, pressure on the neck of the keloid was increased but before complaints of the pain. The pressure gradient was used gradually in increasing fashion till the keloid shed off. The leucoplast was applied over the keloid so that pendulous hanging of the growth may not cause pain and damage to the surrounding tissue.

Case No. 1: In 1988, the story started from the author at the age of 44 years having the polypus keloid on the dorsum of left finger as shown in Figure 12.1. It was excised thrice followed by steroid injection but it reappeared. After great disappointment the author applied the above mentioned technique and on 21st day the keloid shed off with no recurrence till today.

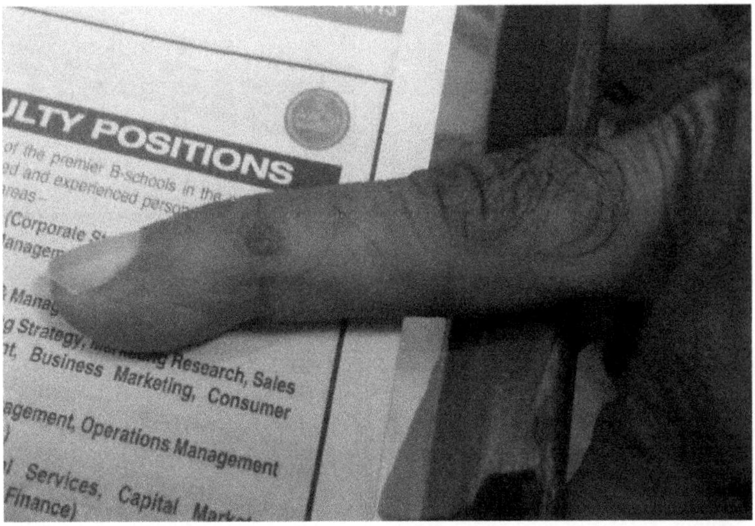

FIGURE 12.1 The keloid removed by pressure gradient technique with no recurrence in 27 years follow-up.

Case No. 2: A male aged about 28 years reported the polypus swelling on the back with a complaint of pain and itching particularly while sweating. The keloid was excised in 2007 and 2008 followed by steroid injection but recurrence was the post operative result. He was treated by above mentioned technique in 2008 and keloid shed off on 28th day. It has been followed till November 2014 with no recurrence. His biopsy was positive (Figs. 12.2, 12.3, and 12.4).

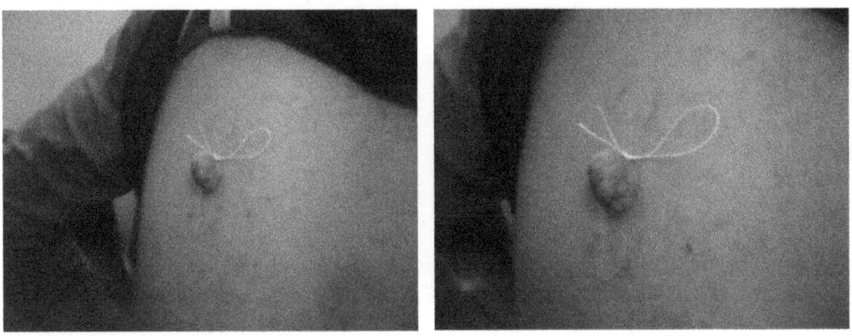

(a) (b)

FIGURE 12.2 The keloid situated on the back tied up using pressure gradient technique and slip loose knot.

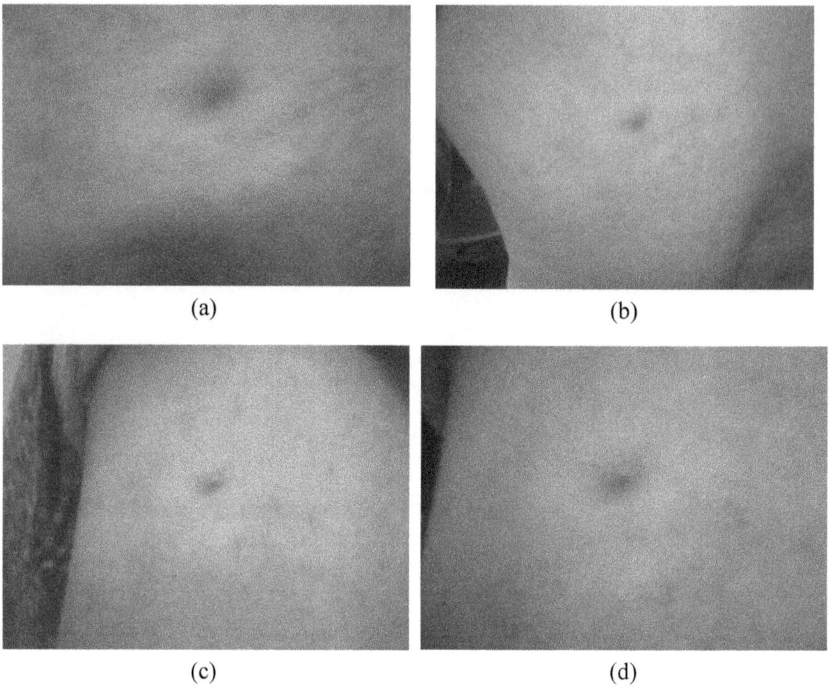

FIGURE 12.3 The keloid shed off on 28th day with scar.

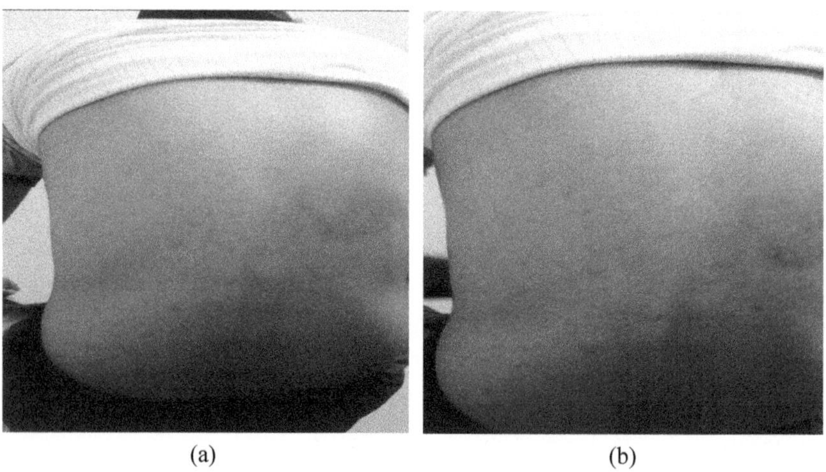

FIGURE 12.4 Post operative status, followed up for six years; showing even no trace of scar.

Case No. 3: A lady aged about 60 years having the keloid on dorsum of right knee and was given excision followed by steroid injection twice within two years. She was treated by author with pressure gradient technique on February 2, 2010 and on 18th day keloid shed off. The follow-up was till August 2014 with no recurrence (Figs. 12.5, 12.6, 12.7, and 12.8).

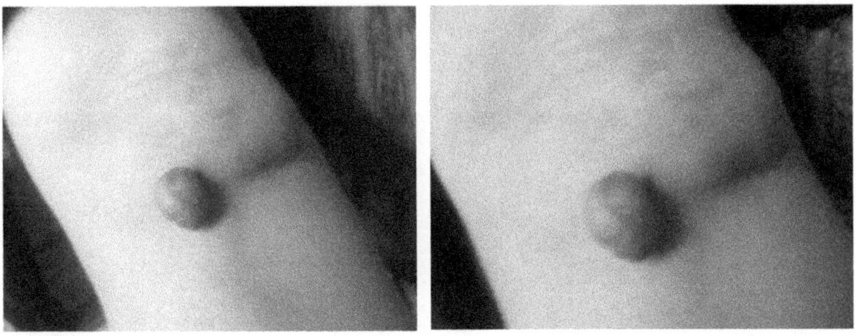

(a) (b)

FIGURE 12.5 The preoperative keloid situated on the dorsum of the knee.

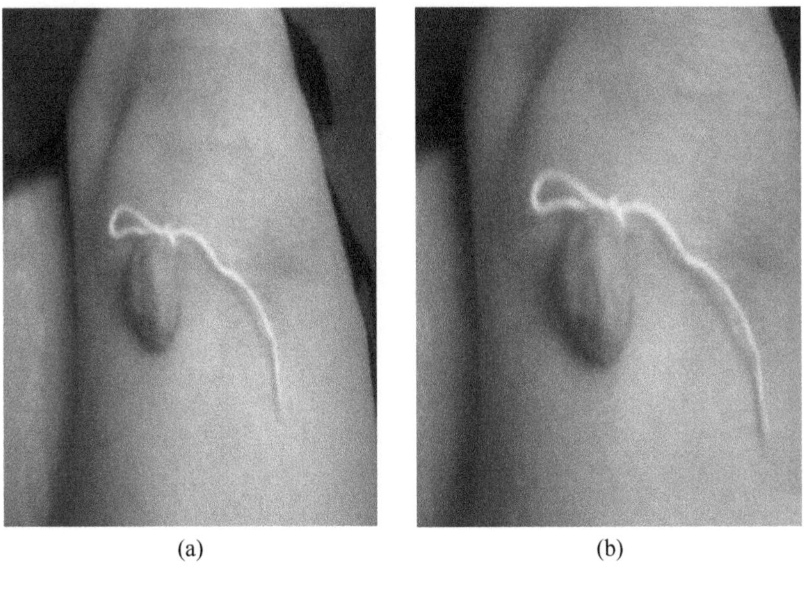

(a) (b)

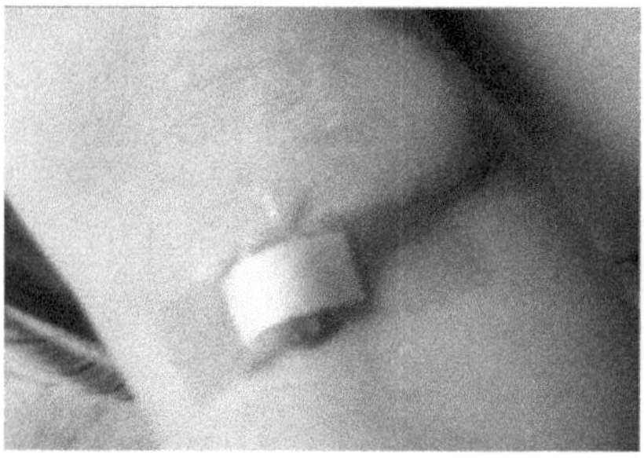

(c)

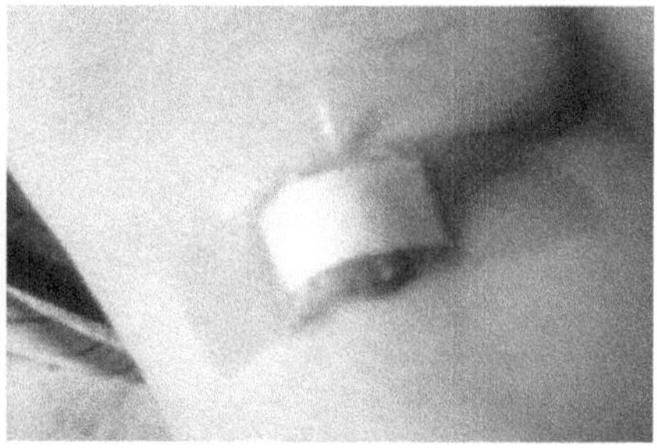

(d)

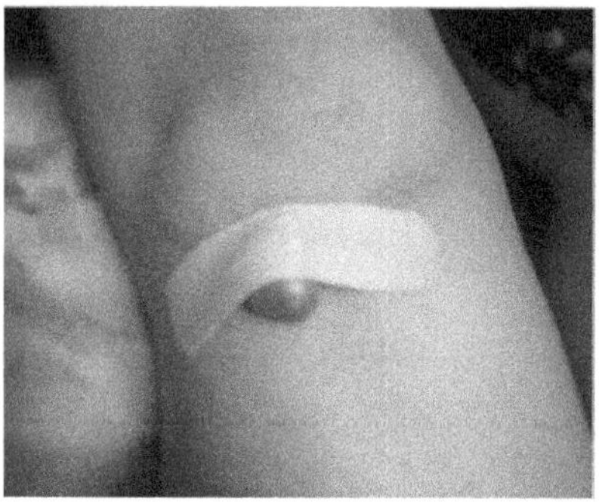

(e)

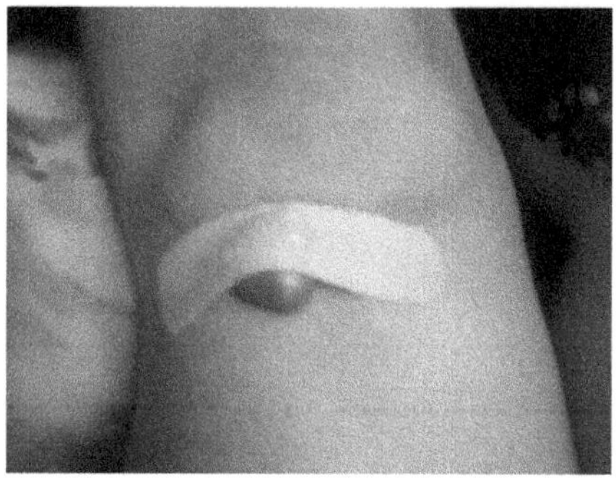

(f)

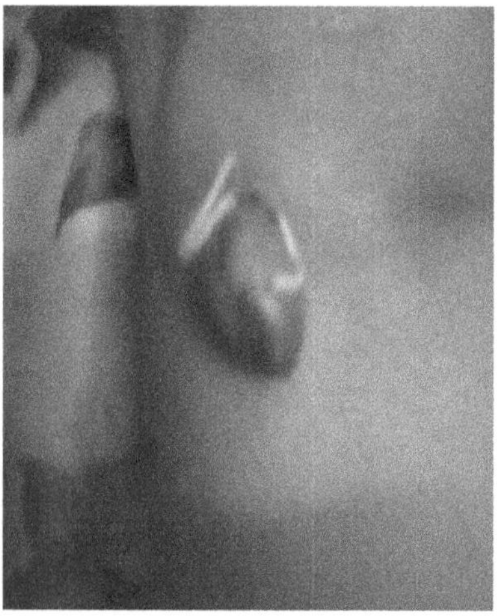

(g)

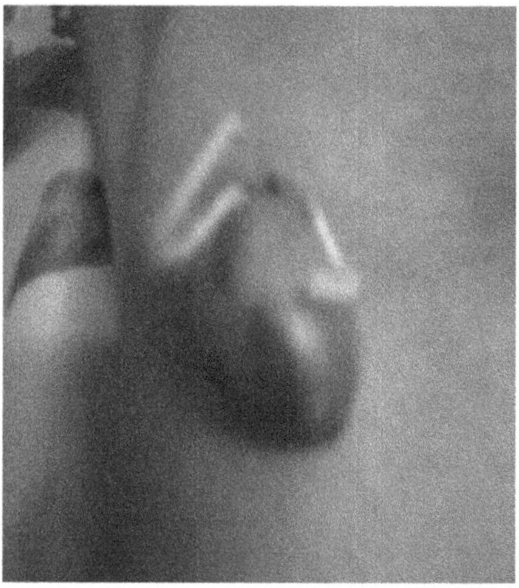

(h)

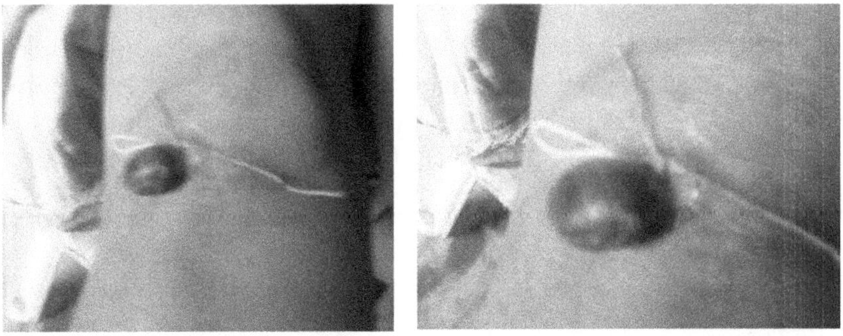

(i) (j)

FIGURE 12.6 Pressure gradient technique applied on the keloid with the help of specific thread showing different stages.

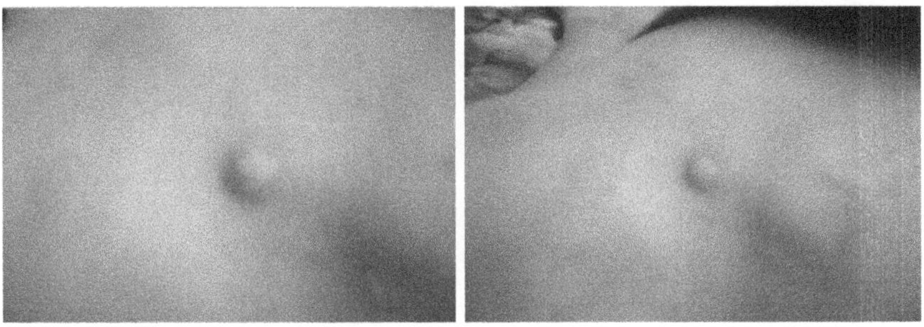

(a) (b)

FIGURE 12.7 The keloid shed off on 18th day leaving a scar.

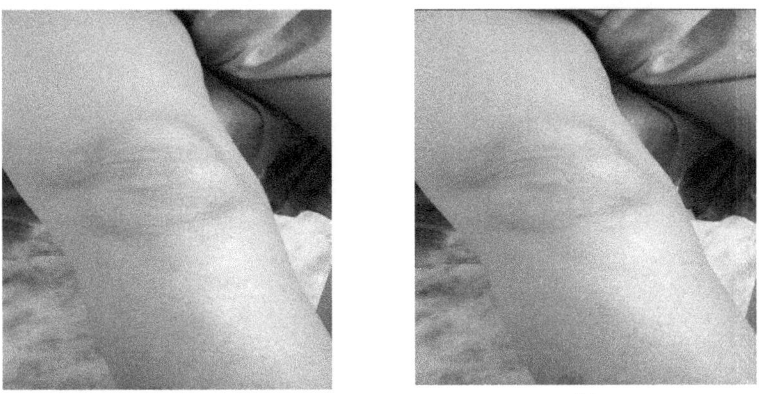

(a) (b)

FIGURE 12.8 Follow-up of 4 years showing no scar supporting the cosmetic reason.

Case No. 4: A man aged about 32 years having keloid below the right ear. He was operated three times in 2011 along with post operative steroid injection but it recurred in February 2012. On March 2, 2012, he was treated with pressure gradient technique and keloid shed off on March 12, 2012. He was followed till October 2014 with no recurrence (Figs. 12.9, 12.10, and 12.11).

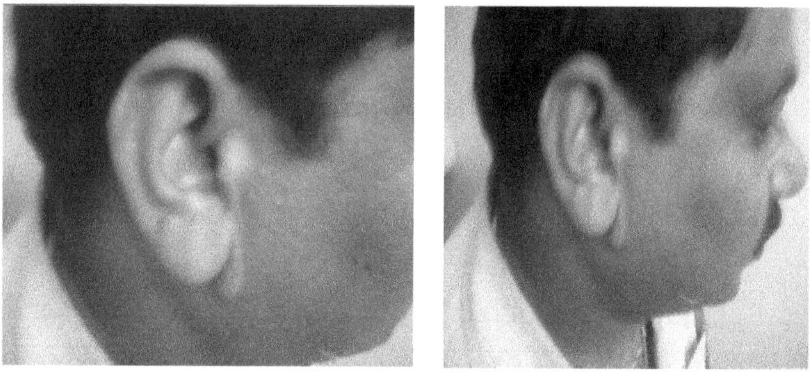

(a) (b)

FIGURE 12.9 Preoperative polypus keloid like condition.

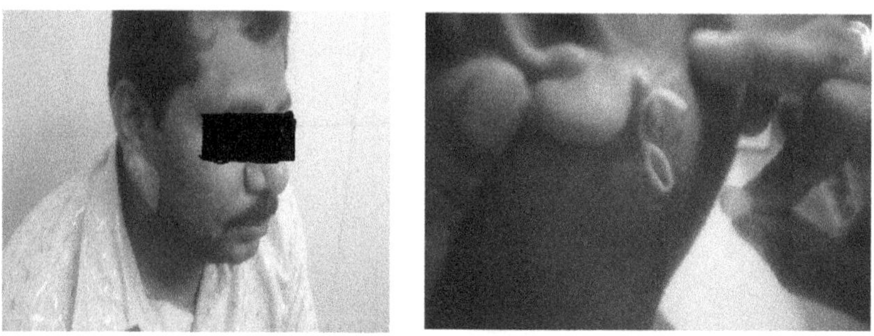

(a) (b)

FIGURE 12.10 Pressure gradient technique applied.

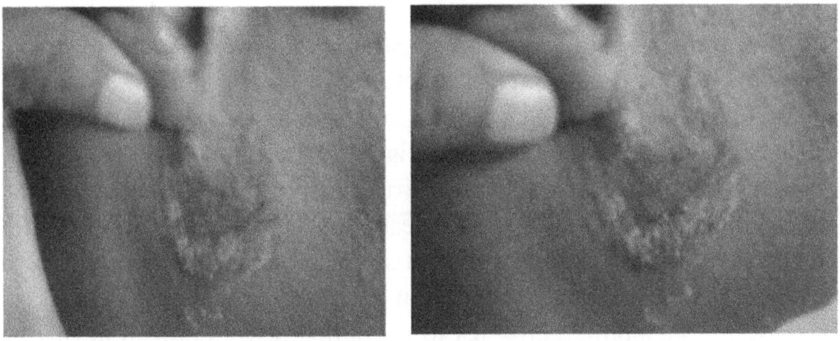

(a) (b)

FIGURE 12.11 The keloid shed off on 10th day.

12.4 RESULT

The modified ligation using pressure gradient technique appears to be 100% successful especially in terms of recurrence. This technique is free from fear of surgery, result oriented, non-hospitalization, non-recurrence, and cost-effective.

12.5 DISCUSSION

All tissues in the body are capable of healing by one of two mechanisms; regeneration is the replacement of damaged tissue by identical cells and is more limited than repairs. In humans complete regeneration occurs in a limited number of cells, for example, epithelium, liver, and nerve cells. In most of the cases repairs take place where damaged tissue is replaced by connective tissue which then forms a scar. Perfusion and oxygenation are the most influential determinants of successful tissue repair. Hypoxia in the tissue leads to the largest obstacle in wound healing. An ischemic gradient initiates the angiogenesis factors which begin the process of neovascularization. This is stimulated by macro phase activity hypoxia resulting from the disruption of blood flow at the time of injury. The role of oxygen in wound healing is complex and yet not fully understood. Neovascularization leads to develop the TcOp2 in the wound, which begins to rise collagen synthesis but only when TcOp2 rises above 20.

In hypoxia, the body sees no ischemic gradient localized to the wound and the wound becomes chronic. Micro Vas and average periwound TcOp2 of less than 20 mmHg leads to risk for early healing failure. For physiological healing, angiogenesis and apoptosis are essential factors. This shows probably the close association between hypoxia (by pressure gradient) and physiological healing. Irrespective of different conventional management, recurrence is the biggest stigma in success of keloid treatment. Conventional remedies in post surgical healing triggers the factors responsible for excessive proliferation of collaterals and micro vessels and increase the metabolic activities to encourage extra deposition of fibroblast to promote unhealthy healing.[18,10] Mechanical compression has been reported in preventive recurrence, after surgical excision of hypertrophic and keloid scars.[19,8] Mechanical compression dressing is thought to reduce oxygen tension in the wound through occlusion of small vessels, leading to reduction in tissue metabolism fibroblast proliferation and collagen synthesis.[18,10]

12.5.1 LIMITATION OF THE TREATMENT

- It is only applicable on cystic and polypus growth having fundus, body, and neck where neck is negotiable.
- Under present circumstances it cannot be applied on the growth of the cavities.
- It is not applicable at present to intravascular growth.
- This cannot be used in intracranial lesions.

12.5.2 APPLICATION OF TECHNIQUES IN ALIKE CONDITIONS

- Nasal polyps
- Extracranial cystic growths
- Anorectal polyps
- Pile masses
- Ear polyps
- Cyst of Bartholin's duct
- Any external polypus growth on the surface of the body

12.5.3 TECHNOLOGIES NEEDED FOR WIDER APPLICATION

- Vascular navigation technology
- The approach to growth in cavities
- The flat keloid growth
- The techniques for intracranial approach

12.6 CONCLUSION

A ray of hope for successful keloid management is peeping through new modified pressure gradient technique of Prof. J. N. Mishra, Lucknow, Uttar Pradesh, India borrowing knowledge from Sushrut. It may be tried on alike conditions also subject to advance techniques for approaching deep tissues.

12.7 MESSAGE

New approach to management of keloid may be the perfect answer in present scenario and this technique may create era of bloodless, painless, and non-infective surgery.

KEYWORDS

- **keloid scar**
- **pressure gradient**
- **non-invasive surgery**
- **silicon gel sheet**
- **surgical excision**

REFERENCES

1. Aköz, T.; Gideroðlu, K.; Akan, M. Combination of Different Techniques for the Treatment of Earlobe Keloids. *Aesthetic. Plast. Surg*. **2002,** *26,* 184–188.

2. Al-Attar, A.; Mess, S.; Thomassen, J. M.; Kauffman, C. L.; Davison, S. P. Keloid Pathogenesis and Treatment. *Plast. Reconstr. Surg.* **2006,** *117,* 286–300.
3. Alster, T. S. Laser Treatment of Hypertrophic Scars. *Facial Plast. Surg. Clin. North Am.* **1996,** *4,* 267–274.
4. Alster, T. S.; Nanni, C. A. Pulsed-Dye Laser Treatment of Hypertrophic Burn Scars. *Plast. Reconstr. Surg.* **1998,** *102,* 2190–2195.
5. Babin, R.W.; Ceilley, R. I. Combined Modalities of in the Management of Hypertrophic Scars and Keloids. *J. Otolaryngol.* **1979,** *8,* 457–460.
6. Bishop, W. J. *The Early History Of Surgery;* Robert Hale Ltd.: London, 1960.
7. Lee SS, Yosipovitch G, Chan YH et al..: Pruritus, pain, and small nerve fiber function in keloids: a controlled study. *J Am Acad Dermatol* **2004**, 51:1002-6
8. Brent, B. The Role of Pressure Therapy in Management of Earlobe Keloids: Preliminary Report of a Controlled Study. *Ann. Plast. Reconstr. Surg.* **1978,** *1,* 579–581.
9. Brissett, A. E.; Sherris, D. A. Scar Contractures, Hypertrophic Scars, and Keloids. *Facial Plast. Surg..* **2001,** *17,* 263–272.
10. Carr-Collins, J. Pressure Techniques for the Prevention of Hypertrophic Scar. *Clin. Plast. Surg.* **1992,** *19,* 733–743.
11. Davison, S. P.; Mess, S.; Kauffman, L. C.; Al-Attar, A. Ineffective Treatment of Keloids with Interferon Alpha-2b. *Plast. Reconstr. Surg.* **2006,** *117,* 247–52.
12. Donkor, P. Head and Neck Keloid: Treatment by Core Excision and Delayed Intralesional Injection of Steroid. *J. Oral Maxillofac. Surg.* **2007,** *65,* 1292–1296.
13. Mafong, E.; Ashinoff, R. Treatment of Hypertrophic Scars and Keloids. *Aesthet. Surg. J.* **2000,** *20,* 114–120.
14. Murray, J. C.; Pollack, S. V.; Pinnell, S.R. Keloids and Hypertrophic Scars. *Clin. Dermatol.* **1984,** *2,* 121–133.
15. Mustoe, T. A.; Cooter, R. D.; Gold, M. H.; Hobbs, F. D. R.; Ramelet, A. A.; Shakespeare, P. G.; Stella, M.; Téot, L.; Wood, F. M.; Ziegler, U. E. International Clinical Recommendations on Scar Management. *Plast. Reconstr. Surg.* **2002,** *110,* 560–571.
16. Vivia, N. *Ancient Medicine;* Taylor & Francis: USA, 2004.
17. Perkins, K.; Bruce, D. R.; Wallis, K. A. Silicone Gel: A New Treatment for Burn Scars and Contracture. *Burns. Incl. Therm. Inj.* **1983,** *9,* 201–204.
18. Sawada, Y.; Sone, K. Hydration and Occlusive Therapy for Hypertrophic Scars and Keloids. *Br. J. Plast. Surg.* **1992,** *45,* 599–603.
19. Stanley, M. J.; Richard, R. L. Use of Pressure to Treat Hypertrophic Burn Scars. *Adv. Wound Care.* **1997,** *10,* 44–46.

CHAPTER 13

COMPLEX ISSUES RELATED TO HUMAN REPRODUCTION IN MODERN SOCIETY

ANN HOLADAY

Anglia Polytechnic University, UK

jivaneesha@gmail.com

CONTENTS

ABSTRACT

The continued existence of any species depends on the survival of the fittest and nature has it's own "weeding out" process to ensure it. So it is for humans. Not so long ago, it was common for women to die in childbirth and for premature and severely disabled babies only to survived if they could do so on their own. However, natural selection is not acceptable in modern-day thinking and it is life at all costs if the baby is wanted and abortion when the child is unwanted.

Adding to this disharmony with nature, women are having babies when they want to have them and not when nature determines they should have them. Modern science has a solution for all reproductive issues, infertile women can get pregnant at almost any age and infertile men can be treated. The laws of nature are not obeyed resulting in a weakening of the human race and overpopulation.

Birth and death are naturally occurring life events. All over the world healthy babies are being born without help from doctors, nurses or medical assistance...it is a natural process. It is not suggested that humanity go back to the days before medical advancements, but to use modern technology to support natural processes rather than creating the imbalances that we see today.

Ayurveda "The Science of Life" works in harmony with nature which is why it is fundamentally important in all issues related to human reproduction including birth control overpopulation, the use of hormones, fertility, pregnancy, childbirth, care of newborns and unwanted children. Of course, modern-day technology and scientific developments in these areas are necessary, but only as supportive measures for the natural process and emergency care. When allopathy is the only option, then childbirth becomes medicalized which is not only prohibitively expensive, but over time, women are at risk of losing their natural instincts and control of their reproductive right.

INTRODUCTION

There has never been a time in recent history when humanity has needed Ayurveda as much as it does today. Humanity is heading towards its own destruction; it is clearly evident that it cannot go on the way it has for the last one hundred years or so. We are slowly but surely destroying the planet on which we live and it may already be too late to save ourselves. Perhaps there is nothing we can do but whatever our fate may be, the answers to life today lie in Ayurveda, "The Science of Life" whether the issues are social, political, environmental, economic, cultural or health.

Ayurveda is an evidence based system which addresses physical, mental and spiritual health of all living beings. The philosophy behind Ayurveda and Yoga has been in existence for thousands of years and developed because man needed to understand life on earth. Ayurveda is described as an Indian tradition because India has managed to preserve its principles, but the knowledge is universal and timeless.

The philosophies of Ayurveda and Yoga are complex concepts, but at the same time are remarkably simple, because they are based on the principle of the five elements which is the origin of all things. Once we realize that the energies of the five elements ether, air, fire, water and earth are everything, every cell of the body, all matter and all living things then we begin to comprehend the magnitude of this knowledge. Understanding the five elements and their evolution from the merging of Prakriti (base substance of the Universe) and Purusha (source of consciousness) is not difficult, but does require a shift in thinking for Westerners.

The pendulum started to swing away from traditional medicine with the discovery of antibiotics for communicable diseases. Nowadays every condition, every disease, acute and chronic are medicalized without any regard for ancient knowledge. Modern medicine has evolved over a relatively short period of time and is scientifically based in which there is extensive knowledge, but very little wisdom. Of course, modern-day technology and scientific developments are vitally important and Ayurveda will never be an alternative to it, but neither will allopathic medicine be an alternative to traditional medicine. This is why the future lies in an integrated system based on the philosophy of "right and appropriate treatment for the patient" not based on a particular system of medicine.

No other area demonstrates the dominance of modern medicine than in aspects of human reproduction where ancient knowledge is critically important. When reproduction is medicalized, we are hand over our right as individual human beings to be in charge of our lives on earth.

13.1 ASPECTS OF HUMAN REPRODUCTION

Aspects of human reproduction for discussion in this paper are birth control and population explosion, cesarean section, hormones, fertility, breast cancer, pregnancy, newborns and unwanted children.

13.1.1 POPULATION EXPLOSION AND UNWANTED CHILDREN

Global human population continues to explode at an alarming rate and at the same time traditional family structure is disappearing.

Human babies are helpless for longer and are more dependent than any other species, yet thousands of babies are abandoned at birth throughout the world, their future at the mercy of fate. Millions of unwanted children are born every year and millions are brought up in by women without male or family support.

The issue of unwanted pregnancies and children is a world-wide problem manifesting in all cultures, religions and walks of life, but is particularly prevalent amongst the poor and underserved. Child trafficking is a multi-million dollar business resulting in prostitution, child pornography, slave labor and violent crime. Children caught in the web of this trend often become the perpetrators and so the cycle continues in ever-increasing circles. Thousands of children are brought up by single women without support, spend their childhood in orphanages or are shuffled around from one foster home to another.

13.1.1.1 CONTRACEPTION

Effective birth control is not acceptable in many cultures and at the same time, a safe alternative to abortion is not available to most women especially poor, single women. Whether we approve of birth control or not, we must recognize that it is a woman's predicament when there is not a man or family support in pregnancy. At one time, men were equally responsible for contraception but over the past forty years or so it has become the responsibility of women. This is partially due to the sexual freedom that women have attained which has given men more freedom from the responsibility of pregnancy. The result of this has meant a huge increase in sexually transmitted diseases (STD's) which were a big deterrent for both men and women when syphilis was life-threatening, but now STD's are easily treated. Nevertheless, STD's are a big issue related to sexual freedom but for most women, the risk of pregnancy is much more of an issue than the risk of STD's.

Long-term effects of using hormones

Most modern women choose oral contraception because it is more reliable. The statistics in the USA show that 77% of women of child bearing age (15–44) is taking oral contraceptives as compared to India, which shows 9% using oral contraceptives. Despite the wide use of oral contraceptives, just under half of the pregnancies in the USA are "unintended" (https://www.guttmacher.org/fact-sheet/unintended-pregnancy-united-states) and abortion is a common method of birth control. Because women are having children much later in life and are sexually active at a younger age, one can assume that many women can be on oral contraceptives for twenty years or more. Furthermore, 38% of post-menopausal women take Hormone Replacement Therapy (HRT) meaning that a large proportion of women are taking hormones for most of their lives. In addition, many are the second or third generation taking oral contraception for twenty years followed by HRT and the long-term effects on humanity as a whole may never be fully realized. However, the effect on the environment is surfacing. Studies of the Pacific NW waters in the US found evidence of pharmaceuticals, particularly hormones, in drinking water and the reproductive systems of fish are being affected. (http://pugetsoundblogs.com/waterways/files/2009/05/).

Hormones and Breast Cancer

In the 1960s, breast cancer was considered to be a degenerative disease and only very rarely did it occur in pre-menopausal women. Nowadays it is not uncommon for women under 30 years of age to be diagnosed with breast cancer. Even though the National Cancer Institute claims only a slight increased risk, there must be a connection between breast cancer, oral contraception and HRT. But instead of advising women against taking hormones, more and more money is poured into research to find the cause of and cure for cancer.

13.1.1.2 RISKS INVOLVED IN FERTILITY TREATMENT

It has been known for a long time that childbirth at a young age is a defense against breast cancer. Many modern-day couples consider having a family much later in life, even when the woman is approaching menopause and more often than not is unable to conceive. Fertility treatment is the normal course for this group which again involves taking hormones which increases the risk of breast cancer. Fertility treatment often results in multiple births. A high proportion of these babies are born prematurely and under natural circumstances would not survive, but with modern technology they can be brought to a normal birthweight. Statistics show that 40% of these babies have cerebral palsy as a confirmed diagnosis and there are other disabilities both mental and physical, which can be attributed to premature birth and medical intervention. News of multiple births in the media celebrates the medical achievement, but rarely is there followup of these children four or five years later.

As *Ms. Jane Denton, Director of the Multiple Births Foundation* writes:

> "The aim of all infertility treatment should be to have one live, healthy baby. The anguish of watching one or more of your children die or live with a severe disability is a situation no parent would wish to face, yet it is a frequent consequence of multiple births that is so often underestimated."

Ayurveda recommends natural methods for treating infertility when both the man and woman spend at least six months detoxifying and rejuvenating so that both the sperm and ovum are in perfect health. Even then a healthy baby is not guaranteed, but every attempt has been made for a positive outcome. Under these circumstances, conception will be natural and the baby is more likely to be normal and healthy.

The current situation is illogical in terms of the natural scheme of things where on the one hand, thousands of babies are being abandoned and on the other, people who would normally be grandparents are going to extreme lengths to have children. Meanwhile, there are thousands of unwanted children without a home, without love, without care and attention. Added to this imbalance is the fact that it is increasingly difficult to adopt a baby and adoptive parents, disillusioned by regulations and laws in their native countries, are seeking adoption overseas, leaving babies in their own countries left without a home.

13.1.1.3 NATURAL CHILDBIRTH AND CESAREAN SECTION

More and more women are choosing or are advised to have cesarean section rather than natural childbirth. The US national C-section rate is over 30%, despite evidence that only 5–10% is optimal. Statistics show that China recorded the highest number of C-sections (46%), followed by Vietnam (36%) and Thailand (34%). The lowest rates were Cambodia (15%) and India (18%) which probably means they are only done when necessary.

The reasons for this trend but are not limited to them and are as follows.

1. There is ***limited awareness*** of the risks involved in cesarean section. Women do not realize C-section is a major surgical procedure incurring risk of infection, blood clots and emergency hysterectomy. Recovery is much longer and more challenging than in natural childbirth. The long-term effect of adhesions can cause pelvic pain, infertility and more serious conditions in future pregnancies, such as ectopic pregnancies and uterine rupture. Babies delivered by C-section are more likely to have complications such as respiratory problems, childhood-onset diabetes, obesity and asthma. (http://www.childbirthconnection.org/?referrer=https://www.google.com/)
2. The average ***hospital payment*** for cesarean is much higher than for vaginal birth, therefore a greater opportunity for profit. In addition, a planned cesarean is easier to schedule and more predictable than a vaginal birth making it more efficient and cost effective for hospital and staff.
3. There is "***low priority***" given to making it easier for a woman to give birth naturally such as "doula care" which provides continuous support during pregnancy and labor. The decision to perform a cesarean is often made during labor because the staff does not know the patient, and cannot revert to care by a doula, which is more time-consuming.

4. Some ***labor interventions*** make a C-section more likely. For example, labor induction, continuous electronic fetal monitoring, epidural too early in labor and epidural analgesics causing fetal distress.
5. Many women who have had a previous cesarean would prefer the option of Vaginal Birth After Caesarean (VBAC), but were not given the choice because health professionals and/or hospitals were unwilling to offer it. Women who have had a previous cesarean, are carrying twins or the fetus in the breech position, are rarely given the option to deliver vaginally.

A healthy mature woman's body is designed to deliver a baby and it is much healthier for a baby to be delivered naturally. Modern science has realized the process of birth as an important part of the journey into the world and of development. The contraction of the head in the birth canal and the secretions that nature provides are all part of the process of life and should not be interfered with unless absolutely necessary. There is pain in childbirth and it should not be avoided by using epidurals simply for a woman's comfort. Pain is always there for a reason and if the woman cannot feel it then she is putting her baby at risk. The interesting thing is that, even if labor lasts many hours, once the baby is born the pain is soon forgotten. I have never heard of a woman not wanting another baby because of the pain of childbirth in the first delivery.

13.1.4 NEWBORNS

In traditional societies such as India, women are able to give 100% of their attention to newborns in the early weeks because they are supported by family, extended family and the women of the village. This period is most important for the mother and baby. The mother will have the opportunity to fully recover from childbirth and it is a crucial time for the baby when human bonding occurs. It is well known in Ayurveda that the first weeks of life are vital and that intense nurturing from the mother is crucial to emotional and mental development. Love is the essential ingredient to complete health and we learn how to love by being nurtured and loved ourselves. There is a short window of time in the early weeks of life when this stage of development happens. A mother not only gives nourishment to her baby through breastfeeding but also conveys her love toward her child. This basic human instinct is critical to wellbeing and normal development and is why loving nurturing and calmness are so important to mental health. Thousands of babies throughout the world never receive love or nurturing and begin their lives with fear, bewilderment, anxiety, stress and loneliness engrained in their personalities which are the problems of modern-day society.

13.1.2.1 VEDIC PSYCHOLOGY

Before going further in this discussion, it is important to understand the Vedic concept of psychology in order to realize the consequences of lack of love and nurturing in babies and children. Vedic texts do not describe "Vedic Psychology" as such, but the Vedic concept of "mind" is profound and easily translates into contemporary thinking. Vedic thought not only considers the body, mind and spiritual self to be connected but interconnected, and the mind not confined to just the functions of the brain.

There are three aspects of "mind" which influence the sub-conscious-

- ***Manas or semi-conscious mind*** can be compared to the computer screen. In a computer, we do not know anything about the files on the hard drive until they come up on the screen and likewise we are not aware of what is in the sub-conscious unless it manifests in the semi conscious mind. Mind takes in information through the senses which are the link to the outside world. Proper and early stimulation of the senses is essential to healthy development. If a baby is abandoned at birth or neglected, the child is at risk for developmental and emotional problems which he or she will have throughout life.
- ***Ahamkara or self-conscious mind:*** The Universe is linked to and exists in all things, therefore there is unity throughout but at the same time, everything has its own individuality and is separate. This separateness is called Ahamkara or ego which gives awareness of self or identity. It is the force or energy which gives individuality or "I-ness." It is why "my" comes into being and is the reason we say "my" heart, "my" body because they belong to "me." Every living thing has this sense of identity which gives every part of every being the intelligence to function. Cells are governed by the self-conscious mind.

- ***Buddhi or conscious mind*** can be compared to the computer processor and is the most important aspect of the mind in the context of development. This is the discriminating mind or intellect and its main function is to process information coming into the mind through the senses. The conscious mind allows us to judge, question, decide and doubt. For example, if we see a mirage which gives the illusion of water, the conscious mind will ascertain whether it is water or not before it decides. When there is doubt, then Buddhi matches the object to an impression in the memory. A healthy, functioning Buddhi is essential to mental health, it is responsible for sleep, cognitive powers and intelligence, and allows us to understand, be aware and discriminate, but it must be used properly.
- ***Chitta - sub-conscious mind*** can be likened to the hard-drive of the computer and is the storage compartment of all life's experiences. It acts like a video camera gathering images as we experience life. These impressions or Samskaras are like scars on the sub-conscious.

Buddhi is the most important aspect to sanity. If it is weak, experiences, especially traumatic experiences, will not be filtered and negative impressions on the sub-conscious will disturb the mind. Once an impression is created, it is almost impossible to remove even though there may be some improvement with therapy.

The discriminating mind (Buddhi) is not developed in young children so impressions (Samskaras) go straight to the sub-conscious (Chitta). Everything is recorded even before birth. It is a known fact that the feeling of "not being wanted" will be transferred to the unborn child which is why pregnant women need protection and should avoid stress. Impressions must be of love and a feeling of being wanted, if they are of trauma, abandonment or of being unwanted, deep impressions are made on the sub-conscious which are the cause of emotional damage and mental disturbances in the child.

The full impact of emotional deprivation is recognized by child psychologists and psychiatrists. Dr. Federici of the US is well known for his study of Rumanian orphanages where children have minimal human contact in the early months. Without the loving nurturing of a mother and the security of being wanted, children are permanently damaged, their lives irrevocably impaired.

The physical cause of these disturbances is explained by Dr. Patrick Luyten as damage to the hypothalamic-pituitary-adrenal-axis (HPA) which is a major part of the neuroendocrine system, controls the reaction to stress and regulates body processes. HPA axis is permanently damaged when a child is emotionally neglected in the early stage of life, and remains so after adoption. Animal studies have shown that damage also occurs when the mother is stressed or traumatized during pregnancy.

13.1.2.2 BABIES IN ORPHANAGES

Babies who begin their lives in orphanages are particularly disadvantaged, they are unwanted before birth and abandoned without any nurturing. Even in the best of orphanages where babies are fed, kept clean and are healthy, there is rarely attention paid to his/her emotional and mental wellbeing. In this environment, babies are permanently damaged. Children institutionalized from birth are deprived of love, proper care and interaction. Emotional neglect directly results in poor growth patterns which is a marker of deprivation. There is an increased risk of emotional, learning, behavioral and anxiety disorders, Attention-Deficit Hyperactivity Disorder (ADHD), depression, language deficits, deficiencies in intellectual abilities (low IQ), severe attachment and autistic spectrum disorders. Lack of healthy stimulation slows development of the brain and affects mental capacity. The activity of the brain is altered on many levels and the chances of neuropsychiatric and neurological issues are high. The consequences of deprivation are profound and lifelong even though there may be some potential for recovery.

After placement in foster or adoptive care, the child will make dramatic developmental strides and the younger the child the better the chances of improvement. His or her IQ increases, language development may reach normal levels and emotional disorders, such as anxiety and depression, will be lessened. However, international research study, BEIP,[1] has shown that the incidence of behavioral and attachment disorders and ADHD do not decrease. In other words, all children who have been institutionalized are affected to some degree and none of them recover completely from institutional care, where the word "care" is meaningless.

Many adoptive children, with specific social and healthcare needs, are at risk of psychopathology; they are unstable, have difficulty in establishing relationships and all too often do not find their way into society. Neurobiological damage persists for years after adoption due to disturbances in the HPA, which regulates stress.[2] As long as children are neglected and abused in the thousands of orphanages all over the world, adoption will never hold the promise of a new life filled with love and opportunity. It will not be the source of happiness which these helpless human beings need. Furthermore, children adopted into cultural environments other than their own ethnicity suffer additional mental and emotional disturbances; in fact, experts see this as a major cause of inner conflict for the child.[3]

In the documentary series[4] it was observed that, where children remain with the mother and extended family with village life for support, there is not the isolation for the baby which exits in modern society and orphanages. Even in desperately poor situations, children are happy because they have love and security which material comforts cannot provide. From my own observations, working with poor and disadvantaged children in India as compared to children in modern society: I notice Indian children are more interactive, full of vigor and curiosity and have more confidence. Perhaps what is most apparent is they are contented and not always seeking attention.

13.1.2.3 BABIES IN FOSTER CARE

Foster care is considered to be a preferable option for unwanted children and when it is an ideal situation, of course it is much better than an orphanage. However, many parents foster children to supplement their income, are often young and have busy working lives. The baby still may not get the nurturing and proper stimulation that he/she needs in the early stages of life. Studies in America have shown that foster care is a breeding ground for the exploitation of children.

13.1.2.4 BABIES IN THE MODERN WORLD

In today's material world, there is not much time for newborns, hardly even time for birth to take place in the natural way. Family and extended family has mostly eroded and many mothers have a career and/or are single parents having to work. Present-day work schedules do not allow for women to devote the time needed during the first weeks of a baby's life. Many women work up to their delivery date, babies are often put into daycare at a very early age where care is by strangers who may differ from day to day, therefore rarely do these babies have consistent twenty-four-hour care. Even in reputable daycare, babies rarely get the one-on-one love and nurturing they need, they are left to cry and not held as much as needed. Furthermore, many newborns are over stimulated due to television, telephones, internet and constant ambient noise because there is not the awareness of the need for calmness and silence. They are often taken to public places, kept up late at night and not allowed to sleep when they need to putting undue stress on the developing mind.

13.2 DISCUSSION

The issue of unwanted pregnancy and children is highly complex and one which society has faced since the beginning of time. It exists in every culture, every religious setting and country. Even though the issue may look different in different settings, the common thread is the fact that women deliver the babies, nurture and feed them. Women worry when children are sick and grieve when they are killed or maimed. Women are at the core of the issue therefore, women are at the core of the solution.

Modern society has drifted away from the natural instincts of our ancestors where there were no alternatives to the support of extended family and where skills of motherhood were passed down from one generation to the next. If humanity as a whole does not revive these skills, then we are at risk of losing this basic instincts which define who we are. There is a critical need to raise the awareness of the fundamental need of babies and young children to be intensely nurtured. This message must reach the public at large, governments, orphanage directors, educators, social workers, adoption and foster care agencies and medical workers. The whole world must learn again the importance of one-on-one intensive nurturing in the very early part of life and the fundamental need for all humans to feel wanted, even before birth.

In the West, it was thought not to be a good thing to hold a baby too much and not to pick him/her up if they cried for fear of spoiling the child. This attitude has spilt over into orphanages and foster care where there are not any mothers and the baby is left in a crib in isolation after birth only to be handled when being fed and bathed. It has been shown that if these children are fortunate enough to have a consistent carer in the early days they are better adjusted in the long run. Even though there is a separation issue when adopted, it is not as serious as never having had any human attachment.

In modern society, the opportunity to devote concentrated time to pregnancy and newborns is less and less possible and more commonly impossible. The extended family is disappearing, families are split up, single women are having babies without support of any kind and, unless they work, they cannot support themselves. Furthermore, unwanted babies are left at birth to a foster home or orphanage.

Nurturing is fundamental to all mammals. It is known that if a puppy has not been with its mother from birth to six weeks, then it will be an aggressive dog unsuitable for adoption. Studies on chimpanzees show that a baby which is not cuddled and held becomes withdrawn, unresponsive and does not develop normally. As Western psychologists and psychiatrists debate the results of negative young life experiences and trauma, the gravity of the situation becomes ever clearer.

In 1946, a young catholic nun in India had a revelation to leave the order and devote her life to the unwanted, unloved and uncared-for. In the 1960s and 1970s, Mother Teresa revolutionized human thought and will be remembered for the founding of hospice which is the protection and care of the dying. Hospice is a concept which the whole world has embraced, now it is time to embrace the concept of protecting and supporting mothers and newborns. Unborn and newborn babies are the future of humanity, the adults who will shape our world. The time is NOW.

"An International Congress" is proposed whose mission is to-

- Promote the healthy development of children all over the world by raising awareness of the need for close nurturing of newborns and young children.
- Protect and support women by:

  a) Providing realistic birth control solutions.
  b) Providing a safe and protective environment for delivering and nurturing a newborn baby.

- Protect and support abandoned and disadvantaged children.

- Reform institutional and foster care by bringing back "grand-mothers" to support orphanages, foster care and adoptive agencies.
- Educate & train mature volunteers as ayurveda doulas who would take the baby immediately after birth and nurture the child until adoption or fostering or support the mother through the initial stages. If the baby is not adopted, volunteers the extended family of the child whether he/she remains in an orphanage or goes into foster care.
- Be the advocate for children from conception to adoption or until the child is independent.
- Eliminate neglect, abuse and child trafficking world-wide.

13.3 CONCLUSION

To fully realize a system which advocates an integrated, holistic approach to all aspects of human reproduction would be labor intensive and require many different levels of expertise. A preliminary proposal of these levels could be:

1. Allopathic and Ayurvedic physicians in partnership to oversee overall management.
2. A practitioner/nurse level in Ayurveda and Allopathy directly under the supervision of physicians, managing diet and lifestyle, providing support and education to patients.
3. Ayurveda doulas under the supervision of practitioner/nurses providing on-going and a continuum of support for pregnant women, newborns pre and post natal care.
4. Mature women volunteers working at a grass-roots level in the communities to identify issues, educate and provide on-going support for single women, pregnant women, babies and young children.

Clearly natural therapies have an important role to play in reproductive medicine. But, it must be integrated with allopathy as there will always be a need for care which holistic medicine cannot provide. However, let us not forget that conception, pregnancy, birth and care of newborns are natural processes therefore on-going care, education and support in all areas of reproduction can be addressed more effectively in an integrated, holistic health setting.

KEYWORDS

- **ayurveda**
- **breast cancer**
- **cesarean**
- **foster care**
- **orphanages**
- **newborns**
- **oral contraception**
- **fertility**
- **human reproduction**

REFERENCES

1. B.E.I.P. "Bucharest Early Intervention Project" **Charles A. Nelson M.D., Nathan A. Fox M.D., Charles H. Zeanah M.D.** This US study compares the development of children living in institutions to the development of formerly institutionalized children living in Romanian foster homes. Both groups are compared to a group of children never-institutionalized living with their biological families. The domains of development studied include brain, behavior, social and emotional development, attachment, cognition, language development and physical growth.
2. **Patrick Luyten, PhD.** Associate Professor and Co-Director of the Psychoanalysis Unit at the Department of Psychology, University of Leuven (Belgium), and Senior Lecturer at the Research Department of Clinical, Educational, and Health Psychology, University College London (UK). Dr. Luyten explains how the HPA functions and how it is damaged if the child is neglected in the early stage of life and how it remains so after adoption.
3. **Prof. Dr. Ronald S. Federici, Psy. PhD.** USA specializes in mental disorders, which manifest in adoptive children. Care for Children International www.drfederici.com Dr. Federici at a symposium of the faculty of Social Sciences at Utrecht University, Netherlands – June 9, 2006, stated: "Even if children are adopted into a disturbed family, it is better than being institutionalized from birth because they experience some level of attachment. If the family is pathological, very poor or even abusive it is preferable to the child being abandoned at birth and living in a hospital or orphanage."

4. A Dutch 15-hour Television Series covering international adoption in Romania, India, China, Haiti, Rwanda, Ethiopia, Korea, and Vietnam in which all data are confirmed by personal testimonies and experiences of adoptive children, adults, and parents. First Series - "Life as it is: Adoption" (10 × 30') by VRT, Belgium. Second Series - "Adoption. Part 2" (10 × 30') by VRT, Belgium. Third Series - "Adoption. Part 3" (10 × 30') by VRT, Belgium.

EXPERTS IN THE FIELD

Dr. Marek Wojciechowski (Pediatrician), University Hospital Antwerp.

Dr. Wilfried Smis (Psychologist), Observatory and Treatment Center.

Dr. Patrick Luyten and Dr. Nicole Vliegen (Clinical Psychologists), University of Leuven. In 2009 began a full scale, long-term research project on international adoption in Flanders.

Annik Lampo, Juvenille Psychiatry, University Hospital, Brussels, at the 2010 International Association for Child and Adolescent Psychiatry and Allied Professions (IACCAPAP) World Congress in Peking, spoke about the problems of early-stage child neglect and adoption. She stressed the need for improved basic care (intensive nurturing) in the birth countries BEFORE adoption and importance of guidance of the adoptive parents AFTER adoption putting emphasis on development, attachment, adaptation, and cultural differences.

Helena Daelman is the author of "Kleur bij kleur. Een kritische kijk op adoptie.

Translation: "Color by color. A critical view on adoption."

Houtekiet/Linkeroever Uitgevers nv 2011 ISBN 978 90 8924 173.

Publications by Dr. Federici

"Help for the Hopeless child": Assessment of the Post-Institutionalized child.

"Post Institutional Autism PTSD" Rumanian Adoptees. Journal of Autism and Development - October 2005–2006, Volume 35.

"Institutional Autism:" An Acquired Syndrome, THE POST May 1997.

"Psychosocial Growth Retardation in Rumanian Orphanages" Federici, Mason, Hines - Journal of Neurodevelopment October 2009.

"Growth Parameters Help Predict Neurologic Competence in Profoundly Deprived Institutionalized Children in Rumanian Orphanages" Federici, Johnson, Aaronson, Pearl, Sbordone, Zeana, et. al. Society for Pediatric Research. December 1998.

Dr. Federici has written many articles, spoken publicly and appeared in the media in the USA and Europe. He is a world-renowned expert due to his research and work with traumatized adoptive children particularly from Rumania. The following is a small sample of his work.

"Learning and Behavioral Concerns of Internationally adoptees Referred for Neuropsychological Evaluation."

"Impact of Stress on Growth in the Internationally Adopted Child."

"Pre & Post Pubertal Growth in Profoundly Deprived Institutionalized Children."

"Long-Term Neuropsychiatric Disabilities in the Post Institutionalized Child."

"Comprehensive Evaluation and Innovative Treatment of the Damaged Internationally Adoptive Child."

"Comprehensive Evaluation of Traumatized Children from Eastern Europe."

INDEX

B

C

For Product Safety Concerns and Information please contact our EU representative GPSR@taylorandfrancis.com
Taylor & Francis Verlag GmbH, Kaufingerstraße 24, 80331 München, Germany

www.ingramcontent.com/pod-product-compliance
Ingram Content Group UK Ltd.
Pitfield, Milton Keynes, MK11 3LW, UK
UKHW021300190926
475701UK00009B/163
* 9 7 8 1 7 7 4 6 3 6 2 1 3 *